Understanding Cancer Immunotherapy

Understanding Cancer Immunotherapy

A Guide for Students, Patients, and Caregivers

Nancy Liu-Sullivan, Ph.D.
Foreword by Ralph Garippa, MSKCC

BLOOMSBURY ACADEMIC
NEW YORK • LONDON • OXFORD • NEW DELHI • SYDNEY

BLOOMSBURY ACADEMIC
Bloomsbury Publishing Inc, 1385 Broadway, New York, NY 10018, USA
Bloomsbury Publishing Plc, 50 Bedford Square, London, WC1B 3DP, UK
Bloomsbury Publishing Ireland, 29 Earlsfort Terrace, Dublin 2, D02 AY28, Ireland

BLOOMSBURY, BLOOMSBURY ACADEMIC and the Diana logo are trademarks of Bloomsbury Publishing Plc

First published in the United States of America 2026

Copyright © Nancy Liu-Sullivan, 2026

Cover design: Chloe Batch
Cover image © Science Photo Library/Getty Images Plus/Thom Leach

All rights reserved. No part of this publication may be: i) reproduced or transmitted in any form, electronic or mechanical, including photocopying, recording or by means of any information storage or retrieval system without prior permission in writing from the publishers; or ii) used or reproduced in any way for the training, development or operation of artificial intelligence (AI) technologies, including generative AI technologies. The rights holders expressly reserve this publication from the text and data mining exception as per Article 4(3) of the Digital Single Market Directive (EU) 2019/790.

Bloomsbury Publishing Inc does not have any control over, or responsibility for, any third-party websites referred to or in this book. All internet addresses given in this book were correct at the time of going to press. The author and publisher regret any inconvenience caused if addresses have changed or sites have ceased to exist, but can accept no responsibility for any such changes.

A catalog record for this book is available from the Library of Congress.

ISBN: HB: 978-1-5381-9156-9
ePDF: 979-8-8818-5550-5
eBook: 978-1-5381-9157-6

Series: Bloomsbury Ethics, 1234567X, volume 6

Typeset by Deanta Global Publishing Services, Chennai, India
Printed and bound in the United States of America

For product safety related questions contact productsafety@bloomsbury.com.

To find out more about our authors and books visit www.bloomsbury.com and sign up for our newsletters.

For Carole Ann Sullivan Cole, my beautiful sister-in-law, whom I never got to meet.
For Susan Topping, theatre artist.
For Helen Lin, professor and linguist.
For Merle Goldman, professor and historian.
For David Apter, professor and historian.

FOR ALL SCIENTISTS AND CLINICIANS WHO HAVE DEDICATED THEIR PROFESSIONAL CAREERS TO CANCER RESEARCH AND CANCER CARE.

FOR ALL FAMILIES WHO HAVE FOUGHT BRAVE CANCER BATTLES ALONGSIDE THEIR LOVED ONES.

Contents

Foreword By Ralph Garippa, Ph.D.	viii
Author's Note	xi
Reader's Note	xiii
Acronyms And Abbreviations	xiv
Chronology	xix
Introduction	1
The Dictionary	3
Welcome to Cancer Jeopardy in Memory of Alex Trebeck	225
Cancer Jeopardy Answers	230
Bibliography	235
Index	241
About The Author	244

Foreword

As high-functioning humans, we consider ourselves prepared and ready for most confrontations. Through experience, we are conditioned to battle through a myriad of situations and conditions. We can usually identify our enemies; they are recognized sooner or later by their actions. This premise also holds true for our health; we constantly guard against minuscule foreign invaders such as bacteria, viruses, and fungal infections, which can wreak havoc on a large scale and perhaps even threaten the entire organism if left unchecked. But we never anticipate a betrayal; something from our inner trusted circle which, for some unknown reason, seeks the advancement of its own survival at the detriment of every other cell in the body. Yet that is exactly what cancer does to us and why it is so difficult to deal with emotionally and medically. After all, these new-on-the-scene mutant cells used to be *one of us*, but now they have gone rogue and, for all intents and purposes, don't listen to the fine physiological tuning signals that bring all our organs and tissues into a steady state of existence. The end result: the boat has been rocked, and in its relentless way, the traitor cells will seemingly not be satisfied as the boat continually takes on more and more water until it sinks. It simply makes no sense; or does it?

In the pages ahead of you, author Dr. Nancy Liu-Sullivan will take the reader on a journey through the A-B-Cs (really the A to Z) of cancer in an approachable way that (for the most part) avoids heavy-duty medical and technical jargon. Rather, she deploys a series of metaphors, similes, and analogies to drag cancer out of the shadows and into an easily understandable light. The use of figurative language prevents the reader from being suffocated under the weight of 5-, 6-, 7-syllable words that have become common in medical terminology. Such a feat is not a task for the novice or faint of heart. Spanning the multiple decades of her career as a cancer student, researcher, and teacher, we are regaled with landmark stories and many one-of-a-kind experiences that approximate the length, breadth, and depth of cancer as it impacts individuals and society. Indeed, there will be a few sections of the book where the reader is presented with fully annotated tables and figures that may remind one of being back in school and grappling with the concepts taught in didactic classroom lectures, but these are intermittent necessary visual aids that will help break down the molecular underpinnings of highly complex biology gone awry.

As scientists, we recognize the central dogma in biology that each organism, in its essence, is defined by its chromosomes and DNA, carefully sequestered in a cell's nucleus and then faithfully copied into RNA and subsequently sent through the nuclear membrane into the cytoplasm. There, the instructions, or shall we say (in the spirit of this book) *photocopied instructions*, are translated into the building block proteins that make up our cells, tissues, and living bodies. Most experts agree that there are over 200 different types of cells in the human body at birth; they are the end result of nine months of brilliantly engineered, precisely directed differentiation from a single fertilized human ovum. These diverse cells divide and regenerate when damaged or to replace aging cells. They obey their spatial boundaries and cooperate with their neighboring cells. After all, one does not normally read about liver cells invading the gallbladder, or lung cells migrating to the brain, or pancreas cells taking up residence in the small intestine. But in cancer, these rules are broken. In fact, cancer co-opts many of the body's maintenance systems in its quest to grow locally (as a primary tumor) and advance systemically (as a metastatic tumor). If law enforcement agencies were describing it, they'd say it's an *inside job*.

In *Understanding Cancer Immunotherapy: A Guide for Students, Patients, and Caretakers*, the reader is informed of the most recent advancements in research and the resulting medical treatments that have been developed to reverse the unfair advantages that cancer cells have taken to mercilessly exploit the host organism. These include:

- immune system, cloaking and uncloaking, wound healing, inflammation;
- mechanisms of accelerated metabolism, feeding requirements of proliferation gone amok, the genesis of tumor-supportive vasculature;
- the microenvironment; the milieu, cell-to-cell communication, and cooperation;
- cell surface topology, receptors, and channels regulating the border;
- the epigenome (proteins which help regulate the on/off of DNA transcription).

Historically, when referring to a solid tumor, both physicians and patients alike use the term "*the tumor,*" as if it were simply a ballooning mass of similar, if not identical (clonal) cells. Nothing could be further from the truth; in fact, single-cell experiments have conclusively shown the tumor to be a multifaceted, multifunctional community of heterogeneous cells. Furthermore, these diverse types of cancer cells communicate via physical connections and humoral (secreted) chemical messages to enhance their chances of survival. A revolt, a rebellion, a cooperating enclave of ne'er-do-wells. According to the American Cancer Society (ACS), as of 2024, the top twelve most prevalent cancer sites are the following, in ascending order: breast, prostate, lung/bronchus, colon/rectum, skin (melanoma), bladder, non-Hodgkin lymphoma, kidney/renal, uterus, pancreas, and thyroid. Most are solid tumors; leukemia and lymphoma represent the hematologic (blood-based, or "liquid") cancers. Of course, prostate cancer is specific to men, while breast cancer is over 100 times more common in women than in men. Several other cancers, however, (for the most part) have a somewhat balanced representation across the two sexes. In general, the cancer mortality rate is approximately 50 percent higher in men than in women, while non-Hispanic Black men have the highest cancer mortality rate (~208 per 100,000) and non-Hispanic Asian/Pacific ancestry women have the lowest (83 per 100,000). In the United States, four cancers in particular (breast, lung/bronchus, prostate, and colorectal) account for nearly 50 percent of all new cancer cases, whereas a similar but not identical group of four cancers (breast, lung/bronchus, colorectal, and pancreatic) account for nearly 50 percent of all deaths. In 2024 alone, over 600,000 people will die of cancer in the United States. Worldwide, nearly 10 million persons will die of cancer-related deaths, with ~20 million new cases being reported.

Not all of the news is bleak. The death rate for many cancers has exhibited a marked drop over the last three decades, primarily due to earlier detection, combination treatments, fewer smokers, chemotherapy after surgery, and better preventive measures including nutrition and exercise. In fact, you may be surprised to learn that the five-year relative survival rate for the following five cancers is at or approaching 99 percent: breast, prostate, testicular, thyroid, and skin (melanoma). Encouragingly, Hodgkin's lymphoma and cervical cancer are not far behind at 92 percent. But as dedicated researchers, physicians, and health care specialists in the battle against cancer, I speak for all by saying we will never even contemplate being satisfied until the survival rates and quality of life are greatly improved for the nearly eighteen million cancer survivors (of all ages) presently in the United States. Over 40 percent of men and women will be diagnosed with cancer at some point in their lifetime, with the cost of cancer treatment exceeding two hundred billion dollars. Both numbers are unacceptably high, and we have all (each one of us) had cancer negatively impact our lives either directly or indirectly, which is why we continue to fight.

Hope is on the horizon, and in some cases, the horizon is already beginning to wash onshore. For example, to date, over 34,000 patients have been treated with chimeric antigen receptor (CAR-T) cellular therapy which was first rolled out by Drs. Carl June and Michel Sadelain for blood cancers but is now making promising inroads against solid tumors. Bone marrow transplants have revolutionized our outlook and perspective on blood cancers over the past five to six decades. Vaccines, which we have grown to accept as commonplace for the prevention of influenza and COVID-19, are now at the foreground of cancer treatment to help circumvent the metastatic spread of the primary tumor once detected and dealt with using radiation, chemotherapy, and surgery. There are more examples, but I shall leave that task to your reading and the pages ahead. Enjoy the journey! Dr. Nancy Liu-Sullivan has graciously opened up the archives of her professional memory and shared her perspective as never before. I am sure that you will soon see cancer in a new, highly comprehensible light. As the ancient Chinese general Sun Tzu once said, *"Know thy enemy and know yourself; in a hundred battles you will never be defeated."*

Dr. Ralph Garippa
Memorial Sloan Kettering Cancer Center, New York, NY

Author's Note

Found in Translation

"Advanced Translation" was my first teaching assignment at Wellesley College's overseas language and culture center. Facing a classroom full of bright American college students from assorted leagues of the Ivy, being stupefied was an understatement. Extending a guiding hand to me was Prof. Helen Lin, chair of the Chinese Department of Wellesley College, Wellesley, Massachusetts.

My next translation desk was at Harvard University Fairbank Center, assisting Prof. Merle Goldman and other scholars over a storied summer at Cambridge, Massachusetts; followed by a more formal, on-stage instantaneous translation event at a conference organized by Prof. David Apter, chair of the History Department, Yale University, New Haven, Connecticut; followed by translating for the revered Toppings: Mr. Seymour Topping who served as managing editor for the *New York Times* and chaired the Pulitzer Prize Committee, and Mrs. Audrey Ronning Topping, an esteemed photojournalist whose works made the cover of the *National Geographic*, *Time Magazine*, and many more.

A few moons later, I found myself at a different type of translation post, analyzing cancer gene expression data sets, trying to discern patterns and discover anomalies that help shine a light on the dark and dank thickly-wrapped cancer enigma. Transitioning from English literature to biomedical science was no walk in the park. Scoring the highest grade in the toughest graduate neuroanatomy class final at Columbia University inarguably served as a confidence booster for the cross-field transition. Still, core biology majors' classes that I skipped to peruse *Beowulf*, *Thomas Hardy*, and *Ernest Hemingway* all had to be made up at both bachelor's and master's levels. I was also extremely fortunate to have found two superb doctoral research mentors, Dr. Dafna Bar-Sagi and Dr. Joav Prives, whose intellectual prowess has instilled a lasting impact on me.

Here and now, nearly one score since the indelible years of graduate school, postdoctoral fellowship at Cold Spring Harbor Laboratory (CSHL), honorable promotion to senior research scientist at Memorial Sloan Kettering Cancer Center (MSKCC), and joining the biology faculty at the City University of New York College of Staten Island, I find myself once again at the translation post, this time translating jargon-replete cancer immunotherapy ideas and implementations to a vernacular comprehensible to the general readership eager to learn more about cancer to fulfill their intellectual curiosity or to become more informed of the devastating disease they themselves or their loved ones are fighting through.

I am indebted to Ms. April Snider, production editor, Bloomsbury, who patiently read all my draft essays, page by page, batch by batch, rain or shine, to help keep the manuscript on track for being "easy to follow" and "jargon free."

My profound gratitude extends to Dr. Ralph Garippa, director and expert on gene editing and drug discovery at Memorial Sloan Kettering Cancer Center (MSKCC), who, despite an extremely hectic research schedule, not only took the time to critique my manuscript but also, with great delight, wrote the *Foreword*.

Equally grateful am I to Prof. Robert Paarlberg, professor emeritus of Wellesley College, adjunct professor of Harvard University's Kennedy School, and a celebrated author, for his input and insight on my sample essays.

My gratitude extends to Dr. Joseph Schwarcz, Professor of chemistry and director of McGill University's Office of Science and Society (OSS). I still recall how I was searching for beyond-the-textbook materials for my pre-med college students and came across a piece on the chemistry of sugars. I emailed Dr. Schwarcz my reflections on sugar in the context of cancer. Dr. Schwarcz replied with a simple but extremely encouraging line, "Interesting! Turn it into an essay for submission." I did, in practically one breath, and titled the mini essay "Cancer's Sweet Tooth," followed by several more, including *Nobel's Sugar Twist*. Publishing at OSS has unquestionably served as an inspirational boost for introducing the important topic of cancer to a larger and broader general audience.

Last but not least, I dedicate my gratitude to Lawrence R. Sullivan, my spouse—professor emeritus of political science and international economy, long-term fellow at the Harvard Fairbank Center and my co-presenter at an invited talk by revered Prof. Ezra Vogel—for his unwavering support of all my cancer research endeavors including, most indelibly, scores of occasions waiting for me (*with yummy diner takeout*): after hours, during weekdays, over weekends, and holidays, in the parking lot by the laboratory on Long Island, Manhattan, and Staten Island.

With all sincerity, I hope this book of 101 storied essays with 106 companion figures and tables organized in alphabetical order serves as a go-to guide for gaining a good understanding of the intricate facets of cancer, the constant tug-of-war between immune cells and cancer cells, and how cancer immunotherapy that unleashes patients' inner immune power to combat cancer has added a pivotal pillar to cancer care. As for *101*, besides being a beautiful prime number, it is also a typical designation for foundational introductory courses. Along a related train of thought: a former physics colleague of my spouse from Wellesley College once debuted an enticing course titled *Physics for Poets*. In a similar spirit, here it is: *Cancer Immunotherapy 101* for our readers from all walks of life drawn by the common pursuit of learning about cancer, why it is tough to treat, and what's going on at cancer immunotherapy forefronts.

Although we cannot make cancer totally disappear owing to the inherent nature of cancer stemming from faulty cell divisions (and cell division being the very apparatus that sustains our very life), with concerted and steadfast efforts in speeding up processes of translating basic cancer discoveries to meds by patient bedside, we *can* reduce cancer to a highly manageable condition, in no uncertain terms!

Sincerely,
Nancy Liu-Sullivan, Ph.D.

Reader's Note

On Aims, Goals, Audience, and the Rationale for the Unique Entry Layout. Unique from conventional cancer treatment, cancer immunotherapy harnesses patient's own immune power to combat cancer. Written with cancer patients and those interested in learning more about cancer immunotherapy in mind, this book guides readers through major cancer immunotherapy platforms along with cancer basics and immune system fundamentals to facilitate better understanding of the forte as well as areas in need of improvement of cancer immunotherapy. To avoid integrally related topics from being separated by the order of sequence of alphabetical letters, multiple mini essays are composed as a series, as exemplified by ***Rhapsody of Ras Trilogy, CRISPR/Cas9 Quartet, p53 Pentalogy***, and ***Risk Reduction of Cancer Hexalogy***. Where appropriate, a ***Food for Thought*** mini True/False Pop Quiz is provided at the end of certain essays that aim at reinforcing core concepts, which also prepares readers for the all-exciting **Immunology Final Jeopardy** at the end of this guidebook. Jargon-free (and jargon-friendly with ***Quick Word Anatomy***, where necessary) and context-rich with a light literary touch at times, the book translates complex cancer facets into a vernacular comprehensible to the general audience.

Nancy Liu-Sullivan, Ph.D.

Acronyms and Abbreviations

AACR	*American Association of Cancer Research*
AB	*antibody*
ACS	*American Cancer Society*
ADP	*adenosine diphosphate*
AG	*antigen*
ALL	*acute lymphoid leukemia*
AML	*acute myeloid leukemia*
AMP	*adenosine monophosphate*
APC	*antigen presentation cells*
APL	*acute pro-myelocytic leukemia*
ASCO	*American Society of Clinical Oncology*
A—T	*adenine bonded with thymine*
ATO	*arsenic trioxide*
ATP	*adenosine triphosphate*
A—U	*adenine bonded with uracil*
BBB	*blood-brain barrier*
BCC	*basal cell carcinoma*
BCG	*Bacillus Calmette-Guerin*
BCR	*B cell receptor*
BM	*bone marrow*
CAF	*cancer-associated fibroblasts*
CAR-T THERAPY	*Chimeric antigen receptor T cell therapy*
CD16	*cluster of differentiation 16*
CD173	*cluster of differentiation 173*
CD19	*cluster of differentiation 19*
CD25	*cluster of differentiation 25*
CD28	*cluster of differentiation 28*
CD3	*cluster of differentiation 3*
CD34	*cluster of differentiation 34*
CD4 T	*T cells that express CD4 = Helper T cells*
CD4	*cluster of differentiation 4*
CD8	*cluster of differentiation 8*
CD8 T	*T cells that express CD8 = Killer T cells = Cytotoxic T cells*
CD80	*cluster of differentiation 80*
CD86	*cluster of differentiation 86*
CH3	*methyl group*
CH4	*methane*
CLL	*Chronic lymphocytic leukemia*
CML	*chronic myeloid leukemia*

CO	*carbon monoxide*
CO2	*carbon dioxide*
CRI	*Cancer Research Institute*
CRISPR/CAS9	*clustered regularly interspaced short palindromic repeats/CRISPR-associated protein 9*
CRRNA	*CRISPR RNA*
CSHL	*Cold Spring Harbor Laboratory*
CSR	*class switch recombination*
CTLA4	*cytotoxic T-lymphocyte–associated antigen 4*
DC	*dendritic cell*
DFCI	*Dana-Farber Cancer Institute*
DNA	*deoxyribonucleic acid*
DOX	*Doxorubicin*
DSDNA	*double-stranded DNA*
DTPA	*di-ethylene-tri-amine penta-acetate acid*
EBV	*Epstein-Barr Virus*
FAB	*antigen-binding fragment [on antibody]*
FC	*crystallizable fragment [on antibody]*
G0	*gap zero [of cell cycle]*
G1	*gap 1 [of cell cycle]*
G2	*gap 2 [of cell cycle]*
GBM	*glioblastoma multiforme*
G—C	*guanine bonded with cytosine*
G-CSF	*granulocytes colony-stimulating factor*
GDP	*guanine diphosphate*
GEF	*guanine exchange factor*
GLUT-1	*glucose transporter 1*
GM-SCF	*granulocyte-macrophage-colony-stimulating factor*
GTP	*guanine triphosphate*
H2O	*water*
HAV	*Hepatitis A virus*
HBV	*Hepatitis B virus*
HCA	*heterocyclic amines*
HCV	*Hepatitis C virus*
HepA	*Hepatitis A infection*
HepB	*Hepatitis B infection*
HepC	*Hepatitis C infection*
HIGM	*hyper IgM syndrome*
HIV	*human immune deficiency virus*
HL	*Hodgkin's lymphoma*
HLA	*human leukocyte antigen*
HLA-A	*human leukocyte antigen class I classical A*
HLA-E	*Human leukocyte antigen class I non-classical E*
HPV	*human papillomavirus*
H-RAS	*Harvey rat sarcoma viral oncogene homolog*

Acronyms and Abbreviations

HSC	*hematopoietic stem cell*
HSV	*herpes simplex virus*
IFN	*interferon*
IFNG	*interferon gamma*
IG	*immunoglobulin*
IGA	*immunoglobulin A*
IGD	*immunoglobulin D*
IGE	*immunoglobulin E*
IGG	*immunoglobulin G*
IGM	*immunoglobulin M*
IL	*interleukin (family or cytokines)*
IL-1	*interleukin 1*
IL-10	*interleukin 10*
IL-12	*interleukin 12*
IL-13	*interleukin 13*
IL-15	*interleukin 15*
IL-2	*interleukin-2*
IL-4	*interleukin 4*
IL-5	*interleukin 5*
IL-6	*interleukin 6*
IL-8	*interleukin 8*
JAMA	*Journal of American Medical Association*
K-RAS	*Kirsten rat sarcoma viral oncogene homolog*
KT CELLS	*Killer T cells CD8-T Cytotoxic T lymphocytes (CTL)*
LN	*lymph node*
LPS	*lipopolysaccharides*
M PROTEIN	*monoclonal antibodies produced in multiple myeloma*
M	*mitosis [of cell cycle]*
MAB	*monoclonal antibody*
MAC	*membrane attack complex (formed by complement proteins)*
MCL	*mantle cell lymphoma*
MHC	*major histocompatibility complex*
MHC-I	*major histocompatibility complex class I*
MHC-IA	*major histocompatibility complex class Ia classical*
MHC-IB	*major histocompatibility complex class Ia non-classical*
MHC-II	*major histocompatibility complex class II*
MM	*multiple myeloma*
MRNA	*messenger RNA*
MSKCC	*Memorial Sloan Kettering Cancer Center*
NCI	*National Cancer Institute*
NHL	*non-Hodgkin's lymphoma*
NIH	*National Institute of Health*
NK	*natural killer cells*
N-RAS	*neuroblastoma-[derived] rat sarcoma viral oncogene homolog*

NSCLC	non small-cell lung cancer
NYULH	NYU Langone Health
NYUMC	New York University Medical Center
O3	ozone
P53	Protein 53; also called TP53 for Tumor Protein 53
PACT	Promises to Address Comprehensive Toxics Act
PAH	polycyclic aromatic hydrocarbons
PAMP	pathogen-associated molecular patterns
PAP	prostatic acid phosphatase
PD1	programmed cell death [receptor] 1
PDAC	pancreatic ductal adenocarcinoma
PD-L1	programmed cell death ligand 1
PENNMEDICINE	University of Pennsylvania School of Medicine
PET/CT	positron emission tomography-computed tomography scan
PRR	Pathogen Recognition Receptor
RAS	rat sarcoma [viral oncogene]
RBC	red blood cells
REM	roentgen equivalent man
RIA	radio-immuno-assay
RNA	ribonucleic acid
RNS	reactive nitrogen species
ROS	reactive oxygen species
S	synthesis [cell cycle]
SCC	squamous cell carcinoma
SCID	severe combined immunodeficiency
SKI	Sloan Kettering Institute
SLE	systemic lupus erythematosus
SSDNA	single-stranded DNA
SV	sievert
T1/2	half life
T1D	type I diabetes
T2D	type II diabetes
TAM	tumor-associated macrophage
TAN	tumor-associated neutrophils
TB	tuberculosis
TCR	T cell receptor
TGFB	transforming growth factor beta
T-H	T helper cells CD4-T cells
TKI	tyrosine kinase inhibitor
TLR	toll-like receptor
TLR4	toll-like receptor 4
TME	tumor micro-environment
TNF	tumor necrosis factor
TREGS	regulatory T cells
T-VEC	talimogene laherparepvec

Acronyms and Abbreviations

U-238	*Uranium 238*
UV	*ultraviolet*
UVA	*ultraviolet A ray*
UVB	*ultraviolet B ray*
UVC	*ultraviolet C ray*
VDJ	*gene segments on antibody*
WBC	*white blood cells*

Chronology

1775: English surgeon Percival Pott observed a link between chimney soot and increased incidence of scrotal cancers, a form of squamous cell carcinoma, among chimney sweepers. This was the first time cancer risks were linked to toxin exposure.

1863: The link between inflammation and cancer was postulated by German physician Rudolf Virchow based on observations that large quantities of inflammation-fighting immune cells resided side by side with cancer cells.

1882: The first mastectomy for breast cancer was performed by William Halstead at Johns Hopkins Hospital, Baltimore, MD.

1891: "Coley's toxin" was developed by William Coley, an American bone surgeon, for the treatment of inoperable soft tissue sarcomas. Dr. Coley, who served at Memorial Hospital (today's Memorial Sloan Kettering Cancer Center, MSKCC), is hailed as the *Father of Cancer Immunotherapy* for his innovative method of using bacterial infection to energize cancer patients' immune power to combat cancer.

1896: Sir George Thomas Beatson, a British surgeon, invented a new form of treatment for removing ovaries in inoperable breast cancer patients. This was the very first attempt at hormonal cancer therapy, also called endocrine therapy. The underlying rationale is to lessen cancer burden by cutting off supply of estrogen produced in ovaries.

1897: Paul Ehrlich proposed "Side chain theory," which describes how the presence of infectious bugs triggers host cells to produce "off shoots" to block out toxins. Later, Dr. Ehrlich refined the term from "side chain" to "anti-toxin" and finally settled on "antibody" as the official name. Based on the globular shape, antibodies are synonymous with "immunoglobulins" (Ig), of which there are five subtypes: IgM, IgA, IgD, IgE, and IgG. Together with Ilya Metchnikov, Dr. Ehrlich received the Nobel Prize for Physiology or Medicine in 1908 for their discovery of how antibodies mediate humoral immunity.

1898: Pierre Curie and Marie Curie discovered radium and polonium, paving the road for radiation therapy as a new pillar of cancer treatment.

1909: Paul Ehrlich proposed the immune surveillance hypothesis that presence of robust immune surveillance can curtail cancer, whereas absence of functional immune surveillance confers a chance for cancerous growth.

1911: Peyton Rous discovered a virus that can cause cancer in chickens. This was the very first time that a virus was reported as a causative agent of cancer.

1915: The link between chemical carcinogens and cancer was empirically demonstrated by Japanese physician Katsusaburo Yamagiwa and his research assistant Koichi Ichikawa. By repeatedly painting coal tar on rabbit ears, the team of scientists successfully induced squamous cell carcinoma in rabbit ears. This milestone experiment also provided supporting evidence for the link between persistent inflammation and cancer postulated by Rudolf Virchow.

1928: Sir George Papanicolaou detected cervical cancer by examining cervical cells under the microscope. The test is coined as "Pap smear."

1937: The National Cancer Institute (NCI) was established when President Theodore Roosevelt signed into law the National Cancer Act on August 5, 1937.

1947: American physician Sidney Farber tested the use of a folic acid antagonist drug (called Aminopterin) in stopping leukemia and achieved, for the first time, temporary remission in 10 out of 16 patients with childhood leukemia. This was the first anti-metabolite drug against cancer.

1948: Astrid Fahraeus demonstrated that only plasma cells produce antibodies. Derived from B cells, plasma cells have since acquired the nickname of "antibody factory."

1949: The FDA approved the first DNA-modifying nitrogen mustard for cancer treatment. Derived from "mustard gas" used in the First World War as a chemical weapon, nitrogen mustard was repurposed to kill cancer cells via DNA mutation. Nitrogen mustard marked the advent of modern chemotherapy.

1950: Richard Doll and Tony Bradford Hill discovered the link between long-term tobacco smoking and lung cancer.

1953: The Cancer Research Institute (CRI) was established by visionary Helen Coley Nauts and Oliver R. Grace Sr. with financial support from Nelson Rockefeller.

1957: Alick Isaacs and Jean Lindenmann discovered interferons (IFN), a class of immune signaling molecules that belong to the family of cytokines.

1957: James Gowans discovered immune cell circulation between the lymphatic system and bloodstream.

1959: Lloyd Old, MSKCC physician and CRI lead scientist, demonstrated anti-cancer properties of BCG, the tuberculosis (TB) vaccine, for the treatment of early-stage bladder cancer.

1960: Rosalyn Yalow and Solomon Bersen developed Radio-Immuno-Assay (RIA) that precisely quantifies minuscule-level antigens such as insulin. Dr. Yalow, a proud graduate from the City University of New York (CUNY) Hunter College, was awarded the 1972 Nobel Prize for Physiology or Medicine.

1961: French physician Jacques Miller discovered thymus, the gland indispensable for immune T lymphocytes' selection and development.

1964: Epstein-Barr virus (EBV) was identified as a causative agent for Burkitt lymphoma, a type of cancer derived from mutated B lymphocytes.

1964: Lloyd Old, MSKCC physician and CRI lead scientist, discovered the connectivity between major histocompatibility (MHC) and leukemia in mouse cancer studies.

1966: Lloyd Old established association between Epstein-Barr virus (EBV) and nasopharyngeal cancer.

1968: Lloyd Old identified cluster of differentiation 8 (CD8) antigen. A biomarker found on the surface of Killer T (KT) cells, CD8 is indispensable in mediating KT activation.

1971: President Nixon authorized the National Cancer Institute (NCI) Director to coordinate and establish national cancer centers as an integral component of the *War on Cancer* initiated by the Nixon/Johnson administration.

1972: Rodney Porter and Gerald Edelman resolved antibody chemical structure and were jointly awarded the Nobel Prize for Physiology or Medicine.

1973: Ralph Steinman at Rockefeller University discovered a new type of immune cells termed dendritic cells (DC) which was later confirmed as a major antigen presentation cell (APC) indispensable for T lymphocyte activation.

1975: Rolf Kiessling, Eva Klein, and Hans Wegzell jointly discovered Natural Killer (NK) cells. Killer T (KT) and NK cells are the immune dynamic duo that eliminate immune dangers such as infected cells and cancer cells.

1976: Cesar Millstein and Georges Koehl successfully produced purified monoclonal antibody (mAb) proteins that made it possible for the development of mAb drugs against a host of diseases including cancer.

1976: Japanese immunologist Tonegawa Susumu solved the mystery of how a limited number of genes could produce richly diversified and pathogen-specific antibodies in the millions by somatic cells. And the answer to antibody diversity stems from rearrangement of the V (variable), D (diverse), and J (joining) segments of immunoglobulin (antibody) gene(s) in the bone marrow during B cell development. Dr. Tonegawa was awarded the Nobel Prize in Physiology or Medicine in 1987.

1976: Robert Gallo and his research group discovered interleukin-2 (IL-2), a versatile immune signaling cytokine.

1979: A year of significance for the discovery of p53 independently reported by team David Philip Lane and Lionel Crawford, team Daniel Linzer and Arnold Levine, and team Albert DeLeo and Lloyd Old. Instrumental to the subsequent characterization of p53 and core components of the p53 signaling pathway are Bert Vogelstein, Carol Prives, Scott Lowe, and many more.

1980: George Snell, Jean Dausset, and Baruj Benacerraf won the Nobel Prize for Physiology or Medicine for their respective contributions to the Major Compatibility Complex (MHC) in mice and in humans termed human leukocyte antigen (HLA). Knowledge of MHC and HLA biology is instrumental for safer organ transplantation and a more in-depth understanding of immune response and regulations.

1982–2024: Ras research has spanned forty-two years with the initial discovery in rat sarcomas in the 1960s, then a hiatus, followed by a series of quantum leaps in the 1980s with the identification of Ras genes in humans which has paved the way for FDA approval of a pair of Ras inhibitor drugs in 2024. Over the past few decades, generations of scientists have worked indefatigably on in-depth dissection and analysis of Ras and Ras family of molecules. Outstanding movers and shakers of Ras basic and clinical studies include Robert A. Weinberg, Julian Downward, Michael Wigler, James Fermisco, Dafna Bar-Sagi, Geoffrey Cooper, Channing Der, Adrienne Cox, Scott Powers, Linda Van Aelst, Frank McCormick, Mark Philips, David Tuveson, Neal Rosen, Christopher Marshall, Allan Hall, and many many more.

1984: A new oncogene called *Her2* in humans (*Neu* in rats) was found to be expressed in ~25 percent of more aggressive breast cancers, laying the foundation for subsequent development of anti-Her2 targeted cancer therapy.

1986: The first recombinant hepatitis B (HBV) vaccine received FDA approval.

1986: Demonstration by Steven A. Rosenberg of patient's own immune cells (isolated from the patient's tumor vicinity, expanded in the lab, and returned to the patient) capable of tackling cancer provides foundational support for cancer immunotherapy.

1991: The FDA approved BCG for treating early-stage bladder cancer based on groundbreaking discovery by team Lloyd Old at MSKCC.

1991: Interleukin-2 (IL-2) therapy was approved by the FDA for the treatment of metastatic melanoma.

1991: James Allison discovered CTLA-4, a protein expressed on the surface of T cells that functions as a T-cell brake (immune checkpoint). When bound by its corresponding ligand called B7 on antigen presentation cells (APC) or cancer cells, it renders T cells inactive, hence unable to tackle cells unwanted by the host body. Ipilimumab (Yervoy), a mAb antibody drug, binds to CTLA-4 to occupy the binding pocket on T cells, which enables T cells to be in activate state. Initially approved for the treatment of melanoma, Ipilimumab has also been granted approval for the treatment of kidney cancer, colon cancer, and liver cancer.

1992: Tasuku Honjo discovered programmed cell death-1 (PD-1), which, akin to CTLA-4, is a T cell brake. Pembrolizumab (Keytruda), a mAb drug that prevents PD-1 inactivation, received FDA approval in 2014 for the treatment of melanoma, followed by additional approval for treating other cancers including lung cancer and colon cancer. In the same year, Nivolumab (Opdivo), an inhibitor drug that blocks PD-1 from being bound and inactivated by its ligand PD-L1, also received FDA approval for the treatment of advanced melanoma.

1992: T cell engineering kicked off at Memorial Sloan Kettering Cancer Center (MSKCC), chartered by Dr. Michel Sadelain. Using a viral vector as a carrier, germane genes were engineered into T cells with the goal of equipping T cells with super immune power to tackle cancer cells.

1993: The first-generation chimeric antigen receptor T cell (CAR-T) therapy that fused a component part of antibody to T cells (hence "chimeric" in molecular nature) was developed by team Zelig Eshhar at the Weizmann Institute, Israel. Although unsuccessful when the platform moved to human studies for lack of durability, the ingenious idea laid the groundwork for subsequent generations of successful CAR-T therapeutic platforms.

1994–1995: Investigations on BRCA1 and BRCA2 showed a genetic link to increased risk of breast cancer, ovarian cancer, and additional cancers.

1995: Lieping Chen discovered PD-L1 as a molecule that keeps immune T cells at bay from attacking cancer cells. In 2016, Atezolizumab (Tecentriq), the monoclonal antibody drug that blocks PD-L1 and PD-L2 (which harbors the same T cell inhibitory function as PD-L1), received FDA approval for the treatment of bladder cancer, liver cancer, lung cancer, and melanoma.

1995: Regulatory T cells (Tregs) was discovered by Shimon Sakaguchi. Tregs play a suppressive role in the immune system to prevent the system from overreacting and causing self-damage.

1996: The US FDA approved the drug that blocks estrogen production (anastrozole) for the treatment of postmenopausal breast cancer.

1996: Discovery of Toll-like receptor (TLR) was reported by Jules Hoffmann, demonstrating the pivotal role of the *toll* gene in mediating a powerful immune response against infectious microorganisms in fruit flies.

1997: The FDA approved Rituximab as a targeted cancer therapy against a cancer protein called "CD20" for the treatment of B cell Non Hodgkin's Lymphoma (NHL) and B cell acute leukemia. In subsequent years, five additional anti-CD20 monoclonal targeted therapy drugs were approved by the FDA. These include mosundtuzumab, oblituximab, ocrelizumab, ofatumumab, and ublituxab.

1998: Bruce Beutler identified a member of the *toll* gene family called *tlr4* as the receptor sensor for a bacterial marker protein called "lipopolysaccharide" (LPS), which translates to plain English as "sugars of sorts." Charles Janeway characterized TLR4 as a prototype of pattern recognition receptor (PRR) which is indispensable in mediating recognition by innate immune cells of antigens displayed on bacterial cells and viral particles.

1998: Trastuzumab (Erhutu) was approved by the FDA. As the first mAb drug against oncoprotein Her2, trastuzumab is used to treat a type of breast cancer that harbors high levels of Her2, also called Her2-positive breast cancer.

1998: Michel Sadelain introduced a co-stimulator molecule called "CD28" into engineered T cells, which, when applied to CAR-T cells, demonstrated unparalleled sustainability. Incorporating CD28 into chimeric T cells was indispensable for the successful second-generation CAR-T therapeutic platform.

1998: The FDA approved thalidomide, a horrific 1950s deformity-causing teratogen, as a repurposed drug to treat chemotherapy-induced nausea in patients who are unable to or choose not to get pregnant.

Although not a drug for cancer treatment per se, the use of thalidomide adds an additional dimension to cancer care.

2001: *FOXP3*, the gene pivotal for transforming nascent T cells into regulatory T cells (Tregs) was identified independently by Alexander Rudensky and Shimon Sakaguchi.

2001: Carl June developed a version of second-generation CAR-T therapy that involves engineering 4-1BB into patient-derived T cells with enhanced T cell activation and stability.

2002: The discovery of the autoimmune modulator (*AIRE*) gene was reported by team Diane Mathis and Christophe Benoist. As an important gene found in T cells from the thymus, *AIRE* plays a pivotal role in making sure that T cells that have a high preference for one's self body cells getting selected out in the thymus. Individuals with a mutation in *AIRE* are afflicted with autoimmune diseases where Killer T (cytotoxic T cells, CTL) cells attack self body cells that require medical intervention.

2003: Michel Sadelain demonstrated in a milestone study how human CAR-T cells equipped with CD19 receptor successfully slayed mouse leukemia cells that harbor CD19 antigen. This is the first demonstration that T lymphocytes could be engineered with a molecular GPS that precisely guides immune cells to find and kill cancer cells, paving the road for engineering other cancer-specific receptors on CAR-T to tackle cancers beyond leukemia.

2006: Gardasil was approved by the FDA. Protecting against two strains of human papillomavirus (HPV), Gardasil immunizes people against HPV-16 and HPV-18.

2006: *The Cancer Genome Atlas* (TCGA) was established jointly by the National Cancer Institute (NCI) and the National Human Genome Research Institute (NHGRI). A comprehensive database consisting of findings from genomic sequencing and molecular characterization studies of thirty-three cancer types, TCGA stores big data sets for cancer researchers to compare, contrast, seek patterns, and anomalies in cancer gene expression with the goal of identifying promising targets to develop new anticancer drugs. A slice of biological trivia: The name *TCGA* happens to echo the four bases of DNA—T (thymine), C (cytosine), G (guanine), and A (adenine).

2010: William Ludwig became the first adult leukemia patient to receive experimental CAR-T therapy at the University of Pennsylvania School of Medicine and remained cancer-free for a decade until succumbing to a Covid-19 infection in 2020.

2010: FDA approved <u>Sipuleucel-T</u>, a therapeutic vaccine for the treatment of advanced prostate cancer.

2012: Emily Whitehead became the first pediatric leukemia patient to receive CAR-T at the University of Pennsylvania School of Medicine.

2013: The FDA approves T-DM, which is an armed antibody-drug conjugate (monoclonal antibody + mertansine) which blocks structural proteins called microtubules in cancer cells, leading to cancer cell destruction.

2014: Gardasil 9 that guards against seven additional HPV strains (besides HPV-16 and HPV-18), received FDA approval.

2015: The FDA approved T-VEC (Imlygic®) for the treatment of aggressive melanoma.

2016: With the mission of expediting cancer science discovery, enhancing research data sharing, and more efficient coordination between cancer research agencies, *Cancer Moonshot* was spearheaded by the Obama/Biden administration. A Blue Ribbon Panel of experts under the Cancer Moonshot Task Force consists of accomplished scientists and physicians including Tyler Jacks (Chair, MIT), Elizabeth Jaffee (Co-Chair, Johns Hopkins), James Allison (MD Anderson), and Charles Sawyer (MSKCC), among a team of accomplished scientists.

2017: The FDA approved two cancer-related diagnostic tests of MSK-IMPACT and FoundationOne. *MSK-IMPACT* stands for Integrated Mutation Profiling of Actionable Cancer Targets in both common and rare cancers. Mutation profiling is conducted by targeted tumor sequencing. Developed in collaboration with Foundation Medicine, *FoundationOne* (also called F1CDx) is a companion lab test that examines patient tumor tissue samples in search of gene mutations or biomarkers that can be matched to an available drug therapy for patients.

2017–2023: A total of six CAR-T therapies have received FDA approval for the treatment of advanced blood cancers. These include <u>Kymriah</u>, <u>Yescarta</u>, <u>Tecartus</u>, <u>Breyanzi</u>, <u>Abecma</u>, and <u>Carvykti</u>.

2023: Memorial Sloan Kettering Cancer Center (MSKCC) and BioNTech co-developed a personalized pancreatic cancer mRNA vaccine termed "individualized mRNANeoAntigen-Specific Immunotherapy" (*iNeST*), also called "Autogene Cevumeran." Phase I clinical trial was completed by May 2023 with highly encouraging outcomes. Working-in-progress (WIP) Phase II clinical trial kicked off on August 30, 2023, and is currently ongoing.

2024: The FDA granted approval of clinical trials for WGc-043, an mRNA cancer vaccine related to Epstein-Barr virus (EBV).

2024: Co-developed by Moderna and Merck, the Phase 2 clinical trial of mRNA-4157-P201 for the treatment of metastatic melanoma received FDA approval, and the trial is ongoing.

2024: Pembrolizumab, the mAb cancer immunotherapy drug that blocks PD-1, received FDA approval for a new cancer treatment regimen in combination with two chemotherapy drugs for the treatment of primary advanced and treatment-resistant endometrial cancer. The protocol starts with two chemo drugs—,carboplatin and paclitaxel, followed by pembrolizumab.

2024: Amtagvi (Lifileucel), the first tumor-infiltrating lymphocyte (TIL) immunotherapy against melanoma, received approval from the FDA. Pioneering this milestone work is Steven A. Rosenberg, chief of the Surgical Division of the National Cancer Institute (NCI).

Introduction

Candid Cancer Talk with a Poet

Nancy Liu-Sullivan

Candlelight book party, *hors d'oeuvres* delectable, conversations charming. A smartly attired gentleman greeted me politely. All pleasant until he learned about my profession as a cancer research scientist. He murmured pensively,

"*CANCER studies?*"

I nodded, proudly.

He paused for a quick second, then burst out in dry laughter, "Ha, Ha!" and vamoosed in the flickering candlelight.

Later at the party, when the guests thinned out, I couldn't contain my curiosity and inquired of our revered author hostess about that unique gentleman's profession.

"*He is a poet.*"

A poet richly endowed with angsty sarcasm? A poet under the sassy influence of *Prosecco* in generous quantities? Or a poet speaking his unfiltered sentiment over the loss of loved ones to cancer and perhaps blaming researchers for not yet finding a cure?

It has been more than a decade since that uncanny event, yet every bewildering detail still remains vivid. I cannot help but wonder, from time to time, about the hidden reasons for that mysteriously mechanical laughter at the mere mentioning of cancer research. Whatever the reason(s), banal or bitter, subdued or scathing, I am to respect, not to judge. And if I were to cross paths with our poet again, I would share with him why an immediate cancer cure is such a tall order, how cancer immunotherapy research has forged ahead with milestone achievements, and how the journey ahead is still long and circuitous.

Cancer harbors unfathomable complexities. Unlike a fractured bone or strep throat, cancer rarely follows a linear path when it comes to diagnostics, therapeutics, or prognostics. The biogenesis of a malignant tumor follows "*gradually . . . then suddenly,*" depicted by E. Hemingway, in a totally different context, of course. The "gradual" aspect typically harbors a series of mutations in critical genes that suppress tumor hints, stunt DNA repair, and stimulate uncontrolled proliferation and metastasis. This devastating mutation trifecta can culminate from assorted risk factors stemming from hereditary origins, environmental sources, certain chronic inflammatory conditions, lifestyle choices, or the simple process of aging.

Unleashing inner immune power to tackle cancer. Okay, you might ask: The human body may be vulnerable to cancer growth, but isn't it also equipped with powerful immune defense networks to shield us?! Fair question! Yet, the reality is less sanguine: Immune cells do strike an initial and furious fight against cancer cells but then evolve to become bystanders as a result of cancer's molecular tricks and traps. To revitalize immune cells, scientists have developed therapeutic platforms that bypass cancer "roadblocks" and have cured incurable cancers.

The book's mission. A collection of 101 stand-alone but at once integrally related essays in alphabetical order, this book aims to guide readers through the terrain of what gives rise to cancer, how cancer escapes immune surveillance, and why cancer immunotherapy is a robust arsenal to tackle cancer. Where possible, closely knit topics are grouped into series in the form of trilogies, tetralogies, pentalogies, and even hexalogies. Jargon-free and in humanized contexts, this book serves as the go-to source for the general audience.

Postscript: A chilly November morning, the sun was barely above the pale horizon. I got into a taxicab at 5:00 AM sharp, heading for my lab at Memorial Sloan Kettering Cancer Center (MSKCC).
"*Going to work this early?*"
The driver, gray-haired with a smile, inquired.
I explained the twelve-hour drug screening campaign scheduled to take place on that day after days of preparation with a team of fellow scientists. I also flaunted our awesome automated processing systems with super cool robotic arms.
The driver nodded,
"*You are doing God's work.*"
That was a heartfelt word of gratitude for all cancer scientists from all corners of the globe who dedicate their careers and intellectual curiosity to gaining a more in-depth understanding of cancer with the collective goal of turning cancer into a curable common medical condition soon!

The Dictionary

A

AN ATLAS OF IMMUNE BIG PICTURE

Endless shoreline basking in the setting sun. You are taking a walk, barefoot. Ouch! You step on a broken shell. Your foot bleeds. Quickly, the area swells up, turns red, feels warm, and is painful. You manage to limp home. You apply hydrogen peroxide and begin to wonder if the wound has gotten infected.

Inflammation and immune workhorse. Yes, inflammation is deemed a sure sign that our immune system is busy working. The cardinal characteristics of inflammation consist of redness, heat, swelling, and pain. Redness and heat arise as a result of increased blood flow to the injured area; swelling is from excess fluids and immune cells (as well as signaling molecules and factors) rushing to the site of action, and pain is due to the release of chemicals that irritate nerve endings. Inflammation is a sure sign that your immune system has swiftly swung into defense actions, which is a good thing. But exactly how does your immune system carry out the mission? Let's take a closer look.

A tripartite immune system. Three mutually reinforcing components make up our immune system that starts with (1) the physical barriers, followed by (2) the first responders, and beefed up by (3) the elite troopers.

1. **The physical barriers** are formed by skin, hair, stomach acid, tears, mucus, and more. The skin is an effective hedge that protects our body against harsh surroundings. The hair (also called cilia) in our nostrils blocks off tiny microbes and bugs. Our saliva and tears harbor strong enzymes against unfriendly bugs. The stomach acid is an even stronger chemical that kills on contact any germs piggybacked from raw or not thoroughly cooked food. The presence of chemical content found in stomach acid, saliva, and tears adds another layer to our immune physical barrier: the chemical barrier.
2. **The first responders** consist of immune cells from the innate arm of immunity, meaning these immune cells are capable of putting up immune defense on their own with no need for special training. They rush to sites of infection to trigger inflammation which helps remove invading bugs. The innate immune cells are quick in kickstarting action, but they are not perfect; they have no memory. The next time the same bug shows up, these immune cells act as if that were the first encounter. To sum up: innate immune cells are swift but ephemeral.
3. **The elite troopers** report to duty if the immune situation becomes overwhelming. These are specialty immune cells from the adaptive arm of immunity. The term "adaptive" implies that these immune cells need crash courses to gather "expertise." There are two designated training camps for each of the two main elite immune troopers: the thymus for T cells and the spleen for B cells. But once trained, special memory T and B cells arise to store everything on their immune memory flash drive in terms of the way, shape, and form of infectious bugs to ensure a more swift immune retaliation the next time the same bugs show up. To sum up: adaptive immune cells are slower in launching into immune action relative to innate immune cells but possess long-lasting memory.

Teamwork. The first responders and elite troopers work in sync. Close communication exists between innate and adaptive immune cells in dealing with unwanted cells, infected cells, and even cancer cells. Let's use the foot injury example described at the beginning of this essay.

INNATE IMMUNITY		IMMUNE "BRIDGE"	ADAPTIVE IMMUNITY	
Physical/Chemical barrier	*First Responders*		*Elite Troopers*	
Skin	Macrophages	Local lymph nodes	Helper T cells (T-h)	B cells
Mucous membrane	Dendritic cells (DC)		Killer T cells (KT)	Plasma cells
Cilia	Monocytes		Regulatory T cells (Tregs)	Antibodies
Tears	Mast cells		Natural Killer cells (NK)	
Salica	Basophils			
Stomach acid	Eosinophils			
Mucus	Neutrophils			
Quick, General, No Memory			*Slow, Specific, Long Memory*	

Image 1 Atlas of immune big picture. Assembled by Dr. Nancy Liu-Sullivan.

Step 1: A cut is inflicted after stepping over a brittle seashell. Bacteria enter the body through the damaged skin. The bacteria waste no time in infecting cells they encounter.

Step 2: The presence of bacteria sends an immediate "danger" signal that alerts macrophages to ingest the uninvited bugs.

Step 3: Macrophages arrive at the scene and start engulfing. Bacteria gone, danger gone, immune halcyon returns. But wait! What about the body cells that have gotten infected by the bacteria? Worry not, for our immune system keeps all things under neat control. Macrophages call for backup immune troopers. They do so by displaying a slice of the bacterium on a protein "silver platter" called "human leukocyte antigen" (HLA) and travel to a nearby lymph node to meet up with immune T cells.

Step 4: Inside the lymph node, macrophage presents the bacterial slice to a type of T cell that bears "CD4" surface biomarker. At the end of "bacterial intel" exchange, CD4 T cell becomes activated and goes on to help macrophage with the next step: To activate Killer T (KT) cells, more formally known as "cytotoxic T lymphocyte cells (CTL), which bear "CD8" surface biomarker. *Of note: To maintain our "jargon-free" convention in this book, we shall use Killer T (KT) to refer to CTL*. Macrophage presents the same bacterial slice to CD8 KT cell, leading to full-fledged KT activation. Having learned about the way, shape, and form of the bacteria, KT is ready to hit the ground running. A question often raised by my immunology class students: Why can't macrophages pass on "bacterial intel" directly to CD8 KT cells instead of going through an extra step via CD4 T cells? The answer: this extra step renders CD8 KT cell activation more efficiently and robustly. For this very reason, CD4 T cells are also called "Helper T" cells.

Step 5A: KT exits the lymph node, wades over the bloodstream, and arrives at the immune battleground replete with bacterial-infected body cells. Using the immune intel KT learned from macrophage, KT swiftly identifies infected target cells, makes multiple selfreplicas, injects toxic chemicals into infected cells to trigger the "death button" of programmed cell death" also termed as *apoptosis*—a poetic word of Ancient Greek origin that describes leaves falling off trees. Here, KT fierce action leads to infected cell annihilation. Upon accomplishing the immune mission, KT cell catalogs the immune intel to its memory bank to prepare future encountering of the infected cells by the same bug.

Step 5B: When it comes to fighting against infectious bugs, there is one additional family of javelins from our adaptive immune sack: B cells. Born in the bone marrow, B cells are dispatched to immune boot camp in the spleen for training. Upon completion of training, B cells are either embedded in lymph nodes which are distributed up and down our body or sent to patrol in bloodstream. Upon encountering invading infectious bugs, B cells develop into plasma cells and plasma cells produce antibodies to help speed up counterattacks against invading microorganisms.

There! Our immune system fends off danger with the robust three-part apparatus, leaving no stone unturned and no bugs unchecked. In subsequent essays of this book, we shall learn the detailed steps of these intricate processes and how they coordinate with one another under conditions of infections and cancer.

Back to the question raised at the beginning of our essay: Is the wound merely inflamed or infected? The general understanding is that for a cut that remains inflamed for more than ten days with exacerbated swelling, redness, warmth, and pain accompanied by high fevers, seek medical advice because these are signs of infection. This is of particular importance for senior folks who are not immunized against tetanus or who received a tetanus vaccination more than ten years ago. Make no mistake: tetanus requires a medical diagnosis and must be treated ASAP. For a minor skin cut, on the other hand, it generally takes a few days to repair, recover, and be good as new.

The tripartite immune system, that is, the physical/chemical barrier, the innate immunity, and the adaptive immunity, is a complex network consisting of intertwined signaling pathways whose actions can often be dependent on biological/physiological contexts and shaped by disease conditions, particularly in cancer. The introduction here is meant to present the immune big picture, or the immune "forest," if you will. Throughout this book, we shall examine assorted immune "trees" that form the grander immune forest, in health and in diseases, including autoimmune conditions, weakened immune system, and of course, cancer—the central topic of this book. I hope you find the essays informative and thought-provoking at the same time.

Food for thought:

1. Saliva, tears, and urine are components of the chemical barrier of our immune system's first line of defense.
   A. True
   B. False

2. Signs of skin inflammatory response include redness, swelling, warmth, and pain.
   A. True
   B. False

ANTIBODY PLAYBOOK (1): THEME AND VARIATIONS

A major class of immune arsenals, antibodies fight off invading pathogens with a five-body squadron, each designated to engage in niche immune tasks. Let's take a look.

IgM. Immunoglobulin M (IgM) comes in two forms: membrane-bound and free-roaming. Membrane-bound IgM is found on the surface of developing B cells that reside in the bone marrow and serve as molecular "gates" termed "receptor" proteins. At maturity, B cells also add another type of immunoglobulin termed IgD. Hence, B cells harbor a set of two gates. Mature B cells are like new college grads who have successfully obtained their coveted diploma but have not yet landed on their dream job, hence "dormant." A chance for mature but dormant B cells to swing into immune action is immune danger from invading infectious bugs. With the assistance of T helper cells, B cells become activated and differentiate into "plasma cells." Hailed as "antibody factories," plasma cells secrete free-roaming antibodies that are matched to the telltale "antigen" that resides on the surface of infectious bug of interest. One major way for these robustly roaming antibodies to take care of immune business is "jamming." Just like jamming radio waves disrupts radio signals, antibody-jammed infectious bugs literally become "frozen" and unable to invade host cells. Antibodies that turn infectious bugs into crippling clumps are termed "neutralizing antibodies." IgM is the champion neutralizing antibody due to its sheer expansive size of five single IgM joining hands to become a five-unit entity or a "pentamer." What happens to clumps of infectious bugs? They get engulfed by macrophages and dendritic cells (DC) from the human host body, a process of literally being chewed up and spat out—an immune response called "phagocytosis." **Quick Word Anatomy:** *Phago* = to eat or consume; *Cyto* = that of cells; together, *Phagocytosis* = ingestion of cells.

IgG. As the most abundant antibody type in the bloodstream, IgG constitutes ~75 percent of all our body's antibody population. During the Covid-19 pandemic, there was a blood test that detected the presence/absence of IgG and IgM antibodies from blood samples as a diagnostic tool. If an individual is tested positive for IgM but has an absence of IgG antibodies against SARS-CoV-2 virus, it means the person is still infected by Covid-19. If IgG is present but IgM is absent, it indicates that the person had an infection but has recovered from it.

Why is IgM/IgG dual antibody test considered a litmus for Covid-19 diagnosis? The answer lies in the timeline! During an infection, IgM is typically produced by the host body in four to seven days and IgG typically emerges in seven to fourteen days and can sustain for up to twenty-five days. Accordingly, the presence of IgM is interpreted as the infection being in early stage and by contrast, the presence of IgG antibodies signals successful overcoming of the infection. Here is a special situation: What if an individual is tested positive for both IgM and IgG?! A plausible answer could be that the individual was infected with one strain of Covid-19 virus but recovered, followed by an ongoing infection from a different Covid-19 strain. As for the role of IgG in combating infectious bugs, akin to IgM, IgG can also physically "jam" the bugs, disable and block them from entering human cells. IgG, by the way, is also the only type of antibody capable of entering the fetus from the mother through the placenta.

IgA. Unlike IgM and IgG found predominantly in bloodstream, IgA resides in the nose, mouth, and throat. A recent study that investigated why young children had very mild Covid-19 symptoms reveals a surprising discovery: the nasal secretions of young children who contracted Covid-19 were chock-full of IgA antibodies. Since Covid-19 is a respiratory infection, the forefront of the battleground is the nasal cavity. High levels of IgA initiate the fight against Covid-19 at the right place and the right time by neutralizing SARS-CoV-2 viruses to block them from passing down the throat, through the trachea, and to the lungs. Exactly why adults cannot hold a candle to young children in producing adequate IgA antibodies in the nasal cavity remains a mystery. Hope more in-depth research helps shed enlightening light.

IgE. A specialty antibody associated with allergic reactions, immunoglobulin E (IgE) antibodies adhere to immune cells in the blood. When an allergen (a substance that triggers allergy such as peanuts or pollen) interacts with an immune B cell, it drives the B cell into an antibody-producing "plasma cell." Each type of IgE antibodies is associated with a specific "brand" of allergen. Allergy-associated immune cells are comprised of "mast cells" and "basophils." Giant and commodious in size and shape, mast cells were so named by the German physician who made the initial discovery. When an allergic reaction mounts, mast cells or basophils become activated and begin to secrete large quantities of allergy mediators, most notably "histamine" but also "prostaglandins" and "leukotrienes." As the primary allergy mediator, histamine dilates blood vessels, leading to local allergic reactions ranging from watery eyes and a runny nose to wheezing (due to narrowing of the bronchi combined with tissue swelling). A much more severe allergic reaction termed "anaphylaxis" can also result from the release of large quantities of histamine from mast cells or basophils activated by IgE binding and reacting to antigens from a "source of danger," be it roasted peanuts, seafood chowder, pet dander, or a bumblebee sting. A systemic (whole body) allergic reaction, anaphylaxis from histamine leads to a sudden and severe drop in blood pressure which requires immediate medical attention.

IgD. Of the five types of antibodies produced by our body, immunoglobulin D (IgD) is the only one whose functions remain largely elusive. The only known function of IgD is its residence on the surface of B cells that, together with IgM, marks the maturation state of B cells, ready to be dispatched from the bone marrow to the spleen, the B cell training camp.

Doggedly, antibodies with assorted specialties survey our body to timely spot dangers and mount powerful immune reactions in the form of clumping to neutralize and cripple infectious bugs in order to preserve our immune integrity. Tiny antibodies sure assume huge immune protective roles! More about antibodies to follow.

Food for thought:

1. Immunoglobulin A (IgA) antibodies are found to be richly endowed in saliva and tears.
   A. True
   B. False

2. Antibodies such as IgG and IgM are capable of neutralizing invading infectious bugs to prevent them from entering our cells. IgE, on the other hand, mediates allergic reactions.
   A. True
   B. False

ANTIBODY PLAYBOOK (2): OUT OF ONE COMES MANY

A more common Latin phrase, *E pluribus unum*, denotes "Out of many, one." When it comes to our immune system manufacturing antibodies, however, the reigning doctrine is *ex uno plures* which translates to English as "Out of one, many." What is the ONE?

Five types of Igs make up humoral immunity. In descending order by size, we have IgM > IgA > IgE > IgG > IgD, as illustrated below, where IgM assumes a five-unit "pentamer," IgA a two-unit "dimer," and IgE, IgG, and IgD each harbor a single unit and hence are referred to as "monomer."

M & M. The largest size of all antibody types, the "M" in IgM stands for "macro." From a different but related angle, "M" could also mean "mother"—a lateral-thinking rendition. Actually, it makes a lot of sense because IgM is the *bona fide* mother source of other types of antibodies. Like a chameleon capable of switching colors, the messenger RNA sequence dubbed as "mRNA transcript" of IgM can also undergo segmental rearrangement like the letters on a scramble game rack. The cutting and splicing activities switch IgM mRNA to that of IgG, IgA, and IgE. After that, following the "central

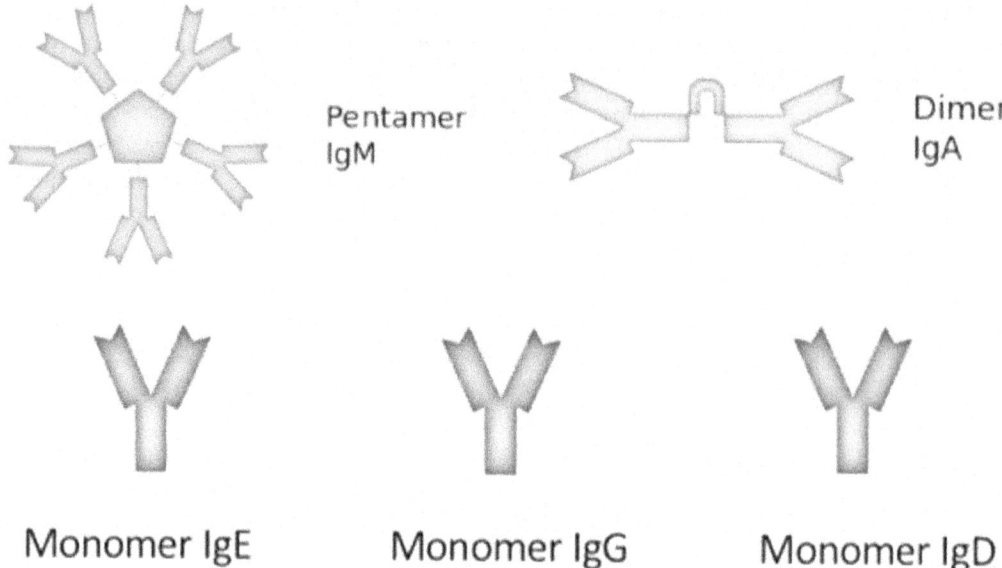

Image 2 Antibody family of five. Wilimedia Commone File: Mono-und-Polymere.svg.

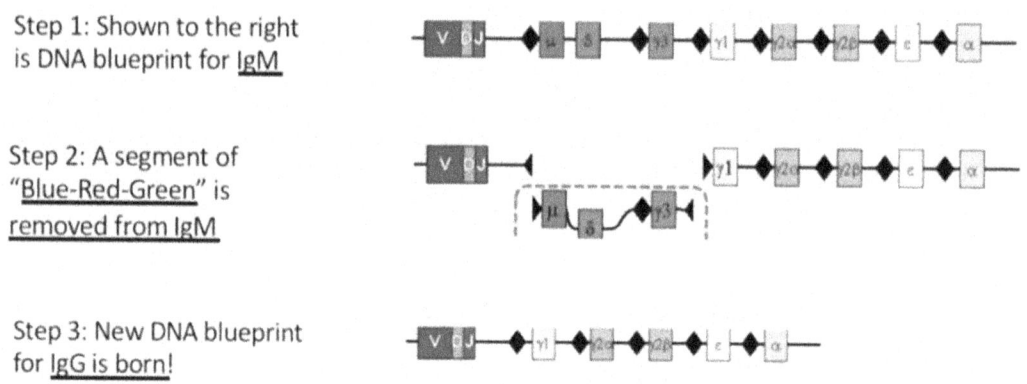

Image 3 Antibody creation by cut-and-paste. Wikimedia Commons File: Class switch recombination .png.

dogma" of DNA → mRNA → protein (coined by Dr. Francis Crick, who, jointly with Dr. James D. Watson, solved the double-helical DNA structure and won the Nobel Prize in 1962), new antibody types are produced beyond IgM, with each antibody-type switch following distinct molecular algorithms. The following figure illustrates the mRNA switch steps:

As shown above, Step 1: IgM mRNA transcript is shown. Step 2: A 3-piece "mu-delta-gamma" segment is removed from the original IgM transcript. Step 3: The remaining IgM transcript is pieced back together, and with this, a brand new transcript that encodes IgG is born! The same removal process of specific segments from the IgM transcript yields additional subtypes of IgG, of which by far four have been identified as IgG1, IgG2, IgG3, and IgG4. Collectively, the excising and reconnecting platform is called "Class Switch Recombination" (CSR) that greatly expands antibody-combating pathogen repertoire.

Diversity delivers success. Imagine the absence of CSR (Class Switch Recombination) where a lone type of antibody, IgM, is the only game in immune town! Imagine the absence of specialized immune functions such as IgA antibodies situated in the nasal cavity to guard against dangerous respiratory infectious bugs like SARS-CoV-2: the bugs would easily sweep through the nasal passage, cross the windpipe, and march into lung tissues to wreak serious havoc! Thanks to CSR, IgA antibodies are derived from IgM to safeguard at the very entrance of the respiratory system to annihilate dangerous bugs at time zero.

To add an additional layer of complexity: antibody diversity also extends to the "mouthpiece" on the two tips of the Y-shaped antibody structure, a region deemed the "antigen binding site," abbreviated as "Fab." As a business slang, "Fab" typically refers to "Fabulous" corporations such as "Fab Seven" in the tech world. In antibody domain, "Fab" denotes "fragment of antigen-binding."

Okay, antigen binding is easy to follow as it describes how an antibody engages an infectious bug by holding onto the representative piece on the bug called "antigen." What about "fragment" in "Fab"? Can an antibody be disassembled into its component parts, like taking apart a *cuckoo* clock? Fair question and there is actually a delectable answer associated with it. It turns out that the almighty Y-shaped antibody with a stem and two branches can be separated into three fragments with the help of a powerful enzyme isolated from a tropical fruit whose name starts with the letter "P." As you must have guessed, the fruit is "papaya," and the enzyme is "papain." Yes, soaking antibody molecules in a solution of papain readily fragments an antibody into its component parts!

Antibodies have also evolved such that the Fab mouthpieces can also undergo molecular rearrangement in the "V-D-J" segment to yield different varieties of Fab with distinct antigen-binding properties, leading to a dramatically expanded antibody binding repertoire! The greater the antibody binding site diversity, the more extensive the antibody capacity to weather assorted bugs, and the better guardians they become in safeguarding the host—us. More to discuss in the next essay.

Food for thought:

1. The "mother" source of antibody subtypes such as IgG, IgA, and IgE is IgM.
   A. True
   B. False

2. Antibody switching class from IgM to IgG, IgA, and IgE originates at the DNA level.
   A. True
   B. False

ANTIBODY PLAYBOOK (3): MATCH MADE IN IMMUNE HEAVEN

The proverbial phrase "match made in heaven" carries with it an enchanting sense of compatibility and happiness. The same sentiment exists in the world of immunology. The two parties are "antigen" and "antibody."

Antigens attract matching partners. The moment an antigen appears under the immune radar, it triggers a reaction. Why? Because it looks "foreign," unlike the familiar "faces" of DNA, molecules, cells, tissues, and organs of the host body. Immune cells are trained to equate "foreign" with "danger," and danger ought to be eliminated. How exactly does an antibody engage an antigen?

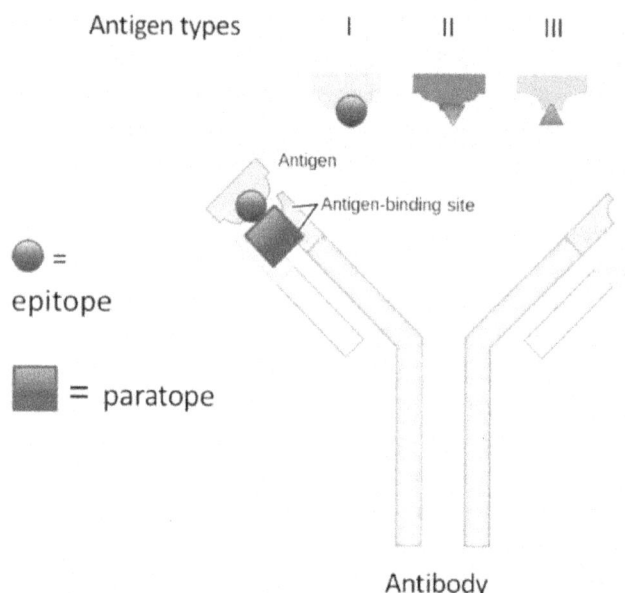

Image 4 Antibody tree structure. Wikimedia Commons File: Antibody.svg

The key-lock scenario. "Anti" suggests "to counteract." Examples include "antiseptic" that disinfects infected skin, "antibiotic" that fights bacterial infection, "antidote" against poison such as snake venom. To join the "anti" rank, here, we have "antibody" that harnesses antigens from infectious microorganisms. A quintessential feature of antibodies is the specificity for a corresponding antigen. How specific? As illustrated below, an antigen must be an exact fit for an antibody, just like a certain key opening a certain lock. As we can tell, of the three types of antigens designated as I, II, and III, only I is a perfect fit for the binding site on the Y-shaped antibody. Unlike the key that opens the lock to your office, where you must fit the entire key into the lock to open your office door, the antibody-antigen interface only requires a representative slice from the antigen called "epitope" that binds and interacts with the corresponding "paratope" region of the antibody.

Antibody diversities are incredibly rich. As discussed in **ASSORTED ALLERGENS FROM SEA TO LAND** (page 13), allergens from pollen and shrimp to pet dander are antigens because they can generate a counteracting antibody specific to the allergen of interest. Other types of antigens come from viruses, bacteria, parasites, and worms. Certain medications can act like antigens as well. Simply put: Antigen varieties are hugely rich. How does our immune system produce so many different varieties of matching antibodies so proficiently and so timely? The secret is recombination.

Letters on an immune Scrabble game rack. Yes, by Scrabble, we mean the famous spelling game, where a string of seven randomly selected letters is arranged in sensible order to form different words. Our immune system follows the same practice in creating diversified antibodies by rearranging different segments; each segment is analogous to an English letter, and different letters form words, as shown in the following figure :

  As shown above, combinations of letters led to the formation of seven different words. If we let the seven letters represent available bricks and mortars that build unique sequences of antibody binding sites on the immune scrabble rack, then the resultant seven words would represent seven possible

Antibody Production Scrabble Board						
A	D	E	S	O	T	Y
Are						
	Dot					
		Eat				
			Soy			
				Ode		
					Taste	
						Yes
Each letter = genetic transcript;			Each word = Antibody sequence code			

Image 5 Antibody Scrabble game. Assembled by Dr. Nancy Liu-Sullivan.

sorts of antibodies, each a perfect fit to a corresponding antigen displayed on the surface of infectious bugs and germs. Of course, the antibody ocean in the human body is vast, capable of generating ~10 billion types of antibodies sufficient to match "antigens" from land, sea, and air. Truly amazing!

Antibody snares and traps. As soon as an antibody "lures" an antigen into the molecular trap, it swiftly neutralizes the danger-replete "foreign" entity. Essentially, a bunch of antibodies round up the unwelcoming antigen in a molecular lattice to prevent it from approaching and invading the host cell. The neutralization strategy is also deployed by Covid-19 counteracting antibodies to cripple Covid-19 viruses from wreaking health havoc in us.

Oh well, unlike the conventional "match made in heaven," there is no "happily ever after" ending when it comes to an antibody matched to an antigen from an invading entity. On the contrary, the perfect match means a perfect kill. Stay tuned for more immune fighting stories.

Food for thought:

1. Antibody binding to antigen is metaphorically depicted as the "key-lock" scenario.
    A. True
    B. False

2. Antibody-antigen binding occurs randomly; that is, any antibody is capable of binding to an antigen.
    A. True
    B. False

ASSORTED ALLERGENS FROM SEA TO LAND

Mrs. Doubtfire, portrayed by the late Robin Williams, brewed wicked mischief. He sneaked into the restaurant kitchen and sprinkled some cayenne pepper powder on the shrimp scampi ordered by Stu, the boyfriend of *Mrs. Doubtfire*'s ex. The moment Stu put a shrimp into his mouth, he choked on it, started coughing, his cheeks turning from red to pale, and most scary of all, he was desperately gasping for air. Did chilly pepper bring upon an allergy in Stu, or was it just a case of irritation? Judging by how, as soon as Stu was cleared of the choked shrimp, he was free of all symptoms, Stu simply had a bad case of irritation. Although extremely rare, chilly pepper can cause an allergic reaction in some folks. Let's dig some more about allergens.

Allergens: Immune system's imagined foes. Defined as substances that cause allergies, allergens can come into contact with us humans via four routes: (1) inhaled (such as pollen from poplars and willows, not to mention canine and feline danders), (2) ingested (peanuts, shrimp, certain meds, and more), (3) injected (melittin and phospholipase from bumblebee stings!), and last but not least, (4) contact by skin (poison ivy or raccoon scratch). Allergens can be totally harmless if our immune system chooses to ignore them, as is the case for most people. However, one man's seafood chowder could be another man's source of misery! For folks who show allergic reactions to any of the assorted allergens listed above, allergies arise not as a result of any horrendous harm from the allergens but due to an overreaction by our very own immune system that imminent danger is taking place. Allergy symptoms arise from immune cells in full activation and secreting a sea of allergy-mediating molecules, most notoriously histamine but also leukotrienes and prostaglandins, as discussed in **AN ATLAS OF IMMUNE BIG PICTURE** (page 5). Here, let's focus on a few representative allergens from sea to land.

Allergens from the sea. For those who suffer from shellfish allergy, food items they ought to shy away from include (but no means an exhaustive list) shrimp, lobster, crab, clam, mussel, scallop, oyster, octopus, squid, and believe it or not, not, escargot! As for fish, bass, cod, and flounder are on the to-avoid list by folks with heightened sensitivities.

Food allergens from the land include eggs, milk, wheat, soybeans, strawberries, peanuts, and tree nuts. Again, this is only the tip of the iceberg.

Indoor and outdoor allergens. This is a long list starting with pollen, Bermuda grass, dust, mold, mildew, dander-tainted canine and feline fur, and beyond.

Certain medications are allergens. According to University of Pennsylvania School of Medicine, common medications that act as sources of allergens consist of seizure medication, certain insulin products, drugs that contain iodine, Penicillin family of antibiotics, including amoxicillin (the first-line medication to treat strep throat), and many more. For detailed information, please refer to https://www.pennmedicine.org/for-patients-and-visitors/patient-information/conditions-treated-a-to-z/drug-allergy.

Life savers. Some allergic reactions are mild and can clear on their own. Other types of allergies, especially food-triggered allergies, tend to be sudden, severe, and associated with "anaphylaxis," a life-threatening situation associated with acute respiratory and cardiovascular symptoms. ***Quick Word Anatomy:*** *Ana* = *w*ithout or against; *Phylaxis* = *p*rotection; together, *Anaphylaxis* = without a protective mechanism. Two types of meds are available for treating allergies. *Benadryl* is an antihistamine med that counteracts the deleterious effect of histamine released into the bloodstream by mast cells or basophils. *EpiPen* is an automatic injection that contains "epinephrine," also called "adrenaline." One jab into the muscles of the upper thigh helps open up airways, making breathing easier, in addition to elevating dropped blood pressure.

Of high importance: The essays presented in this book focus on topics that fall under the category of cancer, immunotherapy, and immune health. This book is *not a source of medical advice*. For professional guidance on allergies and related subject matters, please consult your physician and, when needed, call 911. Also, it is always a good idea to follow guidance from the US Center for Disease Control (CDC). Three representative websites are included here:

- Allergies in Schools Toolkit (https://www.cdc.gov/healthyschools/food)
- Responding to Anaphylaxis (www.cdc.gov/COVID 19)
- Allergy Testing for Persons with Asthma (https://stacks.cdc.gov/view/cdc/80010)

Back to where the Hollywood saga started: Watching poor Stu suffer an acute case of chilly pepper irritation-induced choking, Mrs. Doubtfire put aside his personal vendetta and came to his moral senses. He picked up Stu from behind and successfully performed the *Heimlich maneuver*, a first-aid technique also called abdominal thrusts. The shrimp flew out of Stu's mouth and Stu became fine and dandy again.

Food for thought:

1. Benadryl contains anti-histamine that reverses the deleterious effect of histamine in allergic reactions of bronco-constriction and increased blood vessel permeability.
   A. True
   B. False

2. EpiPen contains adrenaline and is used to treat severe allergic reactions such as anaphylaxis.
   A. True
   B. False

ASPIRIN CURBS EARLY COLON CANCER

Colon cancer is the third leading cause of cancer death. The full name is colorectal cancer (CRC). Alarmingly, a recent report describes an increase in CRC among young people. To the pleasant surprise of many, aspirin, a common item in everyone's medicine cabinet, has been reported to curb early-stage colon cancer. Let's examine more closely.

Colon cancer starts with non-cancerous polyps. A colon (rectal) polyp is a tiny lump of fleshy growth on the lining of the colon or rectum. Most polyps are benign or pre-cancerous, which, if left unremoved, 5–10 percent of polyps do become cancerous in ten to fifteen years, on average.

Polyps can take the shape of a mushroom or just plainly flat. The latter is often more challenging to detect. Although colon cancer diagnosis requires formal medical procedures, polyp size can often be an indicator of disease severity. Typically, polyps greater than 1 centimeter (cm), the diameter of a Cheerio, have a more likely chance to be cancerous than polyps of less than 1 cm.

Early detection is key. Very often, incurable cancers are already late-stage at diagnosis. Early detection can make a world of difference when it comes to treatment and prognosis. Colon cancer is no exception. Accordingly, the three leading professional agencies—the ACS, American Gastroenterological

Association (AGA), and the National Cancer Institute (NCI) have jointly disseminated CRC screening guidelines, as summarized in the following table adapted based on information provided by the Dana-Farber Cancer Institute (DFCI) of Harvard University (https://www.dana-farber.org/health-library/screening-prevention-for-people-with-a-family-history-of-colorectal-cancer).

As shown, while the types of screening tests are the same for everyone, folks with family history of CRC and precancerous polyps are recommended to start screening ten years (at forty years of age) earlier than those without a family history (at fifty years of age). Here is a thought-provoking question: Since certain polyps can become malignant, is it sufficient to have colonoscopy screening every three years? What if a dangerous polyp starts to develop not long after a colonoscopy? The standard answer:

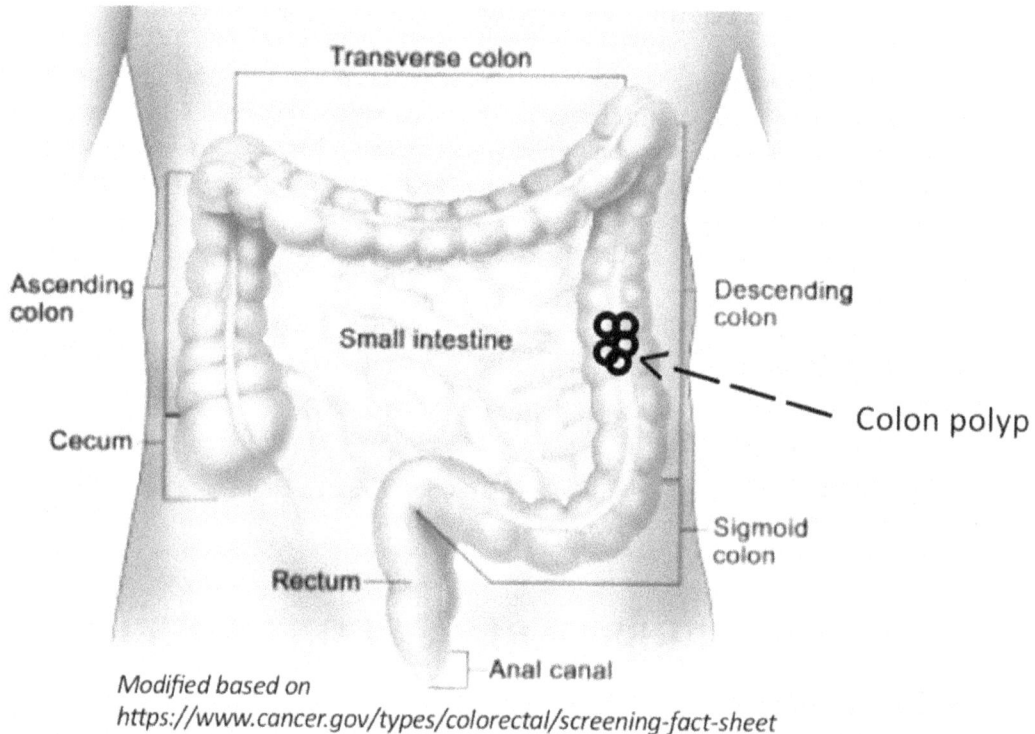

Image 6 Colon polyps. https://www.cancer.gov/types/colorectal/screening-fact-sheet modified by Nancy Liu-Sullivan.

Screening tests	Screening guidelines of colon and rectal cancer	
	With no family history	With family history
Fecal occult blood test	Every year	
Flexible sigmoidoscopy	Every 5 years	
Double contrast barium edema	Every 5 years	
Colonoscopy	Every 10 years	
Screening starting age	50 years of age	40 years of age

Image 7 Colon screening platforms. Assembled by Dr. Nancy Liu-Sullivan.

colonoscopy every three years should suffice since it generally takes ten to fifteen years for a dangerous polyp to become cancerous. For peace of mind, seek guidance from your family Doc!

Colon cancer risk factors. Genetics is a crucial factor that leads to colon cancer. That said, not all individuals with a family history develop colon cancer because colon cancer, like all cancers, is not caused by a single factor. There is always a myriad of factors at play. A high-fat diet, high alcohol consumption, and smoking are all contributing factors. Knowing these factors, a low-fat diet, a healthy lifestyle, and twenty-five to thirty minutes per day of some form of physical exercise go a long way in reducing risks of CRC development. Excitingly, there is a new CRC-curbing recipe in town called aspirin!

Recommended Aspirin regimen. Before delving into the dose and the frequency of aspirin regimen, a recap on the difference between "salicylic acid" (SA) and "aspirin": the former comes from nature (such as cinnamon and turmeric), whereas the latter is the product of chemical modification. The details are described in **ASPIRIN, WEEPING WILLOW, AND CREATIVE CHEMISTRY** (page 18).

The recommended aspirin regimen was established by a group of accomplished medical professionals known as the U.S. Preventive Services Task Force (USPSTF). The mission of this non-governmental organization is to make recommendations to the general public regarding preventive measures in medicine. The Task Force has found that low-dose aspirin is associated with a 40 percent CRC risk reduction. Of note, this reduction only pertains to individuals who meet the study criteria but not for the general population. To translate the recommendations into easy-to-follow terms, I have constructed the following table:

As we can see, the most beneficial group is individuals aged fifty to fifty-nine. But there is a catch: one must take a low-dose aspirin every day for ten years to maximally benefit from the effect. For folks over the age of seventy, the recommendation goes against daily aspirin based on bleeding risks. As for the age group between sixty to sixty-nine, it is up to the individual to decide after consulting their family physicians.

Aspirin keeps early colon cancer at bay. How exactly does aspirin fulfill this onerous task? The first link stems from aspirin's power to reduce inflammation. It is well acknowledged that certain types of chronic inflammation contribute to cancer. Molecules that promote inflammation also boost cancer growth and metastasis. There is a vivid metaphor: *If cancer were a flame, inflammation would be the*

Age	Recommendation
Under 50	NOT recommended
50–59	Low dose, daily, for 10 years
60–69	Personal choice, consult physician
Over 70	NOT recommended

Image 8 Colon screening timetable. Assembled by Dr. Nancy Liu-Sullivan.

oxygen that fans the flame. By curbing inflammation, aspirin nips colon cancer in the bud before it gets a chance to flourish.

New studies have alluded to an additional dimension of aspirin action against early colon cancer: aspirin is beneficial to the good old cancer-restraining bacteria in the gut. It would be interesting to find out if yogurt loaded with billions of health-promoting bacteria over a plate of fresh greens dashed with blueberries and avocado slices could achieve a similar effect or even synergize with aspirin.

As I was putting the finishing touches to this manuscript, another study announced that scientists figured out a specific role aspirin plays against cancer: by restraining platelets. Roaming about in the bloodstream, platelets are potent agents that congeal blood (coagulation). What connects platelets with cancer? It turns out that immune killer T (KT, which bears CD8 molecules on the cell surface) are our elite troopers against cancer cells. Platelets, for not yet known reasons, inhibit KT cells. With aspirin curtailing platelet activities, KTs are free to launch anti-cancer attacks. Of course, a complex disease driven by a multitude of contributing factors, the effect of aspirin on KT is but one of many cancer-curbing angles. One trick carried out by cancer cells to keep KTs at bay is to take a molecular bite at the "NO-GO" protein called "immune checkpoint" on KT surface, leading to inactivation of KT. The detailed description can be found in the T cell essay series (page 187–192).

Food for thought:

1. On average, 5–10 percent of colon polyps can turn cancerous in ten to fifteen years.
   A. True
   B. False

2. Low-dose aspirin regimen has been reported to curb early colon cancer owing to aspirin's capacity of lowering inflammation and of preventing platelet aggregation.
   A. True
   B. False

ASPIRIN, WEEPING WILLOW, AND CREATIVE CHEMISTRY

Some say aspirin is from nature. Others contend it is a human invention. The truth resides somewhere in the middle. Let's dig deeper into the roots of aspirin and how innovative chemistry tinkering endowed a surprising medicinal entity to the magnificent arbor derivative.

It all started with the weeping willow. Some 4,000 years ago, our ancestors ground willow bark into powder and used it to alleviate aches and pains. In its crude form, the powder is a complex sack of chemicals consisting of key ingredients (at low concentrations), non-essential agents, and impurities. To achieve the desired medicinal effect, very large amount of the ground powder needed to be consumed. As is known, all medicines have side effects. The greater the amount, the more serious the adverse effects. Clearly, when it comes to willow bark, to maximize desired potency while minimizing undesired complications, the active ingredient ought to be hunted down!

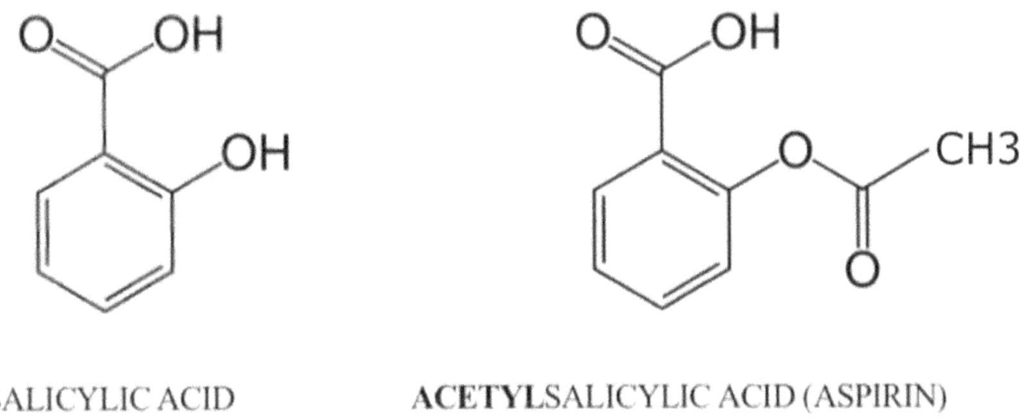

SALICYLIC ACID   ACETYLSALICYLIC ACID (ASPIRIN)

Image 9 Salicylic acid versus acetylsalicylic acid (aspirin). Wikimedia Commons File: Salicylic-acid-skeletal.svg and Wikipedia Commons File: Aspirin-skeletal.svg.

Willow bark's key ingredient uncovered! In 1859, a group of chemists identified salicylic acid (SA) as the key ingredient that enabled willow bark as a pain reliever and inflammation damper. Subsequently, other chemists successfully purified SA and were able to produce synthetic SA in the lab by mimicking the naturally occurring form.

The birth of aspirin. From crude powder to synthetic SA was by all means an impressive stride forward. But there was a big problem. The crude SA contains a chemical group called "phenol" which is a known corrosive used to clear clogged pipes. Ouch! As one can imagine, "phenol" also burns the human stomach lining. A chemist from the German Bayer company, Felix Hoffmann, began tinkering and successfully replaced the toxic "phenol" with a harmless chemical group called "acetyl." Now SA (salicylic acid) with the newly decorated "acetyl" officially became "acetylsalicylic acid" (ASA), which later acquired the more welcoming household name: aspirin. A side-by-side figure of SA and aspirin is illustrated:

A surprise sequel. It turned out that the unassuming "acetyl" that replaced the harsh "phenol" group empowered aspirin with a powerful property: blood thinning! The pioneering work was carried out by Dr. Lawrence Craven, a California country physician from the 1950s. Based on observations that aspirin prolonged the time taken for blood to clot, Dr. Craven proposed the hypothesis of aspirin as a preventive for coronary clots. In a large trial study of 8,000 participants with daily aspirin, none had coronary events. Dr. Craven's vision of aspirin for cardiovascular health was ahead of his time. But how exactly does aspirin thin the blood?

That mechanistic question was tackled a decade later, in the 1960s, by Dr. Harvey J. Weiss, who surmised that aspirin exerted an effect on platelets, which are tiny fragments known to clump together like a "molecular bandaid" to patch together injured tissues. Dr. Weiss demonstrated how platelets aggregated post-injury to the aorta in laboratory rabbits and how the introduction of aspirin dispersed clumped platelets. The mechanism of action of aspirin on anti-platelets was later elucidated as blocking a key molecule called thromboxane A2 (TXA2) in blood clotting (coagulation). Aspirin works by blocking the TXA2 enzyme called cyclooxygenase 1 (COX1). The coagulation signaling cascade and the step at which aspirin interferes is shown in the figure:

As shown on the left, platelet aggregation plays a role in wound healing on one hand, but on the other hand, it could lead to a cardiovascular event in individuals with vascular plaques. The figure on

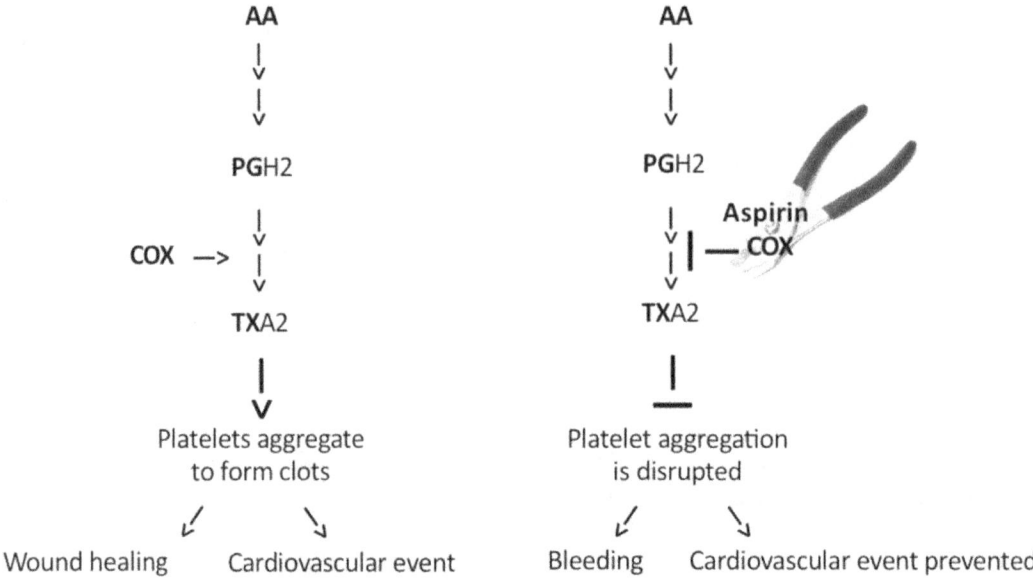

Image 10 Aspirin jams platelet aggregation. Assembled by Dr. Nancy Liu-Sullivan and combined with Wikimedia Commons File: Tool-pliers.jpg.

the right depicts how platelet aggregation is disrupted by aspirin's action. A quick recap of relevant terminologies: AA = arachidonic acid (a fatty acid that activates platelets), PGH2 = prostaglandin H2, upstream of TXA2.

Aspirin has a double edge. The same property of preventing platelet aggregation not only makes it easier to bleed but also bleed longer, especially in the elderly. Accordingly, the FDA has updated its recommendation in April 2022 and warns against daily aspirin routine as a cardiovascular prevention measure based on studies that the risks of bleeding outweigh the benefits for certain groups of people. Mayo Clinic, a leading healthcare professional facility, updated the general aspirin guidelines (based on information accessed in April 2025) summarized below: for individuals aged forty to seventy years who have had a heart attack or a stroke and who do not have bleeding risks, their physician *might* prescribe a daily low-dose aspirin to prevent another cardiovascular event (https://www.heart.org/en/health-topics/heart-attack/treatment-of-a-heart-attack/aspirin-and-heart-disease). For detailed medical guidance, it is always a good idea to consult your family physician.

Food for thought:

1. Aspirin's blood thinning capacity comes from the addition of an acetyl group to salicylic acid, the key ingredient extracted from willow tree bark.
   A. True
   B. False

2. Despite anti-inflammatory and anti-platelet activity, a major side effect of aspirin is bleeding.
   A. True
   B. False

B

BIRDS OF A FEATHER AND FURTHERMORE

One spring semester in a senior-level immunology class at my college, a talented pre-med student asked a question: Immune T cells are trained in the thymus and are called "T" cells, which makes sense. Well, B cells mature in the spleen, so why aren't they called "S" cells? Why indeed! The short answer: chicken.

A mysterious sac in large birds. To the surprise of many, chickens possess a fair share in contribution to immunology. The story is traced back to seventeenth century Italy: an anatomy specialist by the name of Hieronymus Fabricius discovered a sac-shaped organ in chickens which he named the *Bursa of Fabricius*. No one, however, had a clue about the function of the mysterious chicken bursa until the 1950s on the campus of Ohio State University. A Ph.D. student named Bruce Glick was laser-focused on his thesis research project that set out to decipher the function of *Bursa of Fabricius* in chickens. To study the role of an organ (or a gene), scientists remove the target of interest to assess which functions are lost in the organism in the absence of the organ (or the gene)—the so-called "loss-of-function" (LOF) experiments. Bruce did exactly that by subjecting his lab chickens to "Bursectomy." Days and weeks passed, and the chickens (from the Experimental Group) that roamed about with no *Bursa* appeared fine, just like the chickens in the Control group with intact *Bursa*. Befuddling!

Then, something totally unexpected happened. A fellow graduate student needed some chickens to demonstrate to an undergraduate class how chickens mount an immune defense against bacterial infection by producing antibody proteins. That class had been run many times, all with success in that all chickens invariably produced the expected antibodies to combat infection. The batch of chickens, this time, was generously supplied by Bruce.

The lab class failed because 80 percent of the chickens failed to churn out any antibodies despite having been deliberately subjected to a nasty kind of bacteria—an anomalous (unusual) event. Despair not, for anomalies are music to the ears of scientists, and no exception for Bruce. Close examination revealed that the chickens with zero antibodies had all undergone *Bursectomy*. There! A big function of the tiny Bursa finally began to emerge! Simply put: no bursa, no antibodies. The bursa, therefore, ought to be where antibodies are made. Bruce sent the exciting observational study to a slew of academic journals but was turned down one by one for insufficient evidence. Bruce persisted and eventually had the study published.

Another pivotal moment captured in chickens. The antibody-producing revelation about *Bursa* only touched the tip of the B cell immunity iceberg. More questions emerged. The next scientist who picked up the B cell study baton was Dr. Max Cooper, a physician from Louisiana, a decade after the seminal discovery by Bruce. To discern distinctive functions of *Bursa*-bound B cells and thymus-bound T cells in chicken immune defense, Max also applied the "loss-of-function" study design: chickens with or without *Bursa* or thymus, subjected to the presence or absence of irradiation. Patience and meticulous efforts paid off: Max unequivocally demonstrated that B cells contribute to the humoral immune response through antibody production, whereas T cells are indispensable for driving cell-mediated immune defense. Follow-up studies carried out by additional immunologists reveal remarkable joint-venture defense work by B cells and T cells in combating invading infectious bugs.

B cells in blood cancers. The year 2025 marks the sixtieth anniversary of the discovery of B cell's unique contribution to adaptive immunity. Like numerous types of body cells, B cells can also go awry and become cancerous. All cancer cells express ID marker proteins on their surface, ditto B cells. However, since cancer cells were once-upon-a-time normal cells before going rogue, many normal-cell surface markers are also found on cancer counterparts. One such marker on B cells is a molecule called CD 19. A platform of immunotherapy that targets CD 19 was developed and approved by the FDA to treat blood cancers that harbor CD 19.

Wait! You might be asking: If normal B cells also express CD 19, wouldn't the immunotherapy that kills cancerous B cells also annihilate normal B cells?? Indeed! In fact, leukemia and lymphoma patients who have undergone CD 19 immunotherapy also carry zero protective antibodies because all their B cells were thoroughly cleared—a condition called *B-cell aplasia*, as collateral damage from the therapy. But worry not: antibody replacement therapy is on the way! For details, please refer to **CAR-T THERAPY (2): A PHILADELPHIA STORY** (page 51).

As for my pre-med student who raised the "S" cell question, he scored perfectly on MCAT IMMUNOLOGY and equally fabulously on other subjects on the Medical College Admissions Test and is now a proud physician.

Food for thought:

1. Removal of Bursa is bursectomy. Removal of the spleen is splenectomy. Removal of the thymus of thymectomy.
   A. True
   B. False

2. Only cancerous B cells express CD 19 on their surface.
   A. True
   B. False

"BOY IN THE BUBBLE": THEN AND NOW

Same disorder. Two young boys. Nearly half a century apart. Very different outcomes: the second boy is cured, thanks to advancement of science.

Zero immune defense. The first boy was David, born in Texas in 1971. The second boy is Hataalii, born in Arizona in 2018. Despite a time span of forty-seven years, both boys were diagnosed with the same rare congenital immune disorder called "severe combined immunodeficiency" (SCID), caused by a genetic mutation that strikes at the very core of one's immune defense system. To put it bluntly: SCID individuals have zero immune defense and are extremely vulnerable to infections caused by bacteria, fungi, parasites, and viruses. They are particularly prone to lung infections and, sadly, SCID patients do not live to celebrate their very first birthday unless timely medical intervention is successfully carried out. What robs SCID patients of their immune defense?

Mutation is to blame. So far, fifteen different subtypes of SCID have been documented, each with a uniquely debilitating genetic mutation. For example, the critical gene mutated in David is called "*IL2Rg*" (pronounced as interleukin two receptor gamma), whereas the gene mutated in Hataalii is called "*Artemis.*" Generally speaking, SCID is classified as "T-/B+" (pronounced as T negative B positive) and "T-/B-" (T negative B negative). Here, "T" stands for immune T cells and "B" for immune B cells. As indicated, T cells are absent in both groups, whereas B cell presence varies. However, since T cells are indispensable for B cell activation, the absence of T cells, in actuality, renders all patients deprived of both T and B cell immune protection.

David in a bubble. To guard David against infections from bugs and germs in the environment, a special sterile plastic bubble hut was constructed to house David's everyday life, including home schooling until the age of twelve. Then came the decision of transplanting bone marrow stem cells from David's sister. The procedure could have worked to save David's life had it not been met with an unexpected and unfortunate turn: His sister's bone marrow carried an infectious virus called "Epstein-Barr Virus" (EBV). Back in 1964, EBV was identified as a lymphoma-causing virus—the first cancer-causing virus identified. As the stem cells from his sister's bone marrow were transplanted to David, so too were the viruses, although at the time David's medical team was unaware of the silent virus. Deprived of a working immune system, David was unable to fend off the viral infection which rapidly deteriorated to full-blown lymphoma (cancer of the lymphatic system) and took David's life in four months.

A conundrum: How come that David's sister who carried EBV in her bone marrow was able to lead a normal life cancer-free while David quickly succumbed to viral infection-triggered cancer? The answer resides in immune defense: Individuals with a strong immune system are able to keep EBV at bay, whereas those with severely weakened immune systems, such as David Vetter, are unable to.

Despite merely twelve years on planet Earth, David left an indelible dent. Among many contributions to medical science, David's condition shed more light on the in-depth understanding of devastating SCIDs. Of equal importance, the expedited development from EBV viral infection to full-scale cancer provides supporting evidence of a causal link between viral infection and biogenesis of cancer and, in parallel, the quintessential role immune system plays in making or breaking cancer.

Precious freedom to run in the yard. While Hataalii's SCID stemmed from mutation of a different gene called "*Artemis,*" it nonetheless rendered Hataalii without a complete immune system the moment he was born. Thanks to a novel experimental gene therapy treatment innovated by physicians at University of California, San Francisco (UCSF), Hataalii's immune system was successfully restored. No plastic bubble "prescription" for Hataalii. How did the gene therapy work?

Mutation in *Artemis*. The root cause of Hataalii's devastating immune disorder is the mutated *Artemis* gene. To correct the disease, the faulty gene must be corrected. To introduce the correct gene, a molecular vehicle called "vector" was needed. Since viral particles are fast-proliferating species, team UCSF selected *Lentivirus* as the vector to harbor the correct gene. *Lenti* is a French prefix meaning "slow" as "*lentiment.*" The Lentivirus of interest is derived from the Human Immunodeficiency Virus (HIV). No alarm! These are not original HIV viruses but are genetically modified to become "replication incompetent" which means that the viruses are unable to make copies of themselves; hence, no qualms about getting infected with HIV via the gene therapy. To make sure of the correct gene settling down in all body cells in Hataalii, the physicians obtained stem cells from Hataalii. Why? Because stem cells are the "cradle" of all cell types in our body. After introducing the correct gene to Hataalii's stem cells, these engineered cells are returned to Hataalii and start to disseminate gene products from the corrected *Artemis*. Mission accomplished! The experimental steps are illustrated in the following figure.

Step 1: Introduce the **correct copy of the gene** onto a molecular "vehicle" called "vector".	Step 2: Collect **stem cells** from patient's bone marrow	Step 3: Infect stem cells with the virus carrying the correct gene	Step 4: Now patient's stem cells carry the correct gene	Step 5: Return stems cells back to the patient to help grow immune cells in the patient.

Image 11 Stem cell molecular ENGINEERING steps. Assembled by Dr. Nancy Liu-Sullivan.

As illustrated, the correct copy of the *Artemis* gene was incorporated into the Lenti viral vector and was used to "infect" the stem cells obtained from Hataalii. Upon successful infection, the stem cells now carry the correct *Artemis* gene and were returned to the body of Hataalii. As stem cells become mature and get dispatched throughout Hataalii's body, the faulty gene is now replaced by the correct gene. Guided by the correct gene, Hataalii's body is now endowed with a normal immune system that harbors T cells and B cells to help fend off invading infectious bugs.

Today, Hataalii lives like any normal toddler, running, rolling, laughing, and breathing natural air under the sun, thanks to advancement of biomedical science!

Food for thought:

1. Patients of SCID (severe combined immunodeficiency) have zero immune defense systems in their bodies as a result of dysfunctional T cells and B cells.
   A. True
   B. False

2. David Vetter quickly developed lymphoma upon infection by Epstein-Barr Virus (EBV) as a result of non-existent immune defense system in his body.
   A. True
   B. False

C

CANCER TRICKS AND TRAPS (1): SWEET AND SOUR CRAVINGS

Sugar and vinegar whipped with a smidgen of ketchup blended with a sprinkle of soy sauce—out comes savory sweet and sour sauce. Yum! Cancer, believe it or not, also possesses a palate for sweet and sour to sustain its insatiable growth. What's in this cancer "secret sauce"?

Sugar is power. All cells rely on sugar to make cellular gasoline called "adenosine triphosphate" (ATP). Sugar comes in assorted flavors. The sugar craved by cancer cells is glucose, a simple sugar. How do normal cells glean glucose? Easy. The orange juice you have for breakfast, the rock sugar you add to coffee, and the warm milk you savor before bedtime are all sources of glucose after these complex sugars get broken down. Normal healthy cells in our body make ATP from glucose in a three-stage process, as shown in the simplified summary table below: (1) Glycolysis (that yields 2 ATP), (2) Citric *acid cycle* (that also yields 2 ATP), and (3) Oxidative *phosphorylation* (which is the most productive of all stages, yielding 28 ATP). A pretty cost-effective process of 32 ATP from each glucose molecule. Cancer cells, confined by their living environment, preferentially rely on Stage 1 of glycolysis. Why? Glycolysis takes place with no dependence on oxygen. Very poor in oxygen supply, this cancer choice reflects how crucial adaptability that stems from selective pressure is for cancer survival.

Cancer's sweet and sour penchant. The cancer ATP production predilection comes with a catch: Due to low yield, cancer cells must consume a ton of glucose to generate enough ATP. Here is a catch within a catch: Glucose gets broken down to yield "pyruvate." For normal cells, pyruvate enters the next stage of the citric acid cycle. For cancer cells that eschew the next stage, a ton of glucose

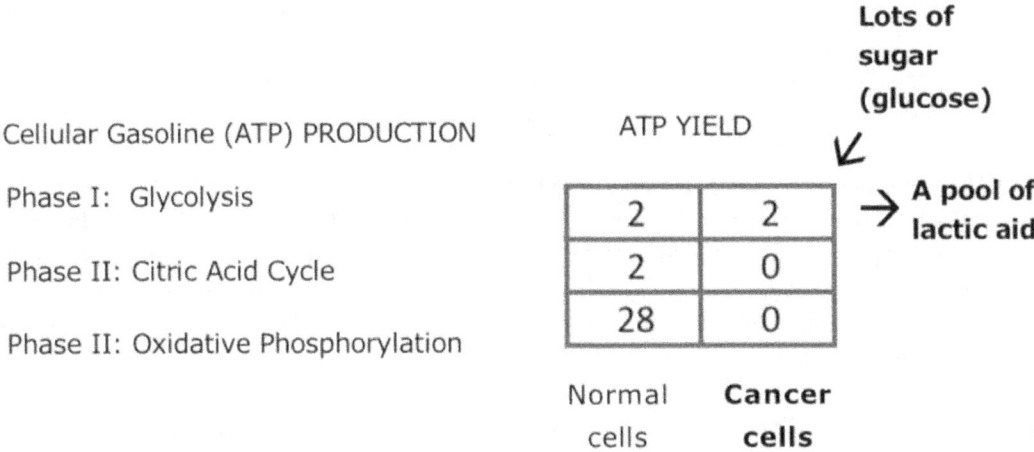

Image 12 Idiosyncratic way by which cancer gleans cellular fuel. Assembled by Dr. Nancy Liu-Sullivan.

generates a ton of lactic acid that gets accumulated in cancer quarters. The **glucose → pyruvate → lactic acid** cascade renders cancer cells constantly bathing in a pool of acids!

Warburg effect. Cancer cells' penchant for breaking down glucose in the absence of oxygen was first observed by Otto Warburg, a German physician-scientist, some two hundred years ago, and it is coined as the Warburg effect. Why on earth do cancer cells favor the no-oxygen way of making cellular fuel when it is so inefficient and generates a ton of acid waste?! Well, it turns out that the waste is turned into a potent molecular defense treasure by cancer cells. More discussion in the next essay.

Food for thought:

1. Cancer cells have a huge appetite for glucose because they rely on only glycolysis to make ATP, which is of low efficiency. This is compensated by large quantities of glucose.
   A. True
   B. False

2. Glucose gets broken down to pyruvate, which is converted to lactic acid. Large amounts of glucose yield large amounts of lactic acid.
   A. True
   B. False

CANCER TRICKS AND TRAPS (2): INUNDATING IMMUNE CELLS IN AN ACIDIC POND

What advantage does a harsh acidic environment provide for cancer? To grasp a good understanding of this question, let's take a step back for a panoramic view of cancer's surroundings.

The tumor neighborhood. Cancer does not exist alone. It takes a village to build the cancer community called "tumor micro environment" (TME). If we imagine cancer as a "house," the TME is the front, back, and side yards. Residing within the confines of the TME are immune cells and support cells. You might say: Great! Is this a case where cancer-fighting immune cells are keeping enemy cancer cells closer? Yes and no. Yes, because immune cells, especially Killer T (KT) cells, are indeed fierce cancer-killing troopers. No, because by and large these immune cells are either corrupted or suppressed by cancer. How does cancer disable host immune system so readily? Acid is to blame.

Acids keep immune cells at bay. The pool of lactic acid immersing the tumor village exerts drastically different effects on TME cellular residents. To begin with, Killer T (KT) cells, the host elite anti-cancer troopers, are literally put into a state of "lethargy" by the acidic milieu, as manifested by no activities. These stagnant KT cells eventually undergo programmed cell death termed "apoptosis," in which the cell's internal death pathway is turned on, fragmenting the cell into a pile of broken pieces followed by subsequent demise.

Corrupting Tregs to do cancer's dirty work. As an added assurance of immune suppression, cancer cells also trick host "regulatory T cells" (Tregs) into cancer enablers. Under normal conditions, Tregs rise up to bring peace and balance to the host immune system that has just completed a battle against infection. Without Tregs, the immune system would continue on a trail of destruction of good body cells, much like the senseless *Don Quixote* portrayed by Cervantes of Spain. Thanks to Tregs, the immune system is prevented from going overboard. Taking advantage of this very immune-suppressing power by Tregs, cancer cells cleverly turn Tregs into immune "gladiators" against host immune cells, be they T cells, B cells, Natural Killer (NK) cells, or macrophages and dendritic cells (DC). You might ask: Okay, cancer converts Tregs to suppressors of immune fighter cells. But, akin to T cells that become active confronting a pool of acids within the tumor microenvironment (TME), shouldn't Tregs cells be also affected by deleterious acids? Thoughtful question! To rescue Tregs, cancer secretes molecules to equip Tregs with a unique capacity to resist and survive the tumor's acrid atmosphere. What are these quiet but powerful molecules?

TGFβ and Foxp3 taking center stage. A versatile signaling molecule, "transforming growth factor beta" (TGFβ) is a cytokine recruited by cancer to the TME to coach Tregs in basic survival skills in harsh acids. TGFβ relies on a sidekick partner called "Foxp3" to help carry out Treg training. An even more seasoned Treg survival coach, Foxp3 guides Tregs to reprogram metabolic energetics. Remember, during glycolysis, glucose gets brown down to pyruvate, which then is converted to lactic acid. And lactic acid is the culprit behind Tregs' survival challenge. To reduce the level and extent of lactic acid, Foxp3 facilitates conversion of lactic acid back to pyruvate, which then enters Stage 2 (Citric Acid cycle) and subsequently Stage 3 (oxidative phosphorylation). Hence, converting toxic acids back to an intermediary product to continue to drive ATP production is a win-win that rescues Tregs out of the unlivable acidic environment and boosts the yield of cellular fuel ATP. To recap:

1. *Cancer activates TGFβ →*
2. *TGFβ activates Foxp3 →*
3. *Foxp3 empowers Tregs →*
4. *Tregs suppress immune cells →*
5. *Cancer escapes immune destruction*

As depicted above, the logistics supply loop to prep Tregs is ready-set-and-go to keep immune cells at bay which paves the way for cancer to survive, thrive, and spread to healthy tissues and organs near and distal. A quick note on cancer metastasis: Pancreatic cancer tends to spread to the liver, melanoma to the brain, and breast cancer to the liver, lungs, and bones. It remains a mystery as to why, while breast cancer metastasizes to other organs, it rarely does spread from one breast to the other. Another topic, another time.

So far, we have explored how acids accumulate as a byproduct of lactic acid production due to cancer's voracious appetite for glucose. There is one additional source that drives cancer acidity, as described in the next essay.

Food for thought:

1. High acidity in the tumor core makes T cells inactive.
    A. True
    B. False

2. Cancer cells transform Treg cells (which calm down an active immune system under healthy conditions) to suppress immune cells and block immune cells from attacking cancer cells.
    A. True
    B. False

CANCER TRICKS AND TRAPS (3): THRIVING IN LOW OXYGEN

In the two previous essays of this series, we learned about cancer's sweet and sour molecular taste buds and how acidity acts as a powerful cancer survival enabler. Here, let us continue to peel the cancer survival "onion" by exploring how oxygen (or precisely oxygen deprivation) is tied to cancer's sweet and sour idiosyncrasies.

Cancer is oxygen-poor. The center of a malignant tumor harbors dark regions, as shown in the figure of mouse glioblastoma multiforme (GBM) cells grown into a three-dimensional tumor sphere mimic by research students in my laboratory at the City University of New York College of Staten Island. The original cell line was a generous gift from Dr. Johanna Joyce, MSKCC.

The dark center (pointed out by arrows) in the tumor core is a sure sign of oxygen deficiency. Cancerous tumors invariably suffer from lack of oxygen (also called hypoxia) due to fast cancer growth outpacing generation of vasculature (blood vessels) for the sorely needed oxygen. ***Quick Word Anatomy***: *Hypo* = under, *Oxic* = oxygen, hence *Hypoxia* = deficiency in oxygen. Hypoxia is associated with a form of cell death termed "necrosis." ***Quick Word Anatomy***: *Nekros* = dead corpse; hence necrosis is translated into plain English as "cell death from within," also coined as "necrotic death."

Cancer's oxygen problem. Oxygen, transported by blood, is the lifeline of all cells of our body. In cases of tissue injuries for normal cells, for example, new blood vessels are formed to beef up blood and nutrient supply to injured areas. For cancer cells that grow incessantly, the demand for new blood vessels is also always high. Mission impossible! Cancer cells are simply unable to satisfy their own

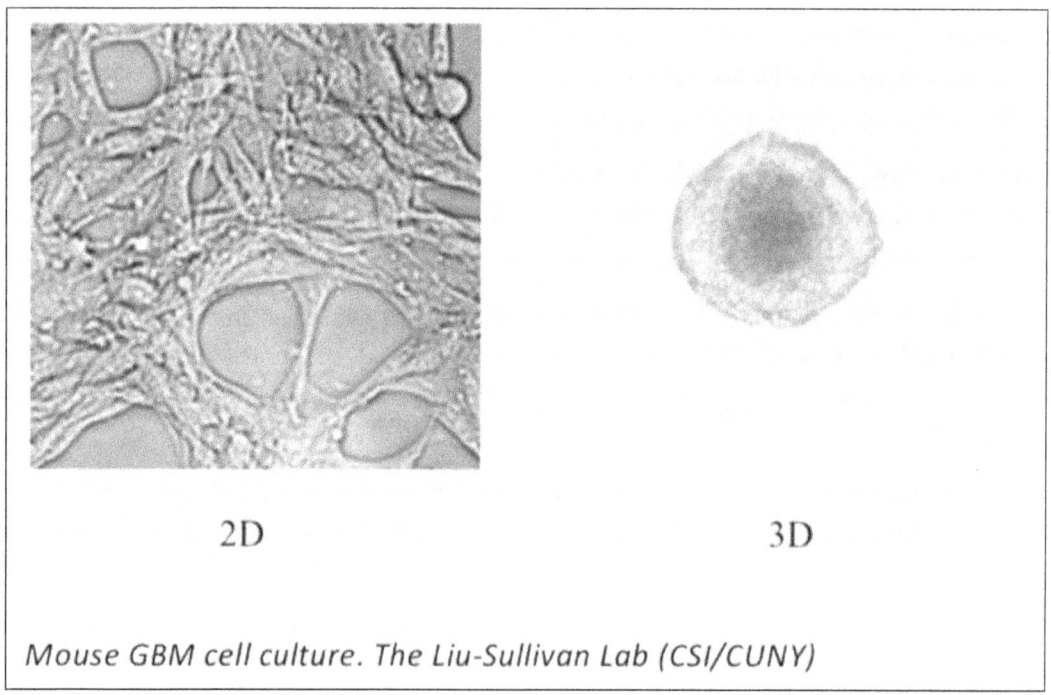

Mouse GBM cell culture. The Liu-Sullivan Lab (CSI/CUNY)

Image 13 Mouse brain tumor in 2d and 3d. Credit to Liu-Sullivan Lab, CSI/CUNY..

demand. At this point, it seems logical to assume that due to sketchy blood supply and inadequacy of oxygen, cancer cells should die off in strolls. Yet, the reality is the opposite: Cancer cells continue to grow and expand in spite of poor oxygen. What's going on? How do cancer cells smooth out the oxygen supply chain quagmire?

No oxygen, no problem. It turns out that cancer has evolved to survive the low oxygen way of living, owing to self-directed adaptations from confronting enormous selective pressure and, here, the pressure to survive. Specifically, sensing a dearth of oxygen, genes that specialize in low oxygen management called "hypoxia inducible factors" (*HIF*) are activated. *HIF* genes come in many subtypes. *HIF-1*, for example, steps up the plate to reprogram cancer cells into low oxygen-tolerant species. Now we have our *Ah-ha* moment: Cancer resorts to making ATP from glucose in the absence of oxygen because cancer is simply a pauper when it comes to oxygen! Hypoxic regulatory genes come to the rescue to allow cancer to make ATP to fuel cellular activities without relying on oxygen while at the same time flooding cancer living quarters with acids to shield cancer by drowning out immune cells—Survival by adaptation, in a twisted fashion. Below is a summary of how cancer evolves to maximize its survival:

1. *Cancer confronts poor blood supply* →
2. *Cancer is oxygen deprived* →
3. *Cancer hypoxia genes are activated* →
4. *Cancer adapts to no-oxygen survival mode* →
5. *Cancer breaks down glucose to make ATP without oxygen* →
6. *Acids accumulate inside cancer cells* →
7. *Cancer cells expel acids to flood the tumor microenvironment (TME)* →
8. *Acids suppress immune cells in TME* →
9. *Acids shield cancer from immune destruction* →
10. *Cancer continues with unstoppable growth and spreading by looping back to Step 1 and all over again and again.*

Amazing how fast cancer research is progressing: as I was in the process of editing this very essay before submitting the revised manuscript to my publisher, a new study reports an exciting observation of how lactic acid (that floods the tumor village) augments tumor resistance against chemotherapy. How do cancer cells achieve this feat? They do so by enhancing DNA repair gene activities to fix cancer cells damaged by chemo drugs. By upgrading the tumor's capacity to repair drug-damaged DNA, cancer cells are able to undo the work of chemo with speedy recovery. Knowing where the problem lies helps pave the way to devise a way to overcome the problem. Let us continue to keep our hopes high.

Rarely is cancer so uncomplicated! With all of the above assorted cancer "survival" schemes said, there is yet one more layer to cancer's self-serving mechanism of defense: a tough cellular fence. Details to follow in the next essay.

Food for thought:

1. Cancerous tumor is deprived of oxygen due to inadequate or incomplete newly built blood vessels.
    A. True
    B. False

2. Cancer cells adapt to low oxygen by turning on genes that help cancer survive in a no oxygen environment. These genes are called hypoxic genes.
   A. True
   B. False

CANCER TRICKS AND TRAPS (4): HARD FENCES MAKE BAD TUMORS

In response to hurricane warning, neighbors lay sandbags around their residence to fend off uninvited flash floods. Cancerous tumors also build a fence, though made up of protein fibers, as an instinctual self-preservation reaction. Let's take a closer look.

Desmoplasia: Cancer's citadel. There is a somewhat esoteric name for the cancer-protective fence: *Desmoplasia*. **Quick word anatomy**: *Desm-* is a prefix rooted in ancient Greek that denotes "connective." *Plassein* is a suffix for "formation." Combining the two parts yields "*Desmoplasia*," which translates to "tumor-insulating fence." The cellular bricks and mortar for constructing the desmoplasia are collagen fibers secreted by a type of cell called fibroblasts. You might be asking: Fibroblasts provide structural support for tissues and participate in wound healing. By no means fibroblasts are cancerous cells. Absolutely right! However, in light of how clever cancer is at gleaning anything and turning it to serve cancer survival, one wouldn't be surprised that here in the tumor microenvironment (TME) cancer degrades fibroblasts to become cancer-associated fibroblasts (CAFs). What's more, working in cahoots with CAFs, cancer also turns immune macrophage cells into "tumor-associated macrophages" (TAMs), which, together with CAFs, cook up a storm of collagens to form desmoplasia.

Exactly how does desmoplasia serve cancer? Desmoplasia blocks radiation therapy that aims at breaking cancer cell DNA, stunts chemotherapy designed to jam up cancer cell division engine, and hinders targeted therapy engineered to disable critical cancer growth and expansion pathways. Not surprisingly, solid cancers notorious for being treatment-resistant are cancers that harbor a thick *desmoplasia*. Sadly, the severity of *desmoplasia* is inversely associated with cancer prognostics: the harder and thicker the *desmoplasia*, the less the length of the patient''''s overall survival rate. An acute example is pancreatic cancer with the full name *pancreatic ductal carcinoma* (PDA), a devastating cancer of the pancreas that has taken the lives of so many including iconic Apple founder Steve Jobs and noted Jeopardy host Alex Trebek. Both fought very bravely. RIP!

The tumor village. To gain a better understanding of tumor desmoplasia, let's pause to zoom out for a forest view of the tumor village. No tumor is an island. Embedded within cancer cells are complex tumor infrastructures of immune cells, in particular tumor-associated macrophages (TAMs), tumor-associated neutrophils (TANs), endothelial cells, epithelial cells, CAFs, and regulatory T (Tregs). The busy community of non-cancer cells that resides in the tumor microenvironment (TME) acts as abettors to promote unrestrained tumor growth and metastasis, as shown in the following figure.

As shown above, the sturdy desmoplastic fence is strategically situated on all sides of the tumor to deflect radiation beams and cancer drugs from entering the tumor proper. This hard tumor-shielding fence ought to be dismantled to allow more efficient delivery of medicinal arsenals to the tumor core. Easier said than done. To know how to tear down the tumor fence, we must decompose the complex desmoplastic network into its component parts in order to understand how the fence is constructed, what sustains nutrient supply chain, and which cell types and signaling molecules are the chief movers

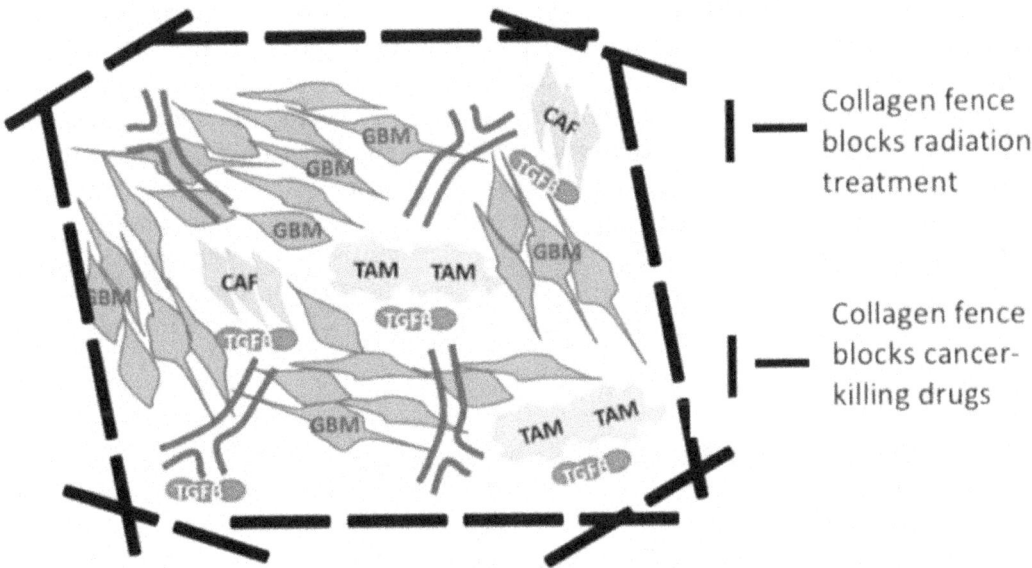

Image 14 Hedge fence for tumor defense. Assembled by Dr. Nancy Liu-Sullivan.

and shakers, which leads us to the milestone discoveries by a brilliant and dedicated pancreatic cancer expert and her proud research team.

Cracking the pancreatic cancer fence code. The leading pancreatic cancer research expert is my very own PhD mentor, the respected Dr. Dafna Bar-Sagi, who, in parallel to running a large research laboratory, guiding a squadron of research scientists and clinical fellows, scrutinizing new data sets, writing grants, publishing papers, giving invited talks nationally and internationally, also at once serving at the helm of the New York University Langone Health flagship as Senior VP and Chief Scientific Officer. Being indefatigable and astute is an utter understatement.

Undeterred dedication has yielded sagacious insights into how pancreatic cancer reprograms metabolic pathways in a cascade of intricately coordinated tumor biology events, as summarized below:

Step 1: Tumor-associated macrophage (TAM) swallows up a whole collagen;
Step 2: TAM breaks apart collagen;
Step 3: TAM obtains arginine, a type of amino acid that serves as a key building blocks of collagen;
Step 4: Increasing levels of arginine serve as a stimulus for the production of reactive nitrogen species (RNS), a potent free radical;
Step 5: Increasing levels of RNS activates pancreatic stellate cells (PSC), a pancreas-specific cell type that plays a pivotal role in structural support;
Step 6: PSC is now in full swing to assemble collagens into bundles and patches;
Step 7: These collagen bundles and patches become the bricks and mortar for a brand *new* collagen fence or desmoplasia to block off anti-cancer radiotherapy, chemotherapy, and targeted therapy.

You might be asking: Wait a minute! What do you mean by "*a brand new collagen fence*?" Fair question. It turns out that the collagen fence around pancreatic tumor is not forever but gets constantly rebuilt and renewed, much like a sea crab continuously shedding off its hard shell and replacing the old with the new. Months ago, as I was drafting the essay titled ***CRAB: THE NAME TELLS A VIVID TALE*** (page 72), I raised a hypothetical question of whether cancer cells also shed their "shell" periodically and if so, could that be a cancer *Achilles heel* that we can leverage to develop an anti-cancer drug? That was a pure thinking-out-loud question before I came across Dr. Bar-Sagi's paper. And now here is one such opportunity to literally capture cancer in its moment of weakness of being between *shells*—with the old hard shell dying off and the new shell still being soft?! As additional pancreatic cancer desmoplasia enigmas get decoded, a more lucid picture shall be in view with promises for a new class of meds that smacks down pancreatic cancer in that moment of molecular and cellular weakness. Looking forward to more unravellings of pancreatic cancer desmoplasia by Team Bar-Sagi!

Food for thought:

1. Collagen fibers form a sturdy fence to protect cancerous tumors.
   A. True
   B. False

2. Cancer transforms normal fibroblasts into CAFs to churn out a ton of collagen bricks to beef up desmoplasia.
   A. True
   B. False

CANCER TRICKS AND TRAPS (5): DYING TUMORS RAISE A STINK

The core of malignant tumors is constantly undergoing "necrosis" (or dirty cell death). The term is said to have been coined by the nineteenth-century German physician-scientist, Dr. Rudolf Virchow.

Death happens in the tumor core. Shown in the following figure is another snapshot of a mouse glioblastoma multiforme (GBM) sphere—tumor in a Petri dish from my research laboratory.

Why does necrotic tumor death selectively concentrate in the core of the tumor? Well, that is a hard-to-reach region for blood supply and oxygen distribution. Oxygen deprivation combined with bathing in caustic acids is a recipe for cellular havoc, and the havoc is manifested as necrosis, a form of messy death initiated inside a cancer cell, marring everything in the cells, including DNA, the genetic material. While intuitive assumption may interpret this dire state of the tumor core as an inauspicious beginning of the end for the entire tumor, closer examination has revealed an astonishing opposite: Tumor necrotic death promotes tumor growth, enhances tumor expansion, and expedites invasion. How odd, and how come?

Creative destruction? To understand how tumor regional demise ends up facilitating overall tumor survival, we need to find out what happens during the necrotic implosion. Studies have shown that dying tumor cells release, among a host of factors, large quantities of potassium, which, together with other key electrolytes (sodium, calcium, and magnesium), maintain cellular metabolism. In the context of dying cancer cells, potassium plays a pro-tumor and anti-immune system role.

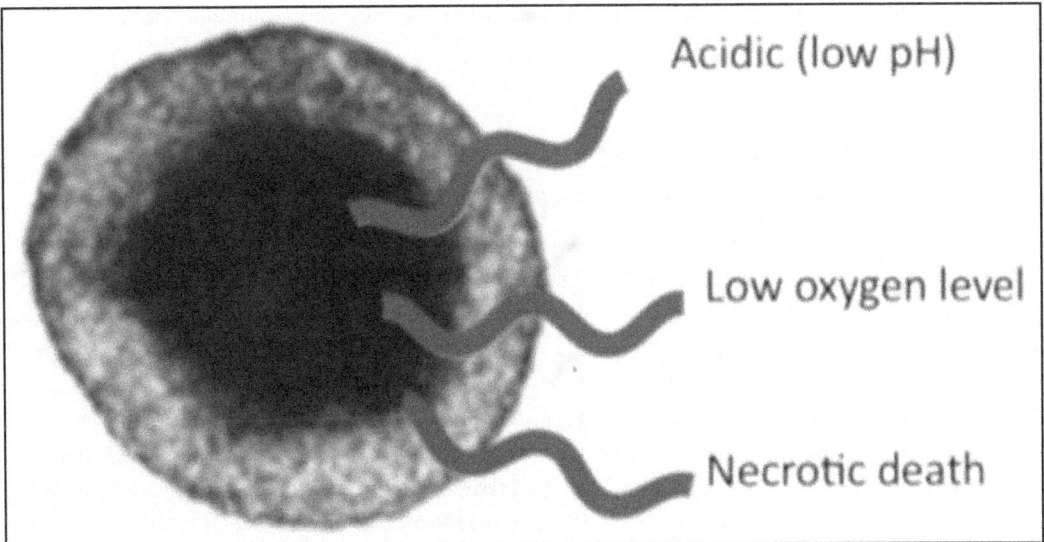

Image 15 Triple whammy confounds tumor core. Credit to Liu-Sullivan Lab, CSI/CUNY.

Specifically, tumor-released potassium weakens immune CD4-T (or helper T) cells, CD8-T (or Killer T) cells, and Natural Killer (NK) cells, all of which are potent anti-cancer immune fighters when functioning normally. In other words, dying tumor cells release potent potassium to cripple cancer-fighting immune cells. How convenient! Akin to the popular "creative destruction" adage in the field of economics where dismantling an old and decrepit structure makes it possible to build anew, tumor necrosis, too, confers a chance for tumors to grow faster with greater metastatic potential. Generally speaking, the extent of tumor necrosis is inversely proportional to cancer patient prognosis where, the more extensive the necrosis, the poorer the prognosis. Thanks to hard-working cancer biologists, an unexpected but mighty important observation has been made where disruption of a blood-vessel-regulatory gene, termed "angio-poietin-like 7" (A-7) in a laboratory rat cancer model has reduced tumor necrosis by up to 99 percent. **Quick Word Anatomy**: "*Angio*" refers to "vessel" and "poietin" for "maker." Both rooted in ancient Greek, the combination means "vessel maker" or, in this context, "blood vessel maker." In light of how A-7 gene in active state plays a critical role in promoting tumor necrosis and how necrosis is unfavorably associated with patient survival, silencing A-7 to suppress necrosis offers a promising possibility for a treatment strategy to prolong prognosis and extend patient lives. For a detailed description, please visit https://www.fredhutch.org/en/news/center-news/2023/02/new-research-insights-into-cancer-tumor-necrotic-core-.html.

Food for thought:

1. Necrotic death severely hampers tumor growth.
    A. True
    B. False

2. Potassium released during tumor necrosis facilitates cancer-fighting immune cells.
   A. True
   B. False

CANCER TRICKS AND TRAPS (6): HAND CAUGHT IN COOKIE JAR

To sustain constant outgrowth, cancer evolves to adapt to surviving in low oxygen and thriving in acidity. Still, ATP, the precious cellular fuel, is hard to glean despite non-stop consumption of glucose. To ensure a seamless glucose supply chain, cancer also commits "cellular thievery." Let's find out how.

Target selection. Cellular fuel is stored in the mitochondrion, a tiny compartment located between the cell membrane and the nucleus. Each cell harbors hundreds of mitochondria as fuel factories. Unquestionably, mitochondria would be the optimal target structure for cancer cells to steal fuel from, but all cells harbor mitochondria. Which cell type is the most ideal target?

One stone, two birds. It turns out that immune T cells in the host are cancer's favorite target for snatching cellular fuel. The manner by which cancer cells carry out the deed bears striking resemblance to airplane aerial refueling, as shown in the following figure:

Shown above, cancer cells extend a hollow tube that pokes directly into the mitochondria of T cells. Why T cells? Recall that two types of T cells coordinate for activation, starting with CD4-T cells being activated in lymph nodes after receiving immune danger "intel" from dendritic cells (DCs). This step serves as the prerequisite for the activation of CD8-T (the so-called Killer T, KT)—Cancer's

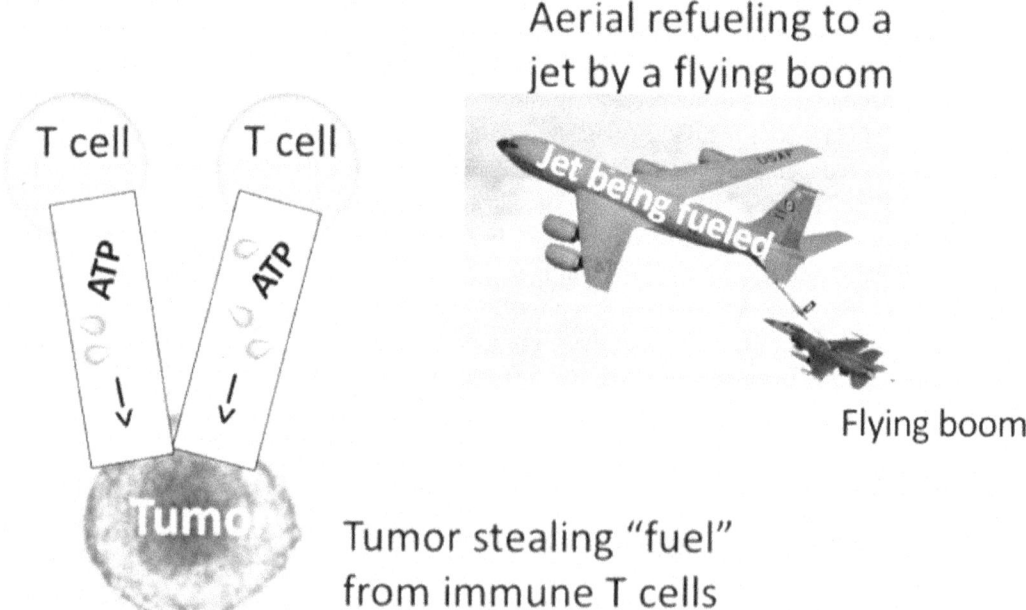

Image 16 Tumor caught in the act. Assembled by Dr. Nancy Liu-Sullivan and combined with Wikimedia Commons File: Kc-135 refuels an F-16 Fighting Falcon.jpg.

arched enemy. Once activated, KT kick-starts immune surveillance and subsequent elimination of infected cells as well as cancer cells. So, it makes perfect survival sense for cancer to go after T cells as a two-pronged scheme: (1) to snatch fuel and (2) to weaken T cells. Another win-win for cancer, not for the better.

Food for thought:

1. Cancer cells constantly confront cellular fuel crisis.
   A. True
   B. False

2. To compensate for ATP supply, cancer cells commit molecular thievery by directly snatching ATP out of the mitochondria of immune fighter T cells.
   A. True
   B. False

CANCER TRICKS AND TRAPS (7): A GAME OF MIA

"*Readyyyyyy, hut!*" The offense team Quarterback shouts out. The Center skillfully snaps the ball to the Quarterback. Let the games begin!

Science imitating sport? Naive about American football, I often wonder about why there is a need for the ceremonial ball snapping from the Center to the Quarterback. Why can't the game start with the Quarterback having the ball in hand? What purpose does the extra step serve? Well, there is neither rhyme nor reason; that is simply the name of the game! Interestingly, a similar situation is found in how immune response kickstarts. Let's sort out the players.

KT AND DC: Immune "Quarterback" and "Center." Akin to American football where the Center snaps the ball to the Quarterback to start the game, the immune Quarterback called Killer T (KT) cell receives a very important piece of intelligence termed as "cancer antigen" from the immune "Center" called dendritic cell (DC) to initiate an immune reaction. Unlike the game of football, this immune "intel" exchange is not for show but for "dough," the dough being a "tutorial" lesson for KT to learn how to accurately identify cancer cells by literally tasting a slice of cancer called cancer antigen. The KT taste bud situated on the KT surface is called T cell receptor (TCR). Now, TCR has a very particular feature: it is unable to spot cancer antigen directly; it can only recognize cancer antigen presented on a molecular silver platter called MHC Class I (MHC-I). The immune tutorial lesson for KT provided by DC takes place in a lymph node. Having mastered the way, shape, and form of cancer cells, KT exits the lymph node with the mission to hunt down cancer cells. This is the first half of the game. The second half takes place where cancer cells reside. The same procedure of KT TCR tasting the cancer antigen shown on MHC-I repeats, except that this time the task of presentation is carried out by cancer cells. Once TCR makes sure that the same cancer antigen on the cancer cell surface matches the cancer antigen KT has learned during the tutorial lesson by DC, KT is swiftly activated and ready to pounce on the cancer cell for speedy annihilation—Game over for cancer. Fantastic, except the above-portrayed first and second halves of the game is the ideal-world scenario. In the world of cancer reality, however, two hurdles exist, both stemming from the same *deliberate* cancer defect.

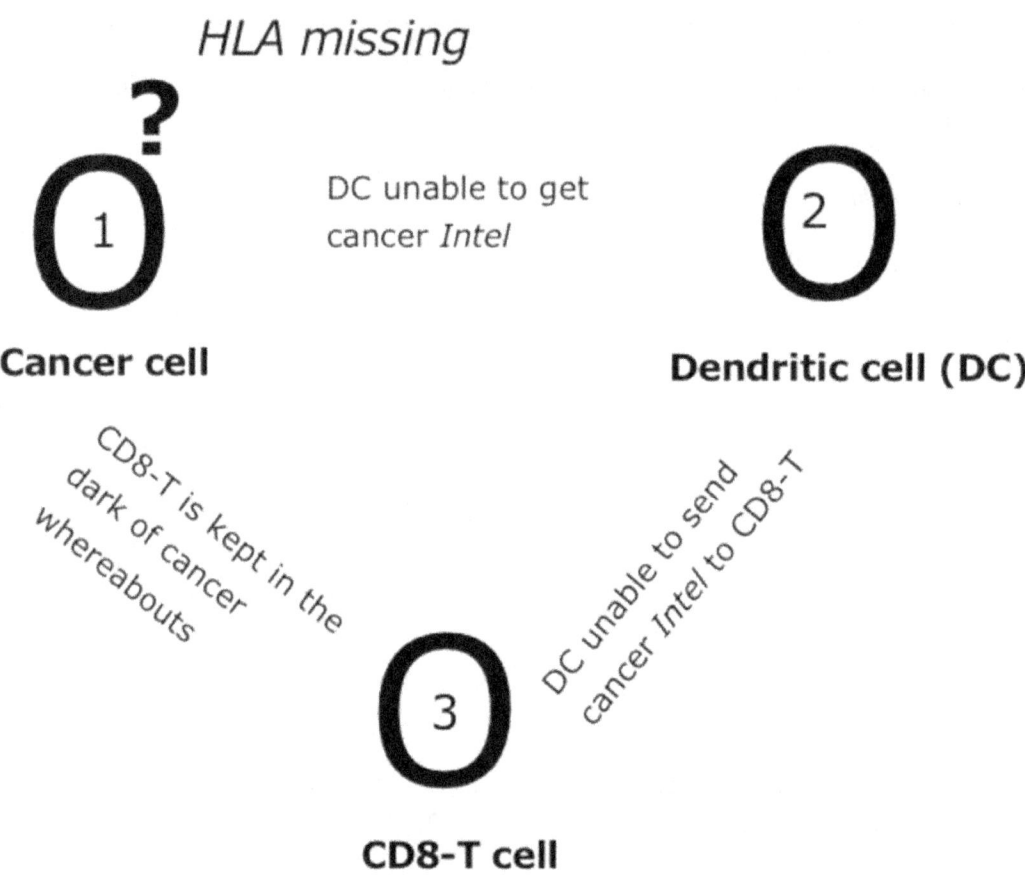

Image 17 Tumor game of hide-and-seek. Assembled by Dr. Nancy Liu-Sullivan.

MHC-I: Silver platter MIA. Both KT interactions with DC followed by KT interactions with cancer cells depend on intact MHC-I, the molecular silver platter that displays cancer antigens. Cunning buggers that they are, cancer cells engage in a game of MIA, that is, to make MHC-I disappear to escape KT attack.

As shown, the absence of MHC (also called HLA) on cancer cells keeps KT cells in the dark, allowing cancer cells to run for dear life. Below is a microcosm of the extent of missing MHC-I on several types of cancer cells. Since the HLA Class I equivalence of MHC-I is associated with human cells, we shall use HLA-I in the following description.

- In colon and rectum cancers collectively termed "colorectal cancer" (CRC), approximately 44 percent of HLA Class I Classical genes are defective.
- In an aggressive type of lung cancer called non-small cell lung cancer (NSCLC), aberrant HLA Class I genes fall within a range of 40–50 percent.
- In aggressive breast cancer, HLA abnormal activities are 40–70 percent.
- In ovarian cancer, HLA defects are 30–60 percent.
- For soft tissue sarcomas (cancers of bones and muscles), HLA flaws cover the most extensive range of 25–80 percent.

Science outwits cancer. All HLA deviation roads lead to one destination: to aid cancer cells in escaping immune surveillance. To get around this cancer molecular subterfuge, scientists have developed innovative T cell therapy to bypass the HLA requirement by equipping Killer T (KT) cells with an artificial molecular "GPS" to enable KT cells to unmistakably spot cancer cells for speedy elimination. Half a dozen such T cell therapeutic treatment platforms have been approved by the FDA at this point. For a detailed description, please peruse the CAR-T THERAPY series (pages 48—67).

Food for thought:

1. Immune Killer T (KT) cells can only recognize cancer antigens when it is displayed on HLA Class I (also called MHC-I) on cancer cell surface.
   A. True
   B. False

2. To bypass the HLA-I dependence on the part of KT, scientists have engineered artificial proteins on KT surface to enable KT to directly recognize cancer cell antigens without HLA Class I or MHC-I.
   A. True
   B. False

CANCER VACCINES (1): CURBING EARLY BLADDER CANCER

"Consumption," the nickname of Tuberculosis (TB), vividly describes how the deadly bacterial infection literally consumes an individual, bit by bit, steadily and progressively, to a state of emaciation and waste. Frederick Chopin, Polish-French virtuoso pianist and composer of *Fantaisie-Impromptu* and many more masterpieces, lamented how he had been working so hard that by the time the composition was finished, it would have finished him. Sadly, Chopin was consumed in 1849, not by his piano *magnum opus* but by tuberculosis (TB) at the tender age of thirty-nine. Today, thank goodness to advancement in medicine, TB is both treatable and preventable.

BCG saved the world. Bacillus Calmette-Guerin (BCG) vaccine was developed at the Pasteur Institute in Paris, France, by Dr. Calmette and Dr. Guerin. BCG became available in 1921 and remains the only vaccine against TB. Relying on a live but weakened strain of the TB-causing bacteria, BCG vaccine is recommended by the World Health Organization (WHO) for countries with high incidence of TB. The United States is not on that list, although sporadic cases do exist.

BCG repurposed to treat bladder cancer. In the 1950s, a medical study campaign was initiated with the mission of testing which cancers could respond to the BCG vaccine and be reduced. The practice of testing an existing med to determine whether or not it could be effective in medical conditions not intended by the existing med is called drug repurposing. A brilliantly bold idea! Also a smart time-saving and cost-saving idea. As widely known, it takes, on average, more than a decade to develop a new drug/meds and the first order of business of a clinical trial is to determine drug/meds safety. Any hint of major adverse effects will disqualify the drug under investigation, for patient safety is and should be the number one concern. After all, if the drug is so potently toxic that it severely handicaps the patient, it would defeat its noble life-saving purpose. I learned that through a first-hand experience: There was once upon a time a multi-million dollar, multi-institutional drug discovery endeavor in which I participated as one of the lead scientists. The drug showed tremendous synergistic effects in eliminating lung cancer cells in petri dishes. During the phase-1 clinical trial, however, one patient developed serious thrombosis, that is, severe blood clotting, and the entire clinical trial was terminated ASAP. The responsible pharmaceutical company, despite the hundreds of millions of dollars invested for the R & D (research and development) of the experimental cancer drug, moved on to new projects. Kudos.

Why is it an ingenious idea to repurpose old drugs for different diseases? Well, the old drugs were already tested to be safe and received official approval (such as the FDA). Accordingly, if an old drug turns out to be efficacious for a different disease, bingo! No worries about drug safety because it has already passed the muster.

Vaccine repurposing carries on. Dr. Lloyd Old, an accomplished physician-scientist at MSKCC, initiated the unprecedented vaccine repurposing screening campaign. Great news arrived: BCG showed high efficacy in eliminating early-stage bladder cancer cells. The findings were later confirmed by fellow scientists at the National Cancer Institute (NCI). It is important to point out that early-stage bladder cancer refers to bladder cancer that has not yet invaded the bladder muscle wall, hence is incapable of spreading or metastasizing. Up to 80 percent of newly diagnosed bladder cancer belongs to this stage and BCG treatment leads to a remarkable 70 percent remission of this cancer.

BCG became the first approved cancer immunotherapy. The idea behind cancer immunotherapy is to unleash the patient's own immune power to tackle cancer. The same logic applies to BCG's anti-cancer action, although the mechanism of action was not unraveled for a decade since its FDA approval in 1990. In the year 2000, scientists at MSKCC began to crack the molecular code of what makes the BCG vaccine work against non-metastatic bladder cancer. It turns out that BCG injected into cancer-inflicted bladders triggers an inflammatory response, putting on high alert a type of immune cell called "CD4-T cells" (also called helper T cells or "T-h" for short). CD4 refers to a protein marker that resides on the T cell surface. Activated CD4-T cells immediately release a powerful signaling molecule called "interferon gamma" (IFNg) that goes on to destroy bladder cancer cells in laboratory mice.

At this point, despite the high efficacy of BCG vaccine against early-stage bladder cancer, and despite an important step in understanding how BCG works taken by MSKCC scientists, two mysteries remain: (1) Exactly how does IFNg eliminates bladder cells in such a swift fashion? (2) Why does the TB vaccine preferentially work against early-stage bladder cancer but not other forms of early-stage solid tumors in the lungs, breast, kidney, or liver? Let's follow up.

Food for thought:

1. The TB vaccine BCG works against early-stage bladder cancer exclusively.
   A. True
   B. False

2. BCG vaccine directly kills early-stage bladder cancer cells on contact.
   A. True
   B. False

CANCER VACCINES (2): PREEMPTING CERVICAL CANCER WITH HPV VACCINES

Delightful news came from the United Kingdom (UK) around November 2023 that after years of judicious effort in vaccination across the British Isles, the rate of cancer inflicted by human papillomavirus (HPV) infection has been leveled out. Hooray! Such impressive progress is not, however, shared by other countries, at least not yet. Hopefully going to school on the British example can help other countries gain a better score on their HPV-associated cancer prevention report card.

Multiple types of HPV. HPV is a double-stranded DNA (dsDNA) virus with infection extending to skin and mucosal cells (cells that line the interior of organs and cavities). More than 200 different types of HPV have been identified based on differences in DNA sequence, also called "genotypes." Of these, sixteen HPV genotypes are classified into the high-risk category, including types 16, 18, 31, 33, 34, 35, 39, 45, 51, 52, 56, 58, 59, 66, 68, and 70. Among these, types 16 and 18 are known to cause 70 percent of all cervical cancers. The statistics on HPV types and associated cervical cancer incidence are summarized in the table below.

HPV vaccines are designed as a prophylactic measure against HPV infection. High-risk genotypes described above are the primary targets. ***Quick Word Anatomy:*** *Pro* = in advance, *Phulax* = to guard; together, *Prophylactic* = To guard in advance. Available HPV vaccines approved by the FDA include Gardasil and Cervarix.

Gardasil. The first-generation HPV vaccine manufactured by Merck, headquartered in New Jersey, United States, Gardasil received FDA approval in 2006. Targeting four types of HPV, namely 6, 11, 16, and 18, Gardasil is a "4-valent" vaccine (4vHPV). *Valent* refers to the number of antigens targeted by vaccines. "Antigen" is the representative slice of the ID card on normal cells, disease-causing bug cells, and cancer cells. A lot of antigens are shared by both normal healthy cells as well as cancer cells while pathogenic antigens are typically unique.

Gardasil 9. The second-generation HPV vaccine, Gardasil 9, was approved by the FDA in 2014. With a much wider range of protective coverage, Gardasil 9 covers HPV 6, 11, 16, 18, 31, 33, 45, 52, and 58. With nine different HPV antigens, it qualifies as a 9vHPV.

Cancer types	Percent caused by HPV
Cervical cancer	91%
Anal cancer	91%
Vaginal cancer	75%
Oropharyngeal cancer	72%
Vulvar cancer	69%
Penile cancer	63%

Image 18 (HPV and cancer). Assembled by Dr. Nancy Liu-Sullivan.

Cervarix. In parallel to 4vHPV and 9vHPV, there is also a 2vHPV (Cervarix) that targets only HPV 16 and HPV 18, manufactured by GlaxoSmithKline (GSK), a UK pharmaceutical company with a major branch located in Prussia, Pennsylvania, United States.

In the US, only Gardasil 9 has been distributed since 2016. Gardasil and Cervarix continue to be in use in other parts of the world.

How does it work? HPV vaccine targets selective slices of antigen proteins found on the surface of the virus. These protein targets are grown in yeast cells cultured in a laboratory. The mature protein then self-assembles to mimic the appearance of the HPV virus. Due to the fact that the HPV protein does not harbor any HPV genetic material (since proteins are the final products of corresponding genes formed by DNA), the protein is incapable of making carbon copies of itself (replication); hence, HPV vaccines that target the HPV proteins do not cause HPV infections in vaccine recipients.

As for how HPV vaccine generates immunity, it follows the same logical developmental steps as other types of vaccines:

- The "target" delivered by the vaccine is recognized by the host immune system as "non-self" and therefore, "dangerous."
- The "target," such as HPV 16, is processed and presented by antigen presentation cells (such as dendritic cells) to CD4-T (helper T) cells in lymph nodes.
- The presentation activates CD4-T cells which then go on to interact with B cells that lead to B cell activation.
- Activated B cells undergo a process called "differentiation" to become specialized plasma cells that produce antibodies specific for the HPV protein. These antibodies are supporting lines of evidence that indicate that the individual has been immunized. Still, the proof ought to reside in the pudding, as discussed below.
- If and when HPV appears on the radar of the now fully prepared host immune system, the HPV-specific antibodies take immediate action to guard the host against HPV infection via an immune process called neutralization.

Efficacy is robust. Data from a clinical trial of Gardasil in male subjects revealed that Gardasil is effective at preventing changes in anal cells from chronic HPV infection. Greater news to follow: data from the clinical trial on Gardasil 9 showed close to 100% efficacy in preventing infections of the cervix, vulva, and vaginal tract in addition to preventing precancerous conditions.

A reasonable question raised here concerns how effective the 2vHPV and 4vHPV vaccines that cover only a fraction of HPV targets are. It turns out that a unique immune response phenomenon called "cross protection" plays an important role in generating a wider repertoire of protection. Specifically, female subjects who received three doses of the 2vHPV vaccine that covers HPV 16 and 18 were found to have mounted immune protection against new infections caused by three genotypes of HPV 31, 33, and 45, even though these are not covered by the 2vHPV vaccine per se.

Of note, HPV vaccines work by developing immunity against prospective HPV infection but do not treat cervical cancer or anal cancer. The notion is that by preventing HPV infection, the vaccines help ward off cancers caused by HPV infection.

In terms of long-term protection, based on data collected so far, Cervarix confers protection for up to eleven years, Gardasil for ten years, and Gardasil 9 for at least six years. These long-term studies are ongoing, and updated data sets are still unfolding.

Food for thought:

1. HPV infection is a risk factor for developing cervical cancer and anal cancer.
   A. True
   B. False

2. HPV vaccines work by training the host immune system to preempt HPV infection, but the vaccines do not treat HPV infection-associated cancers.
   A. True
   B. False

CANCER VACCINES (3): SKIN CANCER DEVOURED BY A VIRUS

From smallpox to influenza to Covid-19, viruses in all shades and shapes wreak health havoc. It turns out that not all viruses are created equal. While most viruses can make us sick, a special class of virus is capable of lending us their viral power to combat cancer. Here, let us zoom in on a cold sore-causing virus that has been engineered into a vaccine to treat a deadly form of skin cancer.

Viruses that slay cancer cells. Viruses that destroy cancer cells are termed as "onco-lytic" viruses. **Quick word anatomy**: *Onco* = tumor, *Lytic* = destroy, together Oncolytic = tumor destruction. So what is this mysterious skin cancer cell-devouring virus? Yes, you've guessed it; it is Herpes Simplex Virus (HSV). The targeted cancer is melanoma—the most aggressive form of skin cancer. The name of the viral vaccine is T-VEC. Approved by the FDA in 2015, T-VEC (abbreviated from talimogene laherparepvec) is the first therapeutic cancer vaccine based on oncolytic virus. As for how the drug name is chock full of strange vowels interspersed with odd consonants, your guess is as good as mine! Name origin aside, why do HSV particles have a predilection for melanoma and how do they dismantle melanoma?

HSV literally blows up melanoma. Viruses are unable to make a living on their own and must hijack the replication machinery of the host to survive and thrive. Capitalizing on this HSV "way of life," scientists designed the HSV-based vaccine to target melanoma. Viruses enter host cells by infection. T-VEC, the HSV-based vaccine, works the same way. Manufactured by Amgen, a California Silicon Valley biotech company, T-VEC is approved to treat advanced-stage melanoma. The vaccine can be injected directly into the skin tumor core or into nearby lymph nodes. Upon entering melanoma cells, HSV viruses unleash their unlimited replication potential to take over melanoma cells with an outcome of tons of viral particles. The physical pressure inside melanoma cells continues to build until it reaches a tipping point and kaboom! Melanoma cells undergo an implosion, an internal explosion initiated from inside melanoma cells, as illustrated in the six-step process below:

Can the HSV vaccine infect cancer patients? Thoughtful question. Well, the naturally occurring HSV virus indeed causes cold sore infections, which can be harmless for healthy people, but for cancer patients, it would be a different story as the viral particles likely further weaken cancer patients' overall state of health and exacerbate cancer. Accordingly, it is of utmost importance to make sure that the vaccine fulfills its role of killing cancer cells without afflicting an adverse infection in patients. A daunting challenge, but it was overcome with great success, thanks to genetic engineering technologies. How was it done?

Well, in politics, there is the slang of "follow the money!" In cancer biology, the equivalence is "follow the genes!" Specifically, genes that empower HSV to implode cancer cells are keepers, whereas genes that bear the potential of causing viral infections are removed or "deleted" from the viral genome (the collection of all genes in an organism) in HSV. There! Tinkering and tweaking of genes have allowed HSV's "wheat" to be maintained but "chaff" to be discarded. With the infection source cleared, T-VEC is ready to hit the ground running against melanoma.

Immune cells pick up the pieces. The ruptured melanoma cancer cells raise a gigantic cellular stink made up of a mixture of chemicals and toxins, all of which are associated with the tumor. These tumor "calling cards" send multiple "danger" signals to the host immune system. Before long, an army of immune cells follows the "danger" signal and arrives at tumor site to clean up destroyed and defeated melanoma cells and their debris.

Results Impressive. In terms of treatment efficacy, the five-year relapse-free survival (RFS) is used as the benchmark. For patients who received T-VEC therapy before tumor removal, the five-year RFS is 22 percent. By contrast, patients who did not receive T-VEC therapy before surgery were observed to have a five-year RFS of 15 percent. Clearly, T-VEC therapy serves to lengthen the five-year cancer-free survival for patients. Of course, there is ample room for improvement to increase the survival rate beyond 22 percent.

Well, HSV is not the only game in town when it comes to oncolytic viruses. Additional promising viral candidates to be explored include adenovirus, measles, Newcastle disease virus, reovirus, and vaccinia. Lots of new grounds to be unearthed ahead of us until one day we reduce cancer to a manageable chronic condition.

Food for thought:

1. T-VEC is the first cancer-devouring viral vaccine used for melanoma treatment.
    A. True
    B. False

2. T-VEC works by having HSV particles replicate and expand exponentially until a breakpoint is reached that causes an internal explosion inside melanoma cells.
    A. True
    B. False

CANCER VACCINES (4): PAP—A BAIT TO FISH OUT PROSTATE CANCER CELLS

We have discussed vaccines that treat early bladder cancer and melanoma. Here, we shall go over another therapeutic vaccine against prostate cancer.

PROVENGE taking on prostate cancer. Manufactured by Dendreon Pharmaceuticals, PROVENGE (Sipuleucel-T) is a type of personalized cancer immunotherapy for the treatment of advanced prostate cancer that is resistant to castration. A platform of treatment, castration can be carried out surgically or via blocking medications. Both aim at reducing levels of testosterone—the hormone that fuels prostate cancer cell growth. For a subset of patients who are castration-resistant prostate cancer (mCRPT), PROVENGE is the treatment option available and is developed as follows:

Step 1: Collecting patient blood: A blood sample from the patient is collected from which dendritic cells (DC) are extracted. By the way, drawing blood from the patient and returning it back to the same patient is an *autologous* medical procedure. **Quick Word Anatomy:** *Auto* = oneself, *Logo* = stud, taken together *Autologous* = related to oneself. In the particular context here, *Autologous* immune cells collected from the patient os returned to the same patient after medical processing.

Step 2: Uploading molecular payload. The patient-derived DCs are cultured in a designated clinical laboratory to incorporate an engineered protein cargo consisting of (1) a potent growth factor piggy-bagged with (2) a prostate cancer-unique molecular ID called *PAP* with the full name as "prostatic acid phosphate."

Since *PAP* is expressed at high levels in the majority of prostate cancer cells but not found in normal prostate cells, decorating DCs with *PAP* enables the DCs to be specific prostate cancer cells. How is *PAP* processed by DC? Engulfing. Specifically, *PAP* gets ingested by DC, placed onto MHC-I in DC, and displayed on DC surface.

What's the potent growth factor on the engineered protein cargo to be introduced to patient's DCs? It is a signaling molecule called "granulocyte–macrophage colony-stimulating factor" (GM-CSF) equipped with a dual function: As a stimulator of DC growth and as a molecular *Key* designed to find the matching *Lock* displayed on the surface of prostate cancer cells. The *Lock* that matches perfectly with the GM-SCF *Key* is the receptor protein for GM-SCF. Now that the intended protein cargo is safely loaded into DCs, these DCs are infused back to the patient. What's next?

Step 3: Engineered DC meet KT in lymph nodes. The DCs that express *PAP + GM-CSF* travel to lymph nodes to inform immune Killer T (KT) cells of *PAP*, the telltale piece of prostate cancer cells, so that KTs become proficient at capturing prostate cancer cells. At the end of the immune tutorial session, KTs exit lymph nodes in fully activated mode, ready to take on prostate cancer cells.

Step 4: Robust KTs taking cancer head-on. Guided by the *PAP* "intel," KT cells successfully locate prostate cancer cells that near the same *PAP* in a complex with MHC-I displayed on prostate cancer cell surface. Having seized the targets, KT cells unleash their "1–2 punch" by secreting two enzyme proteins: The first being "perforin" that literally pokes hole on cancer cell surface to pave the road for the second protein called "grandzyme B." As the name indicates, grandzyme B is too grand in size to enter cancer cells and hence need to rely on perforin the second protein is too large to enter prostate cancer cells by itself, hence, relying on "perforin" action. Upon landing in the interior of prostate cancer cells, Granzyme B initiates a cell death pathway termed as "apoptosis" which reduces the targeted cancer cell to thousands of pieces called "apoptotic bodies," leading to cancer cell irreversible death.

The four-step process of PROVENGE design and engineering is illustrated below:

Based upon encouraging clinical trial outcomes of Provenge extending castration-resistant prostate cancer survival rate of 38%, Provenge was granted approval by the FDA. Terrific! But what about the other 62% of the patients who did not show an immune response despite immune stimulation by PROVENGE. What are plausible underlying factors? MHC-I (HLA Class I) is the first red flag raised.

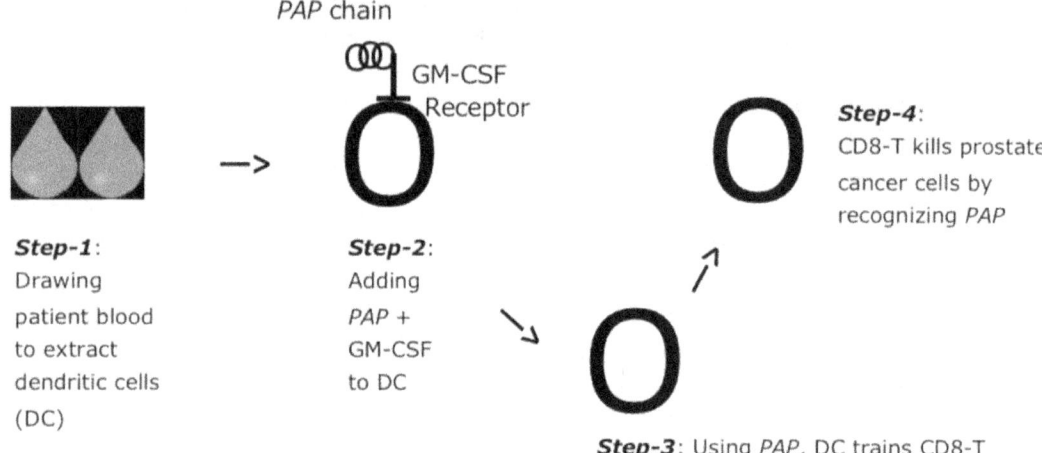

Image 19 Training T cells to hunt down prostate cancer. Assembled by Dr. Nancy Liu-Sullivan and combined with Wikimedia Commons File: Blood Drop.jpg.

Recall in *CANCER TRICKS AND TRAPS (7): A GAME OF MIA* (page 35) we discussed how cancer cells ought to display antigen on the silver platter of MHC-I (HLA Class I) in order for KT recognition and subsequent annihilation. Also recall that to maximize self survival, cancer cells make the deadly silver platter disappear to leave KT in the dark, helpless. For patients who did not response to Provenge, it is plausible that their prostate cancer cells managed to stunt MHC-I (HLA Class I) level to escape KT attack, which is definitely room for improvement. One more note, patients tend to shy away from PROVENGE as a result of the pricy tag of $9,300. Another area with room for improvement.

Food for thought:

1. *PAP* is a cell-surface marker specific for prostate cancer.
   A. True
   B. False

2. PROVENGE relies on engineered patient dendritic cells to stimulate the patient's immune system to combat all types of prostate cancer.
   A. True
   B. False

CANCER VACCINES (5): THE ROAD TO LIVER CANCER JAMMED

Can a chef with hepatitis B (HepB) infection work in a restaurant? The answer is yes, the reason being HepB is transmitted via blood, fecal matter, or bodily fluids. Casual contact such as shaking hands, dining, or eating food prepared by a HepB chef is deemed as safe, so long as the chef adheres to strict hygiene guidelines for hand-washing protocols. In New York City, 311 is reserved to handle complaints from discontent restaurant patrons.

HepB and hepatitis infection. That said, HepB infection is no casual matter for infected individuals. A double-stranded DNA (dsDNA) virus, HepB is the culprit for both acute and chronic HepB infections. According to the U.S. Hepatitis B Foundation, it is estimated that close to 300 million people worldwide are living with HepB infections. Aside from terribly debilitating symptoms, chronic HepB infection can, over time, deteriorate into liver cancer. Fortunately, vaccines that prevent HepB infection are readily available.

Blood-based HepB vaccines: In the early 1980s, the FDA approved the first hepatitis B vaccine developed using hepatitis B surface antigen (HBsAg) derived from the blood samples of people infected with the hepatitis B virus. The antigen particles were killed with harsh chemicals including formaldehyde, pepsin, and urea, followed by heat treatment. Despite the stringent safety records, the blood-derived hepatitis B vaccine always seemed to reserve a din in our heads of *"what if"* safety measures were to suffer from inadvertent oversight? The thought of getting infected with the vaccine that was supposed to preempt the disease defeats the purpose. Accordingly, a new platform that steered clear of using blood products from infected individuals was underway.

Vaccine safety is an inarguably high priority. The product from the new platform came to fruition and received FDA approval in the mid-1980s. The new vaccine applied a genetic engineering technology called "recombinant DNA" for the making of the vaccine. Specifically,

Step 1: Hepatitis B surface antigen (HBsAg) is extracted from hepatitis B viruses.

Step 2: The HBsAg gene is inserted into yeast cells and as yeast cells grow and divide, they also yield a ton of HepB surface antigen.

Step 3: Through processes of converting DNA to RNA, and RNA to protein, the native form of HepB antigen protein comes into shape as a finished protein product that closely mimics the naturally-occurring HepB protein, but with a significant difference: This manmade protein *cannot* make a healthy person sick. This is a masterpiece of genetic engineering that allows scientists to cut/paste or add/delete any gene of interest to suit specific medical needs. There is yet one more molecular trick to make the HepB vaccine safe and powerful.

Step 4: The hepB antigen (HBsAg) is engineered to attach to an aluminum compound termed as "aluminum hydroxide" with the chemical formula of $Al(OH)_3$. What purpose does aluminum serve?

Aluminum: A vaccine enhancer. Durable while at the same time flexible, aluminum is a metal believed to be ideally situated as a vaccine helper, also called an *adjuvant*. **Quick Word Anatomy:** *Adjuvare* (Latin) = to help/aid. How does the presence of aluminum aid vaccines? Aluminum serves a dual function: (1) It slows down vaccine distribution at the site of vaccine injection, which allows time for immune cells to gather and get ready for coordinated action. (2) It also promotes better interaction between disease antigens and host immune cells. Per the US Center for Disease Control (CDC), of the five existing HepB vaccines, all contain aluminum adjuvant except one: *Heplisav-B* with a form of synthetic immune stimulant instead of aluminum.

HepB vaccine report card. The CDC recommends hepatitis B vaccination as a measure to guard people against liver cancer. A large-scale multi-year study consisting of 40,000 subjects with a follow-up of thirty-seven years has reported that hepatitis B vaccination has led to a 72 percent efficacy in curbing liver cancer relapse and 64 percent efficacy in reducing liver cancer deaths. A good score. Of course, HepB vaccines do not kill liver cancer cells but function as a preventive measure: curbing HepB infection curbs the incidence of liver cancer, just like curbing HPV infection with *Gardasil* curbs cervical/anal cancer. A two-step process.

Food for thought:

1. Chronic HepB infection over time increases the risks of developing liver cancer.
   A. True
   B. False

2. HepB vaccines help curb liver cancer by immunizing people against HepB infection.
   A. True
   B. False

CANCER VACCINES (6): IMMUNE WRITING STENTORIAN FROM THE *MESSENGER*

Nested by the beautiful Rhine River, Mainz is known for its magnificent medieval architecture. Summer 2018, several scientists gathered in Mainz at an ancient church hospital and strategized a daring cancer vaccine idea so ahead of its time that no one ever imagined the idea actually coming to fruition just five years later!

A joint venture. Two German scientists of Turkish ancestry, Dr. Uğur Sahin and Dr. Özlem Türeci, both medical doctors and partners in life and in science, share the same passion for developing cancer vaccines. The US team was headed by Dr. Vinod P. Balachandran, an accomplished surgeon-scientist from MSKCC. The topic of the meeting was a joint to develop personalized messenger RNA (mRNA) cancer vaccines. The first priority of this endeavor was aimed at pancreatic cancer, a nasty cancer typically diagnosed at late stage at the time of diagnostics, also known for frequent relapses post-treatment. The objective was to rely on mRNA technology to train patients' own immune cells, starting with dendritic cells (DC), followed by DC training to Killer T (KT) cells to unmistakably spot cancer cells for annihilation. The specific details of the interaction between DC and KT and KT unleashing the 1–2 punch arsenal to tackle cancer cells, can be found in *CANCER VACCINES (4): PAP—A BAIT TO FISH OUT PROSTATE CANCER CELLS* (page 42). Before delving into the elegant details of the mRNA cancer vaccine feat, let's brush up on mRNA basics.

mRNA transcribes the DNA code. As the code of life, DNA forms genes; genes are transcribed as messenger RNA (mRNA), and mRNA decrees directives on how to manufacture proteins. Proteins serve as the building blocks of cells; cells form tissues, and tissues are assembled into organs. Vital organs include the heart, lungs, liver, kidneys, and the brain. Pivotal to the above complex apparatus is mRNA that reliably relays the genetic information to ensure that the DNA code is followed to the "letter," the letters being A, T, G, C for DNA and A, U, G, C for RNA. The progression from DNA to RNA to protein is coined as the "Central Dogma" by the Nobel Prize co-recipient, Dr. Francis Crick (who co-discovered the DNA double helix with Dr. James D. Watson in 1953). The reigning dogma is illustrated in the following figure:

Modification makes RNA stable. Discovered in 1961, RNA took the biomedical community by storm and many jumped on the enticing RNA bandwagon. The intense interest soon subsided because RNA is simply too unstable to be of much clinical utility. While many backed off, one scientist stubbornly stayed the course, despite bleak funding, embarrassing demotion, and a shocking health diagnosis. The scientist is Dr. Katalin Karikó. In 2005, after a long uphill struggle of over two decades, the

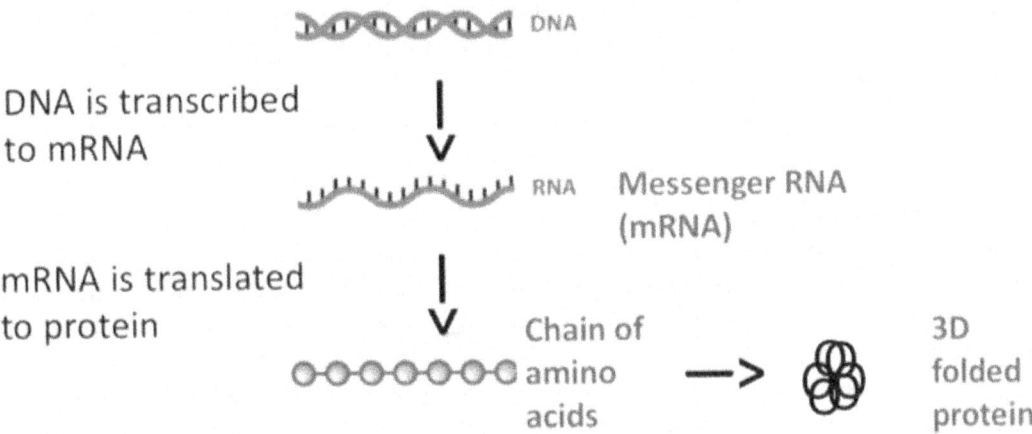

Image 20 Molecular central dogma: DNA→RNA→PROTEIN. Assembled by Dr. Nancy Liu-Sullivan and combined with Wikimedia Commons File: Central Dogma of Molecular Biochemistry with Enzymes.jpg.

crushing RNA obstacle was finally cleared, opening doors for mRNA clinical applications. Having seized the crux of the mRNA instability matter, Dr. Karikó and science partner Dr. Weissman replaced one letter in mRNA and problem solved! For details, please refer to **KATALIN KARIKÓ: LOST FUNDING, GOT CANCER, BUT BEAT BOTH** (page 113).

Vaccines speeding up the clearing of cancer. BioNTech was instrumental in developing mRNA-based Covid-19 vaccines. Spending no time resting on laurels, the team of scientists resumed their endeavor of applying the mRNA technology to the development of cancer vaccines. Unlike the Covid-19 vaccine, where the mRNA of a universal viral antigen—the infamous "spike protein"—is packaged in high-tech fat droplets called "nano lipids" and jabbed into millions of arms to reduce Covid-19 infection severity, cancer mRNA vaccines are *NOT* universal but tailored to individual patients. What's more, instead of a single mRNA, pancreatic cancer mRNA vaccines by MSKCC and BioNTech harbor a total of twenty, yes, twenty patient-unique mRNA sequences for each vaccine tailor-designed for each of the twenty patients enrolled in the investigator-initiated clinical trial at MSKCC. The level of sophistication is dauntingly exquisite. The preparation and implementation processes are described below:

Step 1: Cancer patient's tumor was excised as cleanly as possible and tumor DNA sequenced.
Step 2: Tumor DNA sequencing information helps identify "cancer antigens" *specific* for the cancer patient to allow personalized cancer vaccine.
Step 3: Patient-unique mRNA vaccine is prepared to carry the 20-cancer-antigen payload, per patient.
Step 4: The prepped mRNA cancer vaccine is given to each cancer patient via intravenous (IV) blood infusion after a standard round of treatment with an immune checkpoint inhibitor that helps liberate Killer T (KT) to get ready for the battle against cancer.
Step 5: Patient DC cells process the twenty different cancer antigen mRNA sequences into matched proteins that get displayed on DC surface.
Step 6: Patient DCs travel to local lymph nodes to pass on invaluable patient-unique cancer "intel" to KT cells.

Step 7: The well-trained KTs accurately identify cancer cells guided by cancer antigen map and launch the famously fierce "1–2 punch" that sends cancer cells to their demise.

Step 8: All patients of the clinical trial were closely monitored the moment vaccination was initiated for routine medical care and for collecting valuable patient vaccine response data.

So far so good! Pancreatic cancer is notorious for its bleak five-year survival rate of merely 12 percent. In other words, 88 percent of patients are unable to survive after five years, calling for the high need for more robust treatment strategies. Moreover, pancreatic cancer patients invariably (with extremely rare occasions) suffer from tumor relapse typically one year post-surgery. How to prevent tumor return after surgical removal? A tall order! And now that order has met with encouraging outcomes from the MSKCC phase 1 clinical trial: for patients who received the cancer vaccine, only 25 percent showed tumor relapse, whereas patients who received standard, non mRNA-based pancreatic cancer vaccine had an 87.5 percent tumor relapse rate. Clearly, the tailor-made vaccine has been effective at keeping tumors at bay. Progress so far so encouraging! As the MSKCC lead physician Dr. Vinod Balachchandra remarked, *"The latest data from the phase 1 trial show that we are on the right track."*(https://www.mskcc.org/news/can-mrna-vaccines-fight-pancreatic-cancer-msk-clinical-researchers-are-trying-find-out). As phase 2 clinical trial with an expanded cohort of patient participants begins, we look forward to more encouraging results.

Food for thought:

1. mRNA is the bridge that links the DNA blueprint to the final product of protein.
   A. True
   B. False

2. mRNA pancreatic cancer vaccine clinical trial I has shown a great reduction in patient tumor relapse from 87.5 percent to 25 percent.
   A. True
   B. False

CAR-T THERAPY (1): MAKE IMMUNE DOGS HUNT

Confronting infectious bugs, our immune "dash hounds" mobilize Killer T (KT) cells to put up a fierce fight until danger is cleared. When it comes to cancer, however, the KT canines won't hunt. It turns out that cancer plays molecular tricks to tame KT. How can we strategize to re-energize indolent KT and make them hunt?

KT cells are fierce against infected cells. From air, land, to the sea, germs and bugs are ubiquitous under the sun and under our roof. Worry not, for we are blessed with a powerful immune system for protection. Top on the list of immune elite troopers are Killer T (KT) cells, which take care of business by releasing two sharp molecules: the first one pokes holes in infected cells to pave the way for the second molecule to enter enemy territory and trigger an implosion—the famous KT 1–2 punch! KT usually passes the anti-infection test with flying colors. The problem is cancer: KTs are crestfallen when they are surrounded by cancer cells. How so?

KT under the influence of molecular lethargy. Why are KT cells so effective at killing infectious bugs and infected body cells but not cancer cells? There are several schools of thought: Cancer floods its quarters with lactic acid to drown out KT, cancer dispatches immune "police" Tregs to tame KT, cancer steals energy from KT, and last but not least, cancer disguises its surface ID HLA. Without HLA, cancer antigens can show up under the brightest sunlight, but KT cannot see them because KTs have evolved to only visualize cancer when cancer antigen ID is presented on the HLA silver platter. The details of all the above scenarios have been discussed in depth in the series of *Cancer Tricks and Traps* (pages 25–37). Science is about shedding light on the hidden and exposing the disguised to deepen our understanding of nature and of creatures, including us humans. Indeed, science has found a way to make KT dogs hunt via an innovative CAR-T.

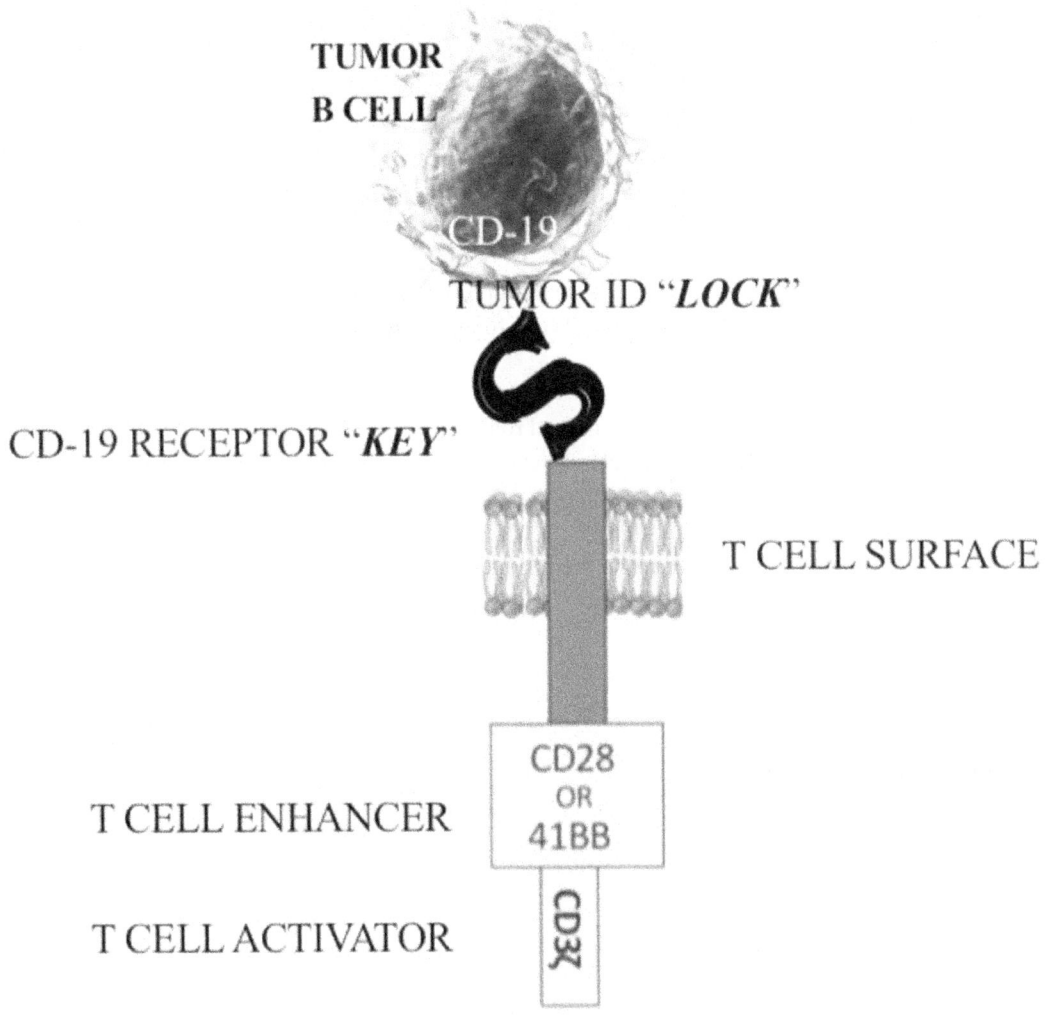

Image 21 2nd generation CAR-T. Assembled by Dr. Nancy Liu-Sullivan and combined with Wikimedia Commons File: Blausen 0624 Lymphocyte B cell (crop).png.

Reigniting KT's killer instinct. To make the KT hunt for blood cancer cells, scientists have devised a molecular make-over by installing a few game-changing protein gears, as shown below in a simplified version of CAR-T design. Since the T-cell makeover involves adding receptor proteins related to cancer antigens to existing T cells, the molecularly tweaked therapeutic platform has acquired the nomenclature of "Chimeric Antigen Receptor-T cell therapy" or simply CAR-T.

1. **CD19: T cell GPS.** How do engineered immune elite T cells find blood cancer cells? They simply follow the molecular GPS in the form of the *key*—the key is called CD19 that recognizes the CD19 *lock* on leukemia and lymphoma cells that conspicuously display a sea of CD19 marker proteins on their surface. What happens after the CD19 *key* opens the CD19 *lock* on cancer cells?
2. **CD3ζ: T cell activator.** An integral part of the intracellular chain within engineered CAR-T cells is "CD3ζ" (pronounced as CD3 zeta) which is instrumental in kickstarting T cell activation. Once the CAR-T cell hits the ground and starts running head on against cancer targets, it needs a molecular helping hand to provide staying power.
3. **CD28 (or 4-1BB): T cell energizers.** Two T cell energizer candidate molecules come into play: CD28 and 4-1BB. Either molecule suffices to provide the needed extra kick for CAR-T. Interestingly, of the two CAR-T therapy drugs approved by the FDA for the treatment of leukemia, one harbors CD28 and the other 4-1BB. The same story describes the two approved lymphoma CAR-T drugs. By the way, CAR-T drugs treat particular subtypes of leukemia or lymphoma but not all subtypes, at least not yet. You might ask: What about the third category of blood cancer termed MM? Are there CAR-T drugs available? The encouraging answer is yes! Two such drugs that have received FDA green light target BCMA—the equivalent of the molecular GPS that leads CAR-T to MM cells for a straightforward reason that BCMA is a loud telltale flag on MM.

Two physician-scientists have played instrumental roles in CAR-T against blood cancer derived from mutated B lymphocytes: Dr. Carl June and Dr. Michel Sadelain. The details are described in ***Les Trois Musketeers*** (pages 115–118).

A five-step ride on CAR-T is illustrated in the following Image:

Step-1	Step-2	Step-3	Step-4	Step-5
T lymphocytes cells are collected from cancer patient.	**T lymphocytes** decorated with CD19R, CD28, and CD3z.	**T lymphocytes** cells are returned to the patient via IV.	**T lymphocytes** cancer cell using CD19R key to match CD19 lock.	**T lymphocytes** activates apoptosis in cancer cells for annihilation

Image 22 CAR-T steps. Assembled by Dr. Nancy Liu-Sullivan.

Step-1: T cells are collected from cancer patient.

Step-2: T cells are engineered with the molecular payload consisting of CD19 receptor, CD3ζ, CD28 (or 4-1BB).

Step-3: Engineered CAR-T cells are returned to the patient.

Step-4: Once in the bloodstream, T cell uses the CD19 receptor "key" to match and open the CD19 "lock" on cancerous B cells.

Step-5: Face to face with cancer cells the arched enemies, CD8-T cells do what they do best: Damage cancer cell surface with a poker enzyme to allow the killer enzyme to enter enemy territory, that is, getting inside mutated B cells to push them over the molecular cliff, a process called *apoptosis* which translates to "programmed cell death." This is the famous "1–2 punch" killing trick by CD8-T also more vividly called Killer T (KT) cells.

CAR-T's good report card. CAR-T transforms indolent immune canines to hunt down cancer cells with vengeance. As for CAR-T cancer therapy performance in leukemia and lymphoma, so far with approximately 50 percent success rates, that is, 50 percent of patients able to reach a milestone of cancer disappearance and stay disappeared—the medical terminology is cancer remission. This is a huge step forward compared to the 10 percent five-year survival rate in patients not treated with CAR-T therapy. Many lives have not only been saved but are living to their full potential. A walking example is Ms. Emily Whitehead, described in the next essay.

Room for improvement. Despite progress made, there is ample room for improvement to increase overall survival percentage in blood cancers, to reduce toxicity, and to extend CAR-T therapy to solid tumors such as melanoma, colon cancer, lung cancer, and brain cancer. The road ahead for CAR-T remains complex and challenging, but with dedication, diligence, and ingenuity, scientists will make it happen. In the next few essays, we shall tour the CAR-T exhibition hall and learn why this therapy is praised as the "living drug."

Food for thought:

1. For CAR-T therapy to work, molecules that robustly activate KT cells and confer staying power are molecularly engineered onto patient T cells.
   A. True
   B. False

2. CAR-T is a single-dose infusion therapy using T cells obtained from the same patient.
   A. True
   B. False

CAR-T THERAPY (2): A PHILADELPHIA STORY

At the age of six in 2012, Emily was diagnosed with an acute form of leukemia. Her physicians exhausted all possible treatment options. Nothing was working. Her cancer kept coming back. Emily's parents refused to give up hope and were steadfast in finding a way.

"CAR-T" arrived from Philadelphia. At the time, an experimental CAR-T therapy was being carried out collaboratively by the team University of Pennsylvania School of Medicine (Penn Medicine) and Children's Hospital of Philadelphia (CHOP). A brand new way of treating cancer, CAR-T aims at revitalizing patient's inner immune power to combat cancer.

Emily became the first pediatric cancer patient to receive CAR-T therapy for the treatment of her recurring acute lymphoblastic leukemia (ALL). The design of CAR-T therapy by Penn Medicine, used by Dr. Stephan Grupp and Dr. Carl June to treat Emily, is the second-generation CAR-T that incorporated "4-1BB" as the co-stimulatory molecule that confers sustainable CAR-T power against leukemia cells.

Cytokine storm is tempestuous. Not long after the engineered CAR-T cells were returned to Emily via intravenous (IV) injection, Emily developed an acute reaction with symptoms of high fever, difficulty breathing, and very low blood pressure—all classical "cytokine storm" symptoms of immune overreaction which, if not treated timely, can deteriorate to life-threatening organ failure. Cytokine storm is also referred to as "cytokine release syndrome" (CRS).

Cytokines are versatile signaling molecules that recruit assorted immune cells to arrive at sites of infection to join the fight. These immune cells, in turn, secrete more cytokines to fuel the fight, which attracts additional immune cells to beef up the fight, and the cycle goes on to build a "perfect" cytokine storm. Even though a cytokine storm is a sure sign that the CAR-T therapy has successfully mobilized Emily's immune cells, the storm itself must be subsided to avoid a life-threatening situation. But where to begin, and which cytokine was the major culprit? Evidence-based medicine provided the answer.

Storm gone, cancer also gone. Medical lab test results came back: A particular type of cytokine called "Interleukin 6" (IL-6) had unusually high levels in Emily's blood. Very, very fortunately, the FDA had just approved a new drug that inhibits the very molecule of IL-6 for the treatment of arthritis. The full name of the drug is "tocilizumab" with the trade name of "Actemra," manufactured by Genentech, a leading pharmaceutical company headquartered in San Francisco. Approved for emergency use, Emily received Actemra treatment, and the cytokines storm was tamed: high fevers corrected, blood pressure normal, *and* all the leukemia cells disappeared! Now in 2025, thirteen years since the pioneering CAR-T treatment, Emily remains cancer-free.

Emily Whitehead Foundation. To support CAR-T development and to benefit more childhood leukemia patients like Emily, Emily's parents established the Emily Whitehead Foundation in 2015. For details, please refer to ***IMAGINE! FRED'S TEAM, JOEY'S WINGS, BAILEY'S WARRIORS, AND EMILY WHITEHEAD FOUNDATION.*** (page 103). Also worth mentioning are the unsung heroes that produced timely lab test results with precision. These are professional medical laboratory scientists (MLS) who work in the hospital Department of Pathology and Lab Medicine, many of whom are my former students, I am very proud to say. They work behind the scenes, and their names are rarely on any front page. Yet, their work is indispensable in assisting physicians in making diagnoses and rational treatment decisions. Hats off to frontline physicians and our medical technology unsung heroes!

Food for thought:

1. Cytokine Storm occurs when immune system gets into a vicious cycle of continuous production of cytokine signaling molecules accompanied by large quantities of immune cells.
   A. True
   B. False
2. Emily Whitehead's cytokine storm was calmed with the help of a drug that suppresses IL-6 activities.
   A. True
   B. False

CAR-T THERAPY (3): FIVE GENERATIONS AND EVOLVING

Having learned the basics of CAR-T therapy, let's take a panoramic view of existing CAR-T models of five generations that target three types of blood cancers: leukemia, lymphoma, and multiple myeloma.

CAR-T blueprint. Below is a very simplified version of the five generations of CAR-T. The first generation *lacked* co-stimulatory molecules such as CD28 or 4-1BB, rendering a very short lifespan for the engineered CAR-T cells. The second generation is equipped with two T cell boosters of either CD28 or 4-1BB plus a T cell GPS (of either CD19 that targets B cell malignancies or BCMA that targets multiple lymphoma). The third generation consists of a combination of CD28 + 4-1BB while keeping all essentials from the first-generation CAR-T. The fourth and fifth generations become more

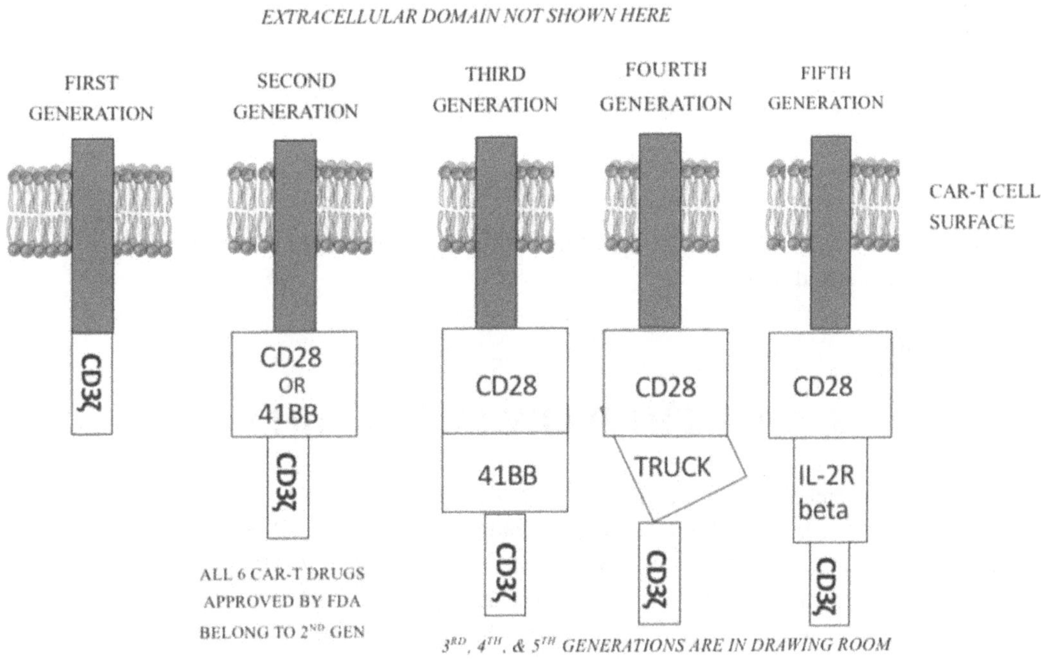

Image 23 CAR-T five generations. Assembled by Dr. Nancy Liu-Sullivan and combined with Wikimedia Commons File: 0302 Phospholipid Bilayer.jpg.

CAR-T Therapies for Blood Cancers (Leukemia, Lymphoma, Multiple Myeloma)					
Brand name	Generic name	Tumor surface target	CAR-T Payload	Pharma & FDA approval year
Kymriah	Tisagenlecleucel	CD19	4-1BB + CD3z	Novartis; 2017
Yescata	Axicabtagene ciloleucel	CD19	CD28 + CD3z	Kite/Gilead; 2017
Tecartus	Brexucabtagene autoleucel	CD19	CD28 + CD3z	Kite/Gilead; 2017
Brayanzi	Lisocabtagene maraleucel	CD19	4-1BB + CD3z	Juno Therapeutics / BMS; 2021
Arbecma	Idecabtagene autoleucel	BCMA	4-1BB + CD3z	Bluebird Bio / BMS; 2020
Carvykti	Ciltacagene autoleucel	BCMA	4-1BB + CD3z	JENSSEN / J & J; 2022

Image 24 FDA CAR-T table. Assembled by Dr. Nancy Liu-Sullivan.

sophisticated with additional T cell stimulators. Only the second-generation CAR-T has received FDA approval. The third and fourth generations are a work-in-progress.

As shown in the table adapted from CAR T Cells: Engineering Immune Cells to Treat Cancer—NCI. https://www.cancer.gov/about-cancer/treatment/research/car-t-cells, January 2024, a total of six CAR-T cancer immunotherapy platforms have received FDA approval. One by one, we'll take a closer look at each CAR-T in essays that follow.

Food for thought:

1. CAR-T is a living drug because live T cells from cancer patients are extracted, engineered, and returned to the patient as live cells.
   A. True
   B. False

2. Five generations of CAR-T therapy drugs have been approved by the FDA that target both blood cancers and solid cancers.
   A. True
   B. False

CAR-T THERAPY (4): KYMRIAH

We described the remarkable cure of Emily Whitehead of her hard-to-treat childhood leukemia in ***CAR-T THERAPY (2): A PHILADELPHIA STORY*** (page 51). In fact, Emily is the first pediatric leukemia patient to receive CAR-T therapy at Penn Medicine and in the whole world since CAR-T therapy was pioneered in the United States. The therapy, "Kymriah," is also the first CAR-T approved by the FDA in 2017, five years after Emily became cancer-free and continues to be cancer-free thirteen years after she was accepted for the Kymriah investigator-initiated clinical trial. Today, Emily is living the life of a normal teenager, finishing up her sophomore year at the University of Pennsylvania.

If you think "Kymriah" is hard to pronounce, try "Tisagenlecleucel," which is the full generic name of this living drug manufactured by genetically revitalizing the cancer patient's own T cells to fight cancer. Developed by Dr. Carl June and colleagues at Penn Medicine, University of Pennsylvania, Kymriah is licensed to the Swiss pharmaceutical company Novartis for manufacturing.

Kymriah SOP: The standard operating procedures (SOP) for Kymriah entail three essential aspects: (1) collecting patient T cells at designated treatment centers, (2) shipping patient T cells to Novartis-authorized manufacturing centers for genetic engineering, and (3) transporting the finished product of Kymriah back to the medical center where a designated healthcare team administers the therapeutically revitalized T cells to combat cancer cells in patients.

Genetic engineering of patient T cells. Pivotal to the Kymriah SOP is the second step of introducing the three core molecules to energize KT cells to "make the immune dogs hunt"! The details are described in *CAR-T THERAPY (3): FIVE GENERATIONS AND EVOLVING* (page 53). The choice of "CD19," "4-1BB," and "CD3ζ" is a rational one and has made wonders in not only curbing blood cancers but enabling 50 percent of the patients to stay clear of cancer, which is not ideal (because it is not yet 100%) but considering the conventional 10 percent of patient survival for five years, Kymriah is undoubtedly a huge step forward.

Special Kymriah manufacturing facilities. After indolent T cells are collected from the patient by medical staff at designated medical centers, the cells are, according to Novartis US headquarters located in Morris Plains, New Jersey, United States, prepared at three Novartis centers in North America and Europe in addition to collaborations under third-party agreements in Europe and East Asia. The table below is a summary:

Special medical centers administer Kymriah. Currently, a total of 167 medical centers or hospitals offer Kymriah treatment. Not surprisingly, New York, California, and Texas stand out with the

Novartis Kymriah Manufacturing	
Novartis	Morris Plain, NJ
	Stein, Switzerland
	Les Ulis, France
Third party agreements	Germany
	Japan
	China

Image 25 Novartis' kymriah. Assembled by Dr. Nancy Liu-Sullivan.

Kymriah Treatment Centers in the U.S.					
NAME	STATE	PHONE	NAME	STATE	PHONE
Banner MD Anderson Cancer Center/Banner Gateway Medical Center	AZ	480-256-6444	Nebraska Medicine	NE	402-559-5600
UCLA Health	CA	888-862-8252	Northshore University Hospital	NY	516-734-8973
UCI Health-UC Irvine Medical Center	CA	714-456-8000	Westchester Medical Center	NY	914-594-2162 (P) 914-493-2276 (A)
City of Hope	CA	833-310-2278	Montefiore Medical Center	NY	718-741-2342 (P) 718-920-4933 (A)
Yale Medical Center	CT	203-200-4362	University of Rochester/Strong Memorial Hospital	NY	585-275-6179
UF Health Shane's Hospital	FL	352-273-9120 (P) 352-733-0972 (A)	Roswell Park Comprehensive Cancer Center	NY	800-767-9355
Holden Comprehensive Cancer Center at The University of Iowa	IA	319-356-8444	NYP-Columbia University Medical Center	NY	212-305-9770 (A) 212-305-4417 (A)
University of Chicago Medicine	IL	844-482-7823	Memorial Sloan Kettering Cancer Center	NY	888-675-2278
IU Health Bone Marrow & Stem Cell Transplant University Hospital	IN	317-944-0920	Oregon Health & Science University	OR	503-494-0305
Dana-Farber Brigham Cancer Center	MA	877-801-2278	Sarah Cannon Center for Blood Cancer at Tri Star Centennial	TN	615-342-7339 (P) 615-342-7440 (A)
Johns Hopkins Hospital Sidney Kimmel Comprehensive Cancer Center	MD	410-502-5487	Texas Transplant Institute at Methodist Hospital	TX	210-575-7800 (A)
Michigan Medicine University of Michigan Medical Center	MI	734-232-7594	The University of Texas MD Anderson Cancer Center	TX	833-368-6382
Mayo Clinic CAR-T Cell Therapy Program: Rochester	MN	507-284-5363	Blood and Marrow Transplant Program at Medical City Dallas Hospital	TX	972-566-4508 (P) 982-566-7288 (A)
The University of Mississippi Medical Center	MS	888-626-1099	VCU Messey Cancer Center Cellular Immunotherapeutics and Transplantation Program In-patient Unit	VA	804-628-2079
UNC Cancer Care	NC	919-445-4208	UVA Stem Cell Transplant Progm	VA	434-924-4333
			UW Health	WI	800-622-8922

Image 26 Kymriah centers. Assembled by Dr. Nancy Liu-Sullivan.

greatest number of Kymriah treatment facilities. The following table was adapted from https://www.us.kymriah.com/treatment-center-locator/ that zeros in on medical facilities that administer Kymriah for both pediatric and adult blood cancer patients.

Side effects. All drugs entail elements of toxicity that manifest in patients as side effects. Not all side effects are on equal planes. CAR-T therapy side effects are particularly pronounced due to the very nature of revitalizing patients' own immune power to combat cancer. As the physiological compass, the immune system guides the body in the right direction in fighting germs to protect it. When artificially excited, such as in CAR-T, the immune system tends to become overwhelmed very quickly, leading to a "cytokine storm." Cytokines are potent signaling molecules that recruit fighter immune cells. More cytokines are released by these recruits, leading to additional recruitment, resulting in immune chaos that ends up damaging healthy cells, tissues, and organs. Organ failure is life-threatening and requires immediate medical attention. In addition, CAR-T therapy by Kymriah is also associated with toxicity to neurological systems. For detailed descriptions of Kymriah side effects, also called "Contraindications," please follow the Novartis guidelines by visiting https://www.us.kymriah.com/

Super steep price tag. Kymriah is marketed at $475,000 for a course of treatment with a single dose. Is the price too dear? Well, it's a very complicated subject not suitable for lengthy discussions here. One thing is for sure—Kymriah is very expensive to prepare—time-consuming and personnel-consuming, not to mention follow-up patient care. For more details, please refer to *HOUSTON, WE HAVE A PROBLEM* (page 99).

Personalized living drug. Each dose of Kymriah is different because it consists of patient-specific T cell products, making the drug a *bona fide* personalized medicine. At the same time, Kymriah, like all other forms of CAR-T therapy drugs, is a living, breathing drug with a full payload of anti-cancer arsenals. All eyes are on next-generation CAR-T equipped with higher potency but reduced toxicities, combined with other treatment modalities to achieve synergistic effects for cancer patients.

Food for thought:

1. The first-ever FDA-approved CAR-T drug is called Kymriah, which is designed by Penn Medicine and manufactured by Novartis.
   A. True
   B. False

2. Emily Whitehead's life was saved by Kymriah, although at the time it was still an experimental drug not yet approved by the FDA.
   A. True
   B. False

CAR-T THERAPY (5): YESCARTA

Legendary former First Lady Jackie Kennedy captivated France during the historic state visit with President JFK in May 1961. Fast forward thirty-two years to 1993, Jackie was diagnosed with non-Hodgkin's lymphoma and passed away the following year after a series of brave battles. While chemotherapy and radiation were the only treatment choices in Jackie's days, lymphoma patients today are blessed with advancements in science exemplified by "Yescarta."

Lymphoma by type. The two distinguishing types of lymphoma are Hodgkin Lymphoma (HL) and Non-Hodgkin Lymphoma (NHL).

HL was first observed in 1832 by Dr. Thomas Hodgkin, an English physician. Subsequently, German physician Dr. Carl Sternberg and American physician Dr. Dorothy Reed independently documented the signature cell type with a conspicuously giant size mutated from immune B cells, also called B lymphocytes. Hodgkin Lymphoma arises in a lymph node and moves from one lymph node to the next; hence, it is easy to trace and treat, relatively speaking.

Non Hodgkin Lymphoma (NHL), by contrast, is much tougher to treat as typically, when diagnosed, it is already late stage. Former First Lady Jackie Kennedy suffered from NHL. Compounding factors, such as the rapid spread of the disease combined with debilitating side effects from radiotherapy and chemotherapy treatment, all gravely weaken patients' immune system, posing very tough battles for patients.

Mutation in B cells. Both HL and NHL arise from mutated B lymphocytes, which are immune cells born in the bone marrow and trained in the spleen to learn how to defend the body by producing antibodies that fight infectious bugs as well as infected self-body cells. When B cells are afflicted with mutations, they grow fast and produce large quantities of totally useless antibodies—useless in the sense that these antibodies are unable to perform tasks of neutralizing infection-causing microorganisms or mediating T cells in killing infected cells or cancer cells. Even worse, these futile B cells take up space in the blood, crowding out red blood cells (RBCs), platelets, and immune cells. Patients suffer from extreme fatigue (due to impeded RBC function from inadequate supply of oxygen to cells and tissues), unusual bruising and bleeding (due to insufficient platelets to carry out blood clotting), and susceptibility to infection (due to severely weakened immune cell activities). In short, mutated B cells wreak serious immune havoc, interfering with normal functions of healthy cells, tissues, and organs. Effective treatment that targets these mutated B cell mutations is in immediate order! Fortunately, we now have Yescarta.

Yescarta is a CAR-T. Approved by the FDA in 2017, Yescarta, with the genetic name of "axicabtageneciloleucel," treats *R/R Large B-Cell Lymphoma* (R/R LBCL), a subtype of Non Hodgkin Lymphoma (NHL) in adult patients. "R/R" stands for "relapsed or refractory," meaning lymphoma that returns after initial remission or lymphoma that is resistant to other types of cancer treatment. Yescarta has achieved 51 percent complete remission (CR) and 21 percent partial remission. A jolly good start!

Yescarta manufacturing centers. Initially developed by Kite Pharma, Inc. (headquartered in Santa Monica, CA), Yescarta is under Marketing Authorization Holder by Gilead Biosciences (headquartered in Foster City, CA). Gilead bought Kite in 2017 prior to Yescarta receiving FDA approval at the end of 2017.

There are multiple authorized Yescarta treatment centers in the United States. For a detailed list, please refer to the link provided by the American Society of Clinical Oncology (ASCO), https://ascopost.com/issues/may-25-2018/treatment-centers-authorized-to-administer-car-t-cell-therapy/ According to a press release by Gilead in December 2022, Yescarta has been approved by pharmaceutical regulatory authorities in Japan to be manufactured at Kite Pharma's El Segundo, California, manufacturing center. The products are to supply Yescarta treatment centers located at six hospitals in Japan.

Major side effects. Similar to CAR-T Kymriah, patients who received Yescarta manifest high fever, low RBC count, low white blood cell (WBC) count, low blood pressure, and difficulty breathing, among a series of other side effects. Accordingly, patients are closely monitored by a specialty healthcare team, the same practice for all CAR-T care.

Yescarta court case. There is an ongoing lawsuit against Kite/Gilead for alleged copyright infringement, with a dramatic jury award of hundreds of millions of dollars to the company Juno but later was rejected by a higher court. The jury is still out.

Food for thought:

1. CAR-T Yescarta is approved by the FDA to treat NHL that has relapsed or is resistant to other forms of cancer treatment.
   A. True
   B. False

2. Like Kymriah, Yescarta manufacturing processes are only carried out at designated medical centers.
   A. True
   B. False

CAR-T THERAPY (6): TECARTUS

As a subtype of Non Hodgkin Lymphoma (NHL), mantle cell lymphoma (MCL) is described as a silent lymphoma which, typically by the time of diagnosis, is already late stage. As a rare blood cancer, MCL tends to afflict predominantly white male individuals between sixty and eighty years of age and accounts for 3–8 percent of all NHL cases in the United States, according to the Leukemia & Lymphoma Society (LLS).

Two CAR-Ts by the same pharma. As the #3 CAR-T immunotherapy approved by the FDA in July 2020 for the treatment of "relapsed & refractory mantle cell lymphoma," abbreviated as R/R MCL, "Tecartus" is manufactured by Gilead/Kite, the same US pharmaceutical company for "Yescarta." Both CAR-Ts rely on the cancer patient's own revitalized immune Killer T (KT) cells to harness the patient's own cancer.

The generic name for Tecartus is Brexucabtagene Autoleucel, and yes, another tongue twister like axicabtagene ciloleucel for Yescarta. So let's stick to the trade names. Notice that both drug names contain "car," as "Yes**CAR**ta" and "Te**CAR**tus." A quick recap: "CAR" stands for "chimeric antigen receptor," which is an artificially designed receptor molecule that gets processed to be displayed on the surface of the patient's own KT cells. The armed KT cells become activated and are expanded to large quantities to find cancer cells for irreconcilable destruction.

Two CAR-Ts: Identical twins but with a twist. Identical twins share 100% of DNA. In a similar vein, twin YESCARTA and TECARTUS share the same "genetic design" in that all the molecular parts used to revitalize cancer patients' Killer T (KF) cells are the same. Like identical twins whose growth environment molds and shapes twin siblings in slightly different ways, the same is true for the two CAR-Ts. Here, Tecartus is bestowed with special "tender loving care" (TLC) in the preparations to tailor the treatment of mantle cell lymphoma (MCL). Before delving into the details of TLC, let's take a look at the unique features of MCL first, which will lead to TLC. Promise!

Mantle cell lymphoma (MCL) and the mantle zone. Speaking of mantles, we are reminded of mantle pieces that decorate fireplaces. The mantle zone within the lymph nodes shares a similar feature to the living-room mantle piece: it forms a ring around the center stage where action is taking place. The action is the flaming fire from the living-room fireplace, while the immune mantle fire takes place in the lymph node, a specially designated zone called the "germinal center" where mutated B cells encounter CAR-T cells. As for MCL diagnostics, the number of lymph nodes affected by mutated B cells determines the stage of MCL, ranging from stages 1–4. The presence of cancerous B cells in a single lymph node is defined as Stage 1 MCL, and the number of affected lymph nodes is proportional to the severity of MCL. For reasons not yet elucidated, mantle cell lymphoma patients are found to have a large number of cancer cells shedding into and circulating in their bloodstream.

Impurity is a dangerous thing. Remember the first step of CAR-T therapy is to collect WBC from blood cancer patients, and from there, T cells are isolated for molecular engineering that fuels T cells with tumor-finding and tumor-fighting power. For mantle cell lymphoma patients, the unusually high number of crowding cancer cells in patient blood poses a considerable challenge: all cancer cells must be methodically and completely teased out so that only pure immune T cells remain for the next step of preparation—a matter of life and death for patients.

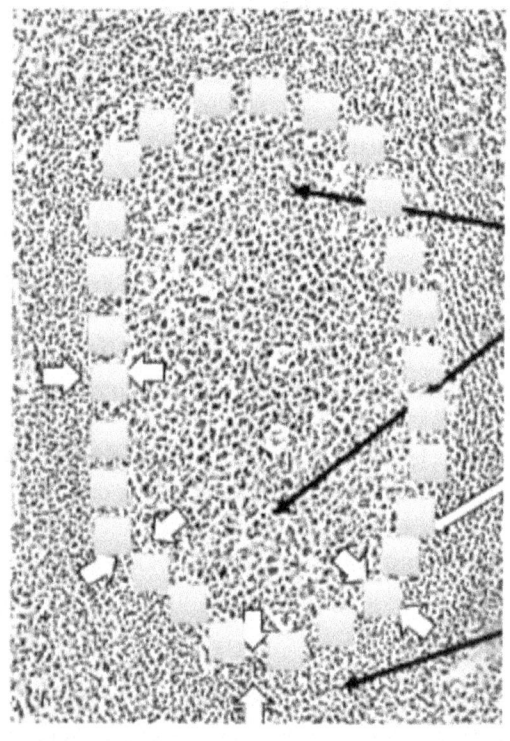

Image 27 Mantle zone. Assembled by Dr. Nancy Liu-Sullivan and combined with Wikimedia Commons Mantle Zone. File: Dark, light, mantle, and marginal zones of a secondary follicle.png.

Tecartus TLC for T cell purity. Filtering all cancer cells out is no easy feat! Aside from the complicated experimental processes required, any cancer cells that fail to be removed from the patient's T cell sample would be "revitalized," which, when returned to the patient's blood, would be analogous to introducing powerful cancer cells back to the patient, defeating the purpose of cancer treatment. A no-no! In fact, there is one documented and very unfortunate case associated with another CAR-T therapy platform where "empowered" cancer cells were inadvertently piggybacked alongside Killer T cells and returned to the patient. The patient had an initial cancer remission but deteriorated over the next six months and sadly passed away. For this precise life-saving reason, scientists at Gilead/Kite designed Tecartus CAR-T therapy with an innovative approach to thoroughly remove all unwanted cells, allowing only the desired T cells to remain. These special cell purification technologies and the encouraging 62 percent of patients experiencing CR of their mantle cell lymphoma upon a single dose of Tecartus infusion led to FDA approval in July 2020 and European Union (EU) approval in December 2020 for the treatment of refractory/relapsed mantle cell lymphoma (R/R MCL) in adult patients, offering a magnificent ray of hope for patients who are not responding to conventional treatment.

Tecartus treatment centers. For detailed information on medical centers authorized for Tecartus treatment, please refer to the following link provided by Gilead/Kite: https://www.tecartushcp.com/car-t-cell-therapy/mantle-cell-lymphoma/treatment-center-locator

Food for thought:

1. CAR-T Tecartus is approved by the FDA to treat relapsed or refractory mantle cell carcinoma, a subtype of lymphoma.
   A. True
   B. False

2. One critical step of Tecartus preparation is to remove all cancer cells from the patient's blood sample to isolate pure T cells before the next step because any cancer cells that slip through the selection would reintroduce the cancer to the patient when Tecartus is infused into the patient.
   A. True
   B. False

CAR-T THERAPY (7): BREYANZI

The fourth CAR-T therapy approved by the FDA for the treatment of large B cell lymphoma (LBCL) is Breyanzi, with the generic name Lisocabtagene maraleucel, which has a more friendly abbreviation as "Liso-Cel."

Similar to the three prior CAR-T therapies (Kymriah, Yescarta, and Tecartus), Breyanzi also targets B cells in blood cancer by inserting of a molecular "key" of the "CD19 receptor" protein that opens the "lock" protein of "CD19" on cancerous B cells in lymphoma. To wit: The CD19 key acts like a molecular GPS to guide CAR-T cells in finding cancerous B cells, followed by a fierce "slash-and-burn" to clear cancer cells.

Breyanzi manufacturing centers. Like all CAR-T therapy products, Breyanzi manufacturing is also strictly regulated and only carried out by designated facilities by Bristol-Myers Squibb (BMS) pharmaceuticals. At the moment, there are four Breyanzi preparation centers in the United States located in Devens, Massachusetts; Bothell, Washington; Warren, New Jersey, and Summit, New Jersey. Breyanzi harbors two unique features. Let's dig deeper.

1 + 1 = > 2. This equation suggests two entities working collaboratively to achieve a goal greater than the simple sum of the two singular entities. The same logic applies to Breyanzi, whose unique preparation stands out compared to the other CAR-T therapies. What is so special about Breyanzi T cell prep? To start with, the general practice of extracting T cells from a patient's blood involves a mixture of T cells taken in random. What is unique about Breyanzi CAR-T is the strictly 1:1 ratio of two types of T cells: those that harbor a surface molecule called "CD8" (also called cytotoxic T cells or Killer T cells) and those that express "CD4" (also called helper T cells) on the T cell surface.

The 1:1 golden ratio has yielded surprisingly productive immune synergy between the two T cell subpopulations, leading to greatly enhanced efficacy of T cells in combating cancer cells while at once reducing adverse effect of "cytokine storm" and therefore reducing chances of putting patients in life-threatening immune overreaction situations.

What makes the ratio golden? Good question! Despite a few preliminary thoughts about why the 1:1 ratio of CD4-T to CD8-T cells leads to the pleasing win-win of higher potency against cancer and reduced cytokine overreaction, scientists are running more experiments to get to the bottom of the mechanism of action. Time will tell! The simplified 1:1 ratio is presented below.

Breyanzi covers the full battlefield. When Breyanzi was first approved by the FDA in February 2021 for the treatment of large B cell lymphoma (LBCL), it was restricted to patients who have received two prior types of treatments but with no effect. Upon second approval in June 2022, Breyanzi received the green light from the FDA to treat LBCL patients who did not respond to only one type of prior treatment. Hence, Breyanzi pretty much covers the full field of the LBCL patient population. This is to the greater benefit of patients: Why wait until after the patients failed to respond to the second type of cancer treatment to introduce Breyanzi? Between the first and second treatments, precious time is lost for the patient. And time is life!

It is not implausible that one day, hopefully soon, when costs dwindle substantially, CAR-T may become the first and standard line for blood cancer and solid cancer treatment.

Food for thought:

1. Breyanzi excels among other platforms of CAR-T in its exquisite 1:1 ratio of CD4-T and CD8-T selection from patient blood samples that has led to enhanced drug potency and reduced adverse effects.
   A. True
   B. False

2. As a summary of all four platforms of CAR-T discussed thus far, every single one targets leukemias or lymphomas that bear B cell mutations.
   A. True
   B. False

CAR-T THERAPY (8): ABECMA

It damages bones, overwhelms kidneys, thickens the blood, inflicts painful aches, and casts life-threatening complications. A devastating blood cancer, (MM has cut life short for many, including General Colin Powell, Stateswoman Geraldine Ferraro, and Roy Schneider, the town police chief in the iconic American movie *Jaws*.

"*BARC*" as a collection of telltale traits. Medical school students are known to have ingenious ways to create mnemonics to ease unimaginable heavy-duty loads of rote memorization. Below is a vivid "*BARC*" depiction for MM, where,

- *B* for "bone" damage and bone pain inflicted by MM;
- *A* for "anemia" caused by a dwindling number of RBC as they are being crowded out by overwhelming numbers of, again, faulty and voluminous "M proteins";
- *R* for "renal" that describes kidney function compromised by the heavy workload of filtering large quantities of dysfunctional, faulty, useless antibodies called "M protein";
- *C* for "calcium" is released into the bloodstream from damaged bones.

Of course, on second look, the above can be rearranged to form a "*CRAB*" mnemonic. Right? When it comes to mnemonic imagination, the sky is the limit.

Plasma cells are "antibody factories." To understand why multiple myeloma (MM) is an incredibly devastating and debilitating medical condition, let's have a quick recap of B cells and their progeny, plasma cells. Born in the bone marrow and "educated" in the spleen, B cells are an integral component of the adaptive arm of our immune system. As illustrated in the following figure: when a B cell encounters an infection-causing bug, it engulfs the whole bug (a process called "phagocytosis"), chews it up, displays a representative piece on its "sleeves," and mingles with another immune cell type called "Helper T cell" (T-h, also called CD4-T). T-h is a practitioner of "trust but verify." Upon confirming with its "molecular antenna" (called T cell receptor or TCR), T-h gives a helping hand to the B cell for full activation. Once activated, the B cell undergoes clonal expansion and transforms to become a plasma cell known as "antibody factories." The antibody molecules produced aim to target the very infectious bug the B cell encountered in the first place. The "Y"-shaped antibodies unleash their fierce anti-bug power to sweep clean all dangers. Important to note: the production of antibodies by plasma cells is carried out on a by-need basis under normal conditions.

Plasma cells gone wild. In Multiple Myeloma, plasma cells become out of control and churn out a cornucopia of antibody-like molecules called M proteins that do not function as normal antibodies. One tends to naturally assume "M" here stands for "myeloma." To quote a famous line from my professor who taught the most challenging graduate class of Neuroanatomy at Columbia University, "*Nice try but no cigar!*" It turns out that "M" has nothing to do with "Myeloma"; rather it refers to "monoclonal." A clone is a carbon copy of the original. As for "mono," it suggests that all identical clones come from the same single source. In the case of multiple myeloma, all the dysfunctional M proteins are the products of a single rogue plasma cell that has gone wild, that is, wildly mutated.

No cure until 2021. Unannounced, MM typically affects people over the age of sixty, more common in men than women and more common in Caucasians. The exact cause remains elusive, no cure was available, and survival rate sadly abysmal for a long while. March 26, 2021, is a day of significance in the history of MM treatment. On this day, the FDA gave approval to ABECMA with the generic name "idecabtagene vicleucel" for the treatment of MM in patients who have had prior treatment but didn't work (hence, their disease is "resistant") or the treatment worked initially but eventually stopped working and the cancer returned (relapsed). Akin to other CAR-T cancer immunotherapy

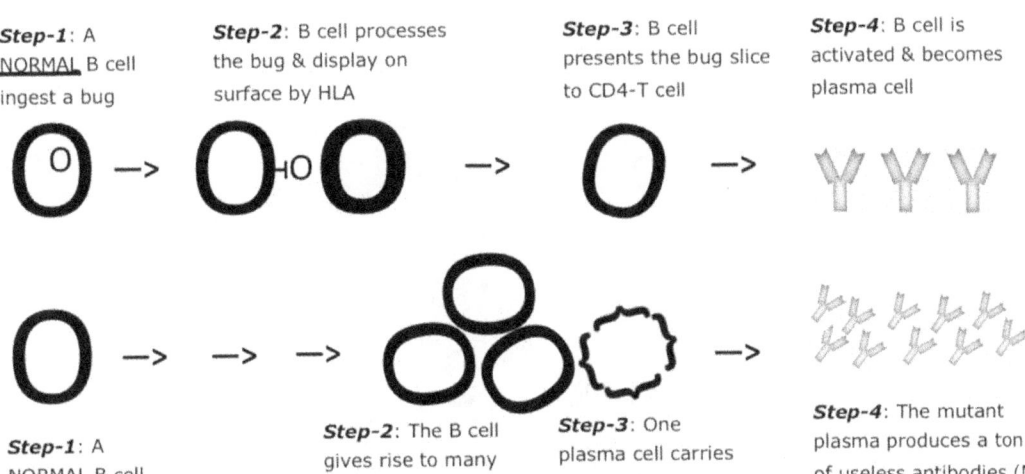

Image 28 B cell journey. Assembled by Dr. Nancy Liu-Sullivan.

drugs, ABECMA is also a living, personalized drug prepared by taking T cells from the patient, engineered with genetic features that guide the molecularly decorated T cells to capture and kill cancerous plasma cells.

Cancerous plasma cell "address." How do trained T cells pinpoint the precise place of residence of cancer-causing plasma cells? Well, a picture is worth a thousand words. The following figure depicts how the T cell "key" finds the cancer cell "lock." The "key" is BCMA, which stands "B cell maturation antigen." Antigen is a molecular ID that tells the identity of cells and is capable of triggering an immune reaction. BCMA is primarily found on the surface of rogue cancerous plasma cells, making it an attractive bull's eye for the living drug ABECMA. Specifically, engineered T cells are guided by the "key" of the BCMA receptor protein to precisely locate cancerous plasma cells by matching to the BEMA "lock." As soon as the key opens the lock, CAR-T cells become activated and begin to secrete the two powerful enzymes of "perforin" and "granzyme-B" to poke holes in MM

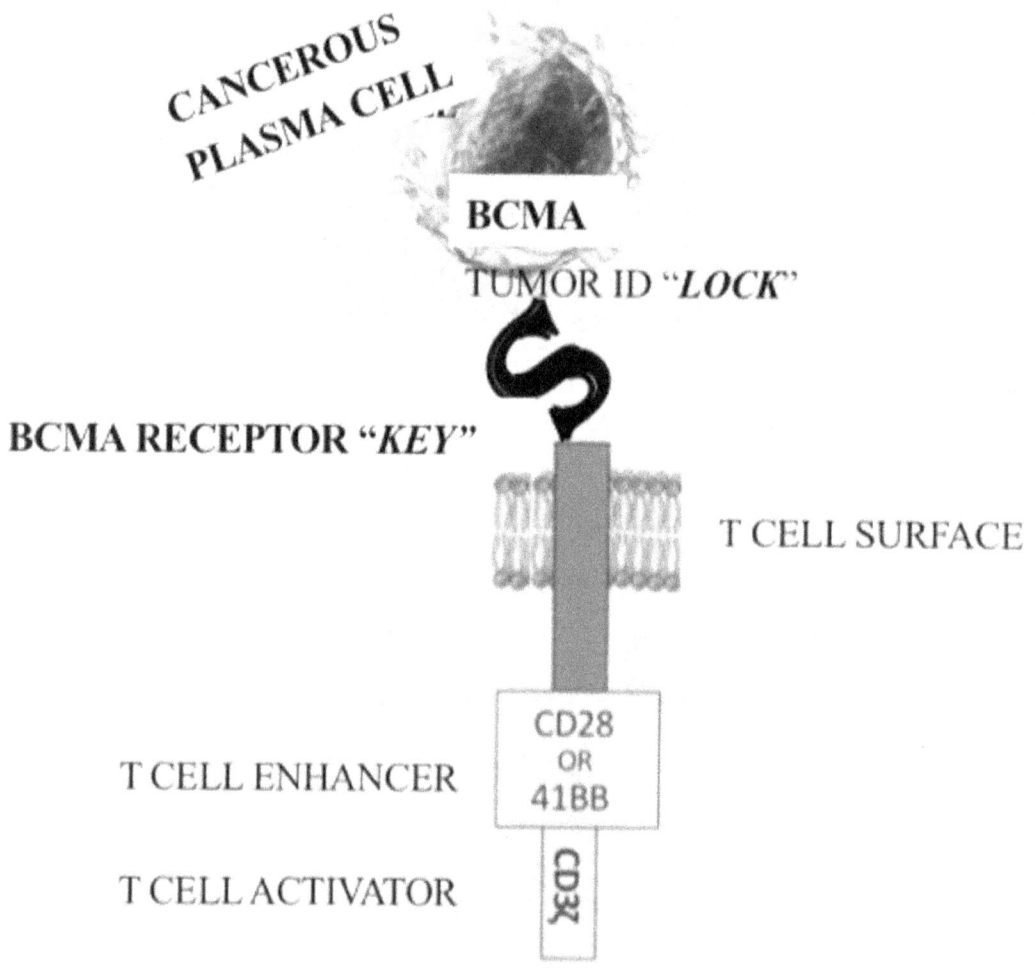

Image 29 CAR-T aimed at MM. Assembled by Dr. Nancy Liu-Sullivan and combined with Wikimedia Commons File: Blausen 0624 Lymphocyte B cell (crop).png.

cells followed by pressing the cell suicide button in MMs for their irreversible destruction. You might wonder: Hmm, this diagram looks familiar. Right! It resembles the figure of the CAR-T drug that saved Emily Whitehead's life from incurable leukemia. But there is one major difference: Emily's drug had a different key (CD19 receptor) on engineered T cells and a different lock (CD19) on leukemia cancer cells. By contrast, ABECMA harbors a different set of key and lock specific for multiple myeloma.

Complete remission (CR) accompanied by a hefty price tag. Designed by the US pharmaceutical pioneer, BlueBird Bio, headquartered in California, and manufactured and marketed by another pharma giant, BMS located in New Jersey, ABECMA has achieved CR in 33 percent and 39 percent of the patients in two separate clinical trials. Those percentages translate to many precious lives saved by ABECMA. As for the cost of this one-time infusion living drug, it is listed as $504,348. Former NBC anchor Mr. Tom Brokaw was diagnosed with MM eleven years ago and is one of the few able to survive more than five years. Having not yet been completely cured, Mr. Brokaw has been living on maintenance therapy to keep cancer cells under control while suffering from the unbearable ramifications of extreme fatigue, a compromised immune system, shortness of breath, and many other debilitating symptoms of daily torment. Hope the new drug can make a decisive difference for Mr. Brokaw and many other MM patients.

Food for thought:

1. ABECMA is the first CAR-T therapy approved by the FDA for the treatment of R/R multiple myeloma.
   A. True
   B. False

2. Like all other forms of CAR-T, ABECMA also costs ~$500,000.
   A. True
   B. False

CAR-T THERAPY (9): CARVYKTI

More than one road leads to Rome. Since the approval of ABECMA in 2021, another CAR-T therapy, also for the treatment of multiple myeloma, received FDA approval in the following year, 2022. The trade name of the newly approved T cell therapy is CARVYKTI, with the generic name as "Ciltacabtagen Autoleucel." Developed by a Chinese pharmaceutical company called Legend Biotech with the global headquarters located in Somerset, New Jersey, United States, CARVYKTI also engineers patient T cells with a molecular "key" called the BCMA receptor protein, a biomarker protein predominantly found on the surface of cancerous plasma cells, but not other body cell types. This makes BCMA a cancer-specific molecule, also a molecular "address" of cancer plasma cell residence.

Game on! The first MM CAR-T therapy ABCEMA approved in 2021 has a complete response rate of around 40 percent. By a pleasant surprise, CARVYKTI demonstrates a 78 percent stringent complete response, abbreviated as "sCR," which is defined as a complete response by the patient to the drug so effectively that no presence of cancer cells can be observed by any platforms of diagnostic tools, including radiation imaging. To wit: after a single infusion of patient-sourced living drug CARVYKTI, close to 80 percent of the patients find their cancer gone! Remarkable, albeit the result was obtained in a clinical trial of ninety-seven participants, among whom seventy-six achieved sCR. Of course, as with all forms of CAR-T, all patients are monitored closely for any post treatment changes.

There! CARVYKTI's complete response nearly doubled that of ABECMA. The race is on! When two pharma companies compete, patients benefit, for healthy competition stimulates innovations, and innovations propel cancer care forward. There is also a slight price differential: $524,833 for ABECMA and $504,344 for CARVYKTI.

Food for thought:

1. CARVKYTI is a CAR-T that also treats R/R multiple myeloma, akin to ABECMA.
    A. True
    B. False

2. CARVYKTI has shown a higher level of emission rate when compared to ABECMA—78 percent versus 40 percent.
    A. True
    B. False

CAR-T THERAPY (10): A WHITE-KNUCKLE RIDE

An innovative technological breakthrough, CAR-T cancer immunotherapy that revitalizes patients' inner immune power to tackle cancer has achieved milestone accomplishments. Many lives have been saved and extended. The ride on CAR-T, however, can be bumpy, some minor, some major.

CAR-T can agitate an immune monsoon. Among many cancer treatment challenges, major immune cells being kept at bay is the most perplexing. As we are thoroughly conversant about at this point of this book, CD8 Killer T (KT) cells are swift and precise in combating infectious bugs as well as infected cells with no qualms. The same KT cells lose their shine and opt to live in quiet co-existence with cancer cells within the tumor microenvironment (TME) as a result of assorted cancer tricks and traps. To rejuvenate KT cells, scientists tinkered with complex molecular components and designed a therapy that enabled tweaked patient KT cells to find cancer cells and finish them off on the spot. On average, ~50 percent of blood cancer patients experience disease remission post CAR-T treatment. However, CAR-Ts also carry with them a molecular catch.

Unintended collateral damage: While fighting glorious battles against cancer cells, CAR-T cells also agitate the patient's entire immune system. Before long, patient immune cells, out of knee-jerk reactions, start to release cytokines which stimulate more immune cells followed by accelerated release of cytokines and additional immune cells; hence, the vicious cycle kicks off, cooking up a cascade of cytokine chaos. How damaging is uncontrolled cytokine unloading to the human body? It triggers high fevers mixed with shivering chills, rapid pulse rate, dangerously low blood pressure, and labored breathing, which, in the absence of timely medical intervention, can quickly lead to multi-organ failure and death. Aside from the immediate and severe side effects of CAR-T therapy, there is also a long-term deletion effect.

CAR-T can trigger secondary cancers. The white-knuckle CAR-T ride bears another and more serious dimension: the emergence of secondary cancers. According to a notice issued by the FDA to CAR-T therapy manufacturers, a "**boxed warning**" must be added to the product description that cancer patient-derived, CD19 and BCMA-targeting CAR-T therapy drugs are associated with increased risks of getting secondary cancers. Of note,note, a "boxed warning" is the highest level of patient safety-related warning designated by the FDA. The purpose is to alert prescribers and patients to severe adverse effects and serious risks associated with specific medications. Below is an example of "boxed warning" unrelated to CAR-T therapy.

A double whammy for cancer patients. Secondary cancers are cancers caused by medical treatment. Chemotherapy and radiation therapy, for example, can be extremely toxic, capable of breaking DNA that leads to cumulative and irreversible gene mutations that cause secondary cancers over time. For chemotherapy, radiation therapy, or chemo-radio combo, the typical secondary cancer is cancer of the skin. As for CAR-T therapy that relies on modified immune T cells to tackle cancer cells, up to the end of January 2024, the FDA has received twenty-five cases of secondary cancers in patients who have completed their CAR-T treatment. Typical secondary cancers associated with CAR-T are cancers derived from mutated T cells of either T cell lymphoma or T cell leukemia. For patients who have developed secondary cancers, they are also confronting the possibility of their primary cancer becoming resistant to CAR-T therapy or a primary cancer relapse. Adding insult to injury!

A silver lining. Despite the stringent FDA boxed warning requirement, the overall risks for secondary cancers are low, at least at this point in time: Out of 27,000 patients who have received CAR-T treatment, there are twenty-five cases of secondary cancer, which is less than 0.1 percent. A new study reported by Stanford University Medical Center describes 6.5 percent of secondary blood cancers among the 724 cancer patients who received CAR-T treatment from 2016–24 and the study

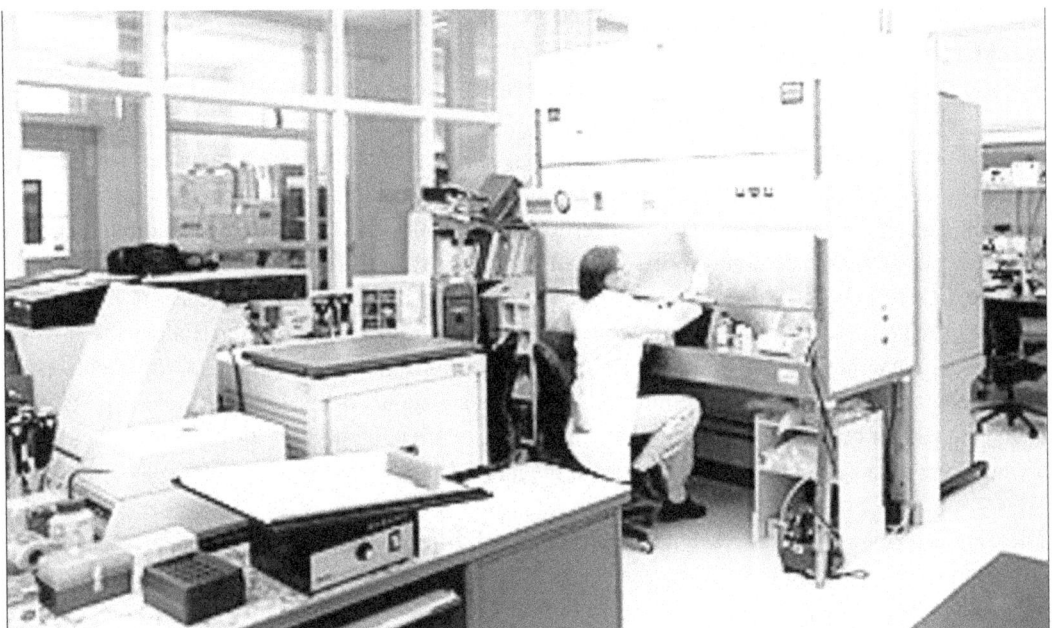

Image 30 FDA laboratory. Wikimedia Commons File:FDA Bldg 64—Lab (5160771733).jpg.

concludes that CAR-T therapy poses a "low risk of second tumor." Well, low risk is better than intermediate or high risks. That said, patients are flesh-and-blood people, not statistics. A silver lining of the current situation is that it provides impetus for scientists to go back to the drawing board to design and develop more optimal CAR-T therapy with maximal efficacy and minimal adverse effects. Meanwhile, the very idea of revitalizing cancer patients' own immune systems to combat cancer remains a very sound idea!

Food for thought:

1. Radiation therapy and chemotherapy can lead to secondary cancer of the skin for cancer patients.
    A. True
    B. False

2. Secondary cancers associated with CAR-T treatment are manifested as blood cancers involving T cells.
    A. True
    B. False

COLD CAPPING, ELEGANT AND COOL!

A group of friends shaving each other's heads to stand by their pal who will undergo chemotherapy—many folks have either heard about it or even gone through a similar experience themselves. A telltale manifestation of the potent side effect, hair follicle loss is almost synonymous with the very word of chemo. An innovative way to minimize the loss of hair follicles has become part of the chemo treatment regimen. Let's find out why it is such a cool idea!

A cold welcome to chemo. As one of the five pillars of cancer treatment, chemotherapy delivers potently toxic chemical drugs to the tumor core. The other four pillars, by the way, are radiotherapy, surgery, targeted therapy, and immunotherapy. A great majority of chemo drugs work by damaging cancer cell DNA to halt malignant tumor growth; some even annihilate entire tumors. Since cancer cells grow uncontrollably faster and in larger quantities than normal cells, more cancer cell DNA gets damaged by chemotherapy. Despite lesser damage compared to cancer cells, normal cells do harbor vulnerabilities in certain fast-dividing body cells such as hair follicles. As a chemo "collateral" damage, hair follicle cells also have their DNA wreaked havoc upon, leading to patient hair falling out. Despair not, for where there is a will, there is a way. Since chemo drugs follow the flow of circulation, if the blood flow is slowed down, it would limit the amount of chemo drug delivered. Translating the same logic to the clinics, physician-scientists have developed a "cold cap" to cool down the temperature of the scalp, which effectively restricts blood flow to the hair follicles and dwindles the amount of chemo drug present at the hair follicles.

The cool idea can work wonders. Studies that compared chemo patients undergoing chemotherapy with or without the cold cap show that more than 60 percent of patients in the cold cap group experienced 50 percent less hair fallout from chemo. You might ask: Why not 100%? Thoughtful question. According to experts at MSKCC, the effect and extent of hair loss reduction by the cold cap depend on three contributing factors: how much, how frequently, and the type of chemo. For details, please refer to https://

www.mskcc.org/cancer-care/patient-education/managing-hair-loss-scalp-cooling. Although the cold cap does not work wonders for everyone in reducing chemo-associated hair fallout, there is a silver lining for all patients: the cold cap confers a faster and fuller hair recovery rate after chemo.

How does cold cap work? The general practice of cold cap therapy is to have the patient put on a cold cap cooled to 32 degrees Fahrenheit. As for the duration, it is 30 minutes before chemo starts, followed by the entire chemo session, followed by 90–120 minutes post-chemo. The cold cap is connected to a computer monitor to ensure the correct duration and precise temperature.

Silky long hair and elegant as ever, Princess Kate Middleton has candidly shared with the public her experience of preventive chemotherapy. Discussions among concerned and caring physicians naturally led to the topic of chemo and cold cap. Delightful that Kate has successfully completed preventive chemo, good as new and fair as ever!

Food for thought:

1. Chemotherapy targets fast-dividing cells such as cancer cells. The treatment leads to patient hair follicle fallout because hair follicles divide and grow at a very fast speed.
   A. True
   B. False

2. A special cool cap helps slow down hair follicle fallout or promotes faster hair re-growth after chemo.
   A. True
   B. False

COLEY'S CANCER TOXIN

An accomplished bone surgeon at Memorial Hospital on the upper east side of Manhattan, New York, in the 1880s, Dr. William Coley treated many patients. One particular case caused Dr. Coley too many sleepless nights. What transpired from this unusual event led to a paradigm shift in cancer care. Let's take a closer look.

An elegant young lady in her early twenties had a minor hand injury from a train ride. Unexpectedly, the injury worsened that eventually led to the diagnosis of sarcoma, a cancerous growth of the bone. The cancer quickly spread and took her life. Determined to get to the bottom of the devastating disease, Dr. Coley scrutinized medical archives, and one case caught his eye: the patient's cheek sarcoma grew to the size of a hard-boiled egg and was deemed "hopeless." Then a miracle ensued. The patient contracted a deadly *erysipelas* bacterial infection and developed high fevers that persisted for days. As the patient's fever subsided, so did the tumor on his cheek. By the time the patient completely recovered from the infection, his tumor also completely disappeared. Seven years later, after finally tracking down the guy in lower Manhattan, New York City, Dr. Coley saw a healthy middle-aged man leading an ordinary workman's life and was still cancer-free!

The mystery link. Infection gone; tumor gone! Dr. Coley immediately speculated an immune connection: dormant before but energized to fight the bacterial infection, and during that process, cancer cells became the unexpected "collateral damage" on the gory immune battleground. The domino events started with one leading to the next: *severe bacterial infection → high fevers →*

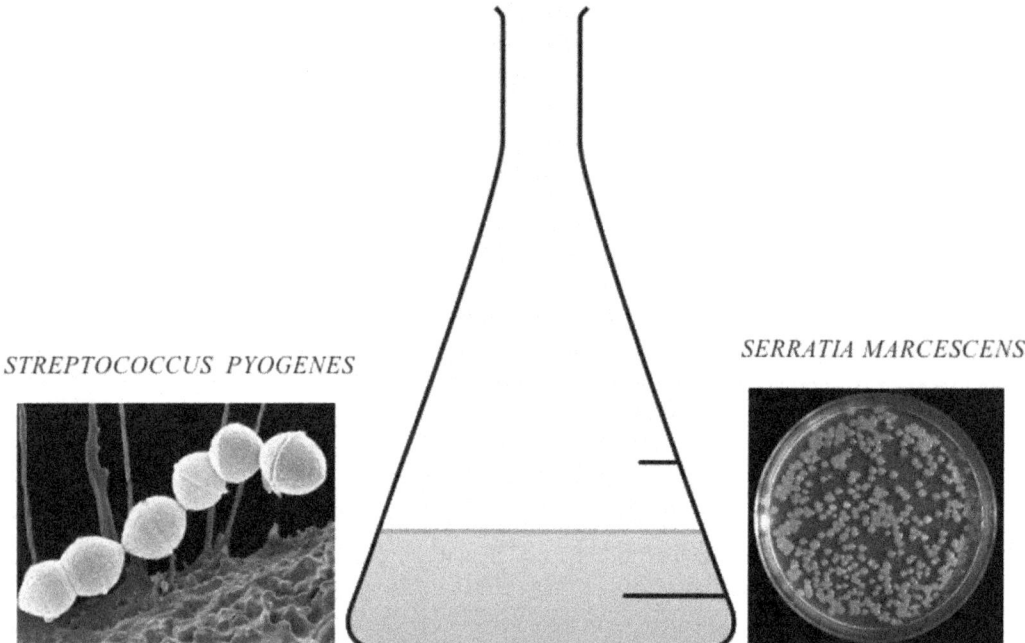

Image 31 Coley's Cancer Toxin. Wikimedia Commons File: Conical flask.svg. File: Streptococcus pyogenes (Group A Strep) (52602981880).jpg. File:Serratia marcescens.jpg.

mobilized immune cells →→ *destruction of deadly bacteria and cancer cells*. The key link, as surmised by Dr. Coley, ought to be the high fevers. What if we purposefully induce an infection accompanied by high fever to wake up immune cells to fight cancer? Dr. Coley started preparing safe dosages of the bacteria that cause erysipelas infection. That was 1891, forty years before the Empire State Building emerged on the Manhattan skyline, to put things in perspective.

Dr. Coley's first try was a triumph. The patient received the bacterial injection, got infected, and developed high fevers as expected. Like the workman's story, Dr. Coley's first patient from this mini clinical trial achieved an amazing fruition: infection gone, sarcoma also gone! This was no random event. Over the next thirty plus years, Dr. Coley recruited large cohorts of cancer patients for further testing. To ensure safety, he also replaced the crude bacterial soup with a safer and more standardized formula consisting of a virus and bacteria combo with a new name: "*Coley's toxin*." The success attracted attention from physicians near and far, all excited about treating inoperable tumors with Coley's toxin.

Setbacks and reflections. Clinical trials today are stringently protocoled with the gold standard of "*randomized, double-blind, and placebo-controlled.*" Clinical trials in the United States are carried out at designated cancer centers approved and generously funded by the National Cancer Institute (NCI) under the US National Institutes of Health (NIH). It wasn't quite the case in Dr. Coley's time.

The effort to test Dr. Coley's toxin around the turn of the twentieth century was a very different picture: no standardized protocols, no funding, and no federal oversight. Indeed, later it was revealed some physicians followed Dr. Coley's toxin formula to the word, some resorted to close resemblance while a host of others improvised their own renditions. It is no surprise that the trial outcomes were all over the map, ranging from highly effective to mildly effective, zero effect, or negative effect. There was no way for Dr. Coley, a single physician, to have organized large-scale testing centers with streamlined protocols and rule-based practices. It was simply logistically impossible at the time. These setbacks led to censorious doubts over Coley's toxins. Scathing remarks were also tossed at Dr. Coley personally. The early twentieth century also marked the discovery of radioactivity, and radiation treatment soon took the world by storm. Dr. Coley's toxins became yesterday's flower.

One believer persisted. While most embraced the new pillar of radiation for cancer treatment, one individual remained confident that the new path carved out by Dr. Coley was a promising one. The brave lady was Helen Coley Naut, the daughter of Dr. Coley and a trained PhD biologist. Helen combed through thousands of pages of medical notes—her father's legacy—and noticed a pattern of cure in patients treated with Coley's toxin by Dr. Coley personally. With the help of a few influential philanthropists, Helen established, in 1953, world's very first institute dedicated solely to research and development of immunological studies for cancer care: Cancer Research Institute (CRI) headquartered in Manhattan, not far from the Empire State Building. CRI attracted leading oncologists and scientists as participants and as leaders, "CR[I]ing" loud and clear of the sound idea in tackling cancer relying on cancer patients' own inner immune powers. One of the earliest proofs of concept demonstrations is the repurposed TB vaccine BCG against non-metastatic bladder cancer, pioneered by Dr. Lloyd Old, who, like Dr. Coley, was also an accomplished physician at MSKCC although nearly a century apart. This was 1959. For Dr. Old's legendary life and science, please visit *The Old Man and the Vaccine* (page 196). The storied history of the CRI, its leadership, and scientific milestones are depicted in JILL O'DONNELL-TORMEY: THE CHOICE THAT MADE A TRANSFORMATIONAL DIFFERENCE. (page 110).

Food for thought:

1. Dr. William Coley pioneered the idea of treating cancer by energizing the patient's own immune system.
   A. True
   B. False

2. Dr. Coley's legacy lives on at the CRI.
   A. True
   B. False

COLORS OF CANCER

One midafternoon after I took care of some inter-office business at the Memorial Hospital Building of MSKCC, I paid a visit to the Gift Shop, which was a few doors down the corridor on the northeast corner of the hospital lobby. The instant I entered the shop, I was captivated: the elegance of carefully curated item choices was impeccable, the serene background music of Johann Bach's *Prelude in C* was soothing, the aroma of cappuccino from the side deli was delectable, but I was most enticed by the idea that all Gift Shop revenues are devoted to cancer research at MSKCC. I made a habit of doing all my holiday shopping at the Gift Shop. The thought that every penny dedicated to research helps dilute the hidden guilt of being spendthrift.

One particular item on display at the Gift Shop is the ribbons of cancer: *Soft pink* for breast cancer, *light blue* for prostate cancer, *dark blue* for colon cancer, *yellow* for bone cancer, *green* for liver cancer, *white* for lung cancer, *black* for skin cancer, *orange* for leukemia, *light purple* for pancreatic cancer, *dark purple* for gynecological cancers, *gray* for brain cancer, and many more. Adding to this growing list is also *lavender*, perhaps the most significant of all, the symbol of Cancer Survivors.

Located west of the main lobby of Memorial Hospital at 1275 on First Avenue, Manhattan, the Gift Shop also offers online shopping to extend support for cancer research. Additional venues to make contributions for MSKCC include the annual Cycle for Survival. By sending a simple email to *CycleforSurvival@mskcc.org*, you will be connected to a research lab for rare cancer research, and your donations will go directly to the laboratory. Money is a means to an end. Let ample amounts continue to flow into cancer research.

Established in 1884 on the upper west side of Manhattan, MSKCC is *the* very first center dedicated to cancer care in the United States. As a direct fruition of the groundbreaking National Cancer Act (NCA) signed into law by President Richard Nixon in 1971, MSKCC (along with Roswell Park Cancer Institute and MD Anderson Cancer Center) became one of the three comprehensive cancer centers designated by the National Cancer Institute (NCI). Here and now in 2025, more than half a century since the 1971 Act, there are seventy-two comprehensive cancer centers supported by the NCI working in synergy on basic bench research that translates into patient bedside meds. These remarkable events are meticulously documented in the book of *Centers Of The Cancer Universe* co-authored by oncology physician and cancer research leader Donald L. Trump, M.D., and science journalist Eric T. Rosenthal. Collectively, the War on Cancer declared in 1971 has been instrumental in elevating cancer care to the next level. Indispensable to the progress is funding for cancer research: In the inaugural year in 1971, NCI had a budget of $1.59 billion. In 2024, the NCI budget is $7.2 billion.

To tackle the complex diseases harbored by complex mutations at genetic and epigenetic levels, it takes a village when it comes to funding to fuel the engine of research. To this end, numerous non-governmental organizations (NGOs) have also played important roles, as exemplified by the CRI and the ACS. A summary table of representative NGO institutes and foundations is presented below. All hands on deck to conquer cancer!

Food for thought:

1. There are seventy-two comprehensive cancer centers throughout the United States, the fruition of the 1971 Cancer Act by President Richard Nixon.
    A. True
    B. False

2. A special cancer support symbol is lavender, dedicated to all cancer survivors.
    A. True
    B. False

CRAB: THE NAME TELLS A VIVID TALE

Shielded by a thick shell, armed with two sharp claws and eight kicker legs, crabs are notoriously clumsy when it comes to crawling forward but extremely dexterous when moving sideways, vividly resembling how cancer cells breach cell-cell barriers and melt molecular fences to invade healthy territories. To cancer biologists, crab symbolizes every name in the book of cancer. At a glance at the pair of the following figures, one cannot help but be marveled at the striking physical resemblance between the crab (on the left) and the cancerous tumor (on the right).

| REPRESENTATIVE NON-GOVERNMENTAL CANCER FOUNDATIONS IN THE U.S. ||
ORGANIZATION NAME	WEBLINK
American Cancer Society	cancer.org
American Institute for Cancer Research	aicr.org
Cancer Research Institutes	cri.org
Cycle for Survival	cycleforsurvival.org
Dancing While Cancering - The Maddie Kramer Foundation	dancingwhilecancering.org
Emily Whitehead Foundation	emilywhiteheadfoundation.org
Fred's Team	fredsteam.org
Leukemia & Lymphoma Society	lls.org
Livingstrong Foundation	livingstrong.org
Lustgarten Foundation	lustgarten.org
MSKCC Giving	giving.mskcc.org
National Breast Cancer Foundation	nationalbreastcancer.org
New York Cancer Foundation	nycancerfoundation.org
Ovarian Cancer Research Alliance	ocrahope.org
Pershing Square Sohn Cancer Research Alliance	psscra.org
Prevent Cancer Foundation	preventcancer.org
Prostate Cancer Foundation	pcf.org
Simons Foundation	simonsfoundation.org
Staten Island Breast Cancer Research Initiative	csi.cuny.edu/alumni-community/community/sibcri
Susan G. Komen for the Cure	komen.org
Zoey's Wings	zoeswings.org

Image 32 Foundations and charities. Assembled by Dr. Nancy Liu-Sullivan.

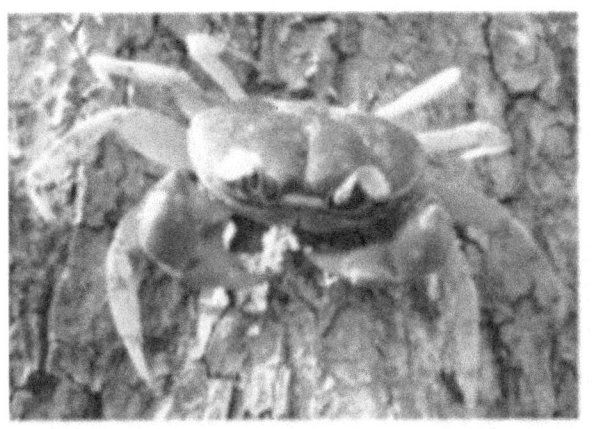
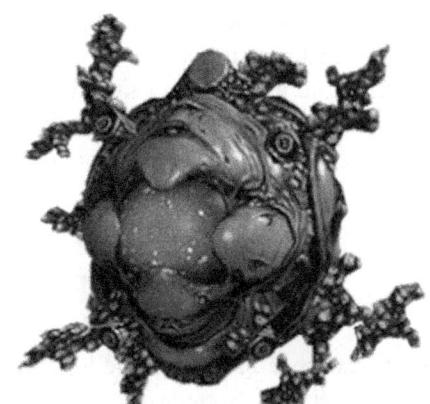

A sea crab   An infested malignant tumor

Image 33 CRAB qua crab. Wikimedia Commons File:Gecarcinus quadratus (Nosara).jpg.

Cancer is shielded by a hard "shell." Like the crab that wraps itself in a hard shell, a cancerous tumor also builds a sturdy fence to shield the tumor community collectively called the "tumor microenvironment" (TME). As a pro-survival tool, the tumor shell serves to block off chemotherapy drugs and therapeutic radiation. For a detailed description, please refer to *CANCER TRICKS AND TRAPS (4): HARD FENCES MAKE BAD TUMORS* (page 30).

Cancer excels at additional fronts. In the seminal paper published in the year 2000, followed by a sequel a decade later in 2010, Dr. Robert Weinberg and Dr. Douglas Hanahan scrutinized thousands of research observations for trends and patterns and distilled ten cancer hallmarks. Below is a brief recap with my rendition to dilute the jargon for ease of understanding for our readers.

(1) *Gas pedal stuck in place* to enable unstoppable cancer cell growth.
(2) *Death-defying chromosome ends* to ensure DNA immortality.
(3) *Dismantling normal cell turnover* to confer cell immortality.
(4) *Shying away from tumor suppressors* to sustain uninterrupted cancer growth.
(5) *Constant mutations* to guarantee tumor successful evolution.
(6) *Creative gathering of cellular fuel* to propel cancer forward.
(7) *Constructing new blood vessels* to pave the road of invasion.
(8) *Migrating out of original site* to carve out new tumor territories.
(9) *Promoting inflammation* to help fan the flames of cancer growth.
(10) *Escaping immune action* to preserve undeterred cancer growth.

Fortunately, for each cancer trait described above, we have one or a few drugs as therapeutic interventions. Regrettably, what is available in our cancer drug cabinet is still a dearth. The advent of artificial intelligence (AI) offers hope for multi-dimensional as well as in-depth queries to both expand our understanding of cancer and to design better drugs with maximal efficacy and minimal toxicity. Let us remain "glass half full"!

Shedding the old shell. One feature uniquely crab is that the crab shell has zero elasticity and does not expand. This poses a serious problem when the crab's body exceeds the dimensions of the shell. No worries for crabs, for they have evolved to be capable of replacing the old hard shell with a new and soft shell to support the crab's growing needs. Allow imagination to run wild: It would be interesting to find out if a cancerous tumor also "sheds" its hard protective shell. If so, and if the window of cancer's "between shells" moment is captured precisely, this could be leveraged as a new tool to zap cancer in its moment of weakness.

CRISPR/Cas9 QUARTET (1): GPS-GUIDED MOLECULAR SCISSORS

Stingrays shove their tail spine to jab venom into the intruders. Skunks raise a stink to scare off uninvited critters. Bacteria, too, have evolved to equip an awesome self-defense apparatus with the acronym CRISPR, against their prime invaders called "phages," defined as viruses that infect bacteria.

CRISPR: Invader intelligence database. Human cells often fall victim to infection by bacteria, the most infamous of which is a toxic strain of *E. coli*, leaving a destructive trail of compromised intestinal lining and bloody diarrhea. At the same time, bacteria can also be the target of infection, mostly by "phage." For self defense, bacterium unleashes its immune arsenal called CRISPR. After winning the first battle over phage invaders, CRISPR makes a copy of a telltale snippet of the phage DNA and stores the valuable viral "intel" on bacterial "DNA memory chips" to save for a rainy day. CRISPR consists of arrays of methodically organized phage DNA sequences, each in a designated grid, each marking a different type of phage. When the same phage dares to show up for the second time, the bacterium quickly retrieves the stored DNA copy from its "database," locates the phage with the matching sequence, and chops it up for good.

A closer look at CRISPR. What guides CRISPR to the phage? How does CRISPR "know" where to cut among a sea of phage DNA sequences? And what tool does CRISPR use to do the cutting? This leads to the three core components of CRISPR.

Component #1: **Guide RNA** (or *gRNA*) is the GPS system that guides the defense machinery to the phage of interest. CRISPR in bacterial cells harbors a two-part gRNA called "crRNA" and "tracrRNA," respectively. To sum up: *gRNA = crRNA + tracrRNA*. You might be asking: Wait a minute! Bacteria store phage *DNA* in its CRISPR Bank. So where does g*RNA* come from? Thoughtful question! Before exploring why the switch from DNA to RNA in CRISPR, let's quickly recap how DNA and RNA are related in general.

Rule-based matchmaking in DNA:

- DNA has two parallel strands with unique directions: The *coding* strand goes 5' → 3' and the *template* strand has the polar opposite direction of 3' → 5'
- DNA is built by four bases consisting of A, T, G, and C with strict matching rules where A is matched with T and G is matched with C, as follows:
  A T G C (DNA *coding* strand of 5' → 3')
  T A C G (DNA *template* strand of 3' → 5')
- For RNA, base T does not exist but is instead substituted with U, as follows:
  T A C G (DNA *template* strand)
  A U G C (RNA strand)

Now, let's go back to the question of why phage DNA involves RNA activities. It turns out that while the CRISPR bank stores phage DNA, when a particular phage DNA is needed for cutting, the bacterial host goes through a step of converting the phage DNA to RNA termed "CRISPR RNA" or *crRNA*. It also occurs that crRNA needs an assistant termed "tracrRNA." Why do bacteria go through this seemingly cumbersome conversion step? Plausibly, it is the product of evolution.

Component #2 PAM is the flagging system that demarcates where the matching phage DNA sequence starts. PAM stands for "protospacer adjacent motif."

Component #3 Cas9 is a pair of molecular scissors that cuts up the phage DNA on target. With the entire genome destroyed, the phage is gone, so is phage-induced infection in the defending bacteria. Mission accomplished for bacterial immune defense against invading viruses.

So here you go regarding the CRISPR blueprint: a pair of scissors (*Cas9*) guided by a GPS system (*gRNA*) arrives at phage RNA site. Cas9 then locates the red flag raised by *PAM*, followed by a decisive cut through phage DNA, leading to the demise of phage.

The full name of CRISPR: As a brilliant bacterial immune defense apparatus, CRISPR stands for *Clustered Regularly Interspaced Short Palindromic Repeats*. Seriously?! Sounds like a tongue twister par excellence! That said, let's demystify CRISPR with our word anatomy as follows, starting with the central word "repeats," since all words that appear before "repeats" are modifiers of "repeats."

Quick Word Anatomy:

- **Repeats** serve as "molecular hedges" that separate one phage DNA sequence from another.
- **Palindrome** describes the structural feature of the "repeats" that can be read forward and backward while maintaining the same letters of sequence in either direction. English vocabulary examples include "gag," "civic," and "radar."
- **Short** is another added modifier for "repeats" which are not only palindromic but also short in length.
- **Interspacer** is the actual phage DNA sequence(s) stored between the "repeats." Collectively, the "interspacers" and "repeats" form part and parcel of the bacterial phage "database." What is interesting is that new generations of bacteria do not need to have encountered each and every type of phage on their own from scratch; the phage memory is passed on from generation to generation. The following figures illustrate how "interspacers" are stored between "repeats," with each spacer designated with a number representing a different type of phage DNA.

Le voila! We have now disassembled complex CRISPR to its component parts. To recap, CRISPR = Clustered, regularly interspaced, short palindromic repeats. Easy as pie, *n'est pas*?

To describe how CRISPR is used for gene editing in human cells, let's borrow a lesson in English grammar. The following sentence has the correct word order in terms of "subject," "verb," and "object" but harbors an error in syntax or meaning. Let's mimic CRISPR editing to correct the error, as follows:

Step 1: Identify the error, "SUMMER" and direct Cas9 to the error by guide RNA (gRNA consisting of crRNA + tracrRNA) followed by stemming out the error by Cas9, shown in the following figure:

Step 2: The error "SUMMER" is successfully removed, leaving a gap in DNA sequence.

Step 3: The gap is filled up with the correct DNA as "WINTER" also called "donor DNA" that gives rise to the correctly expressed gene first and the correctly expressed protein eventually.

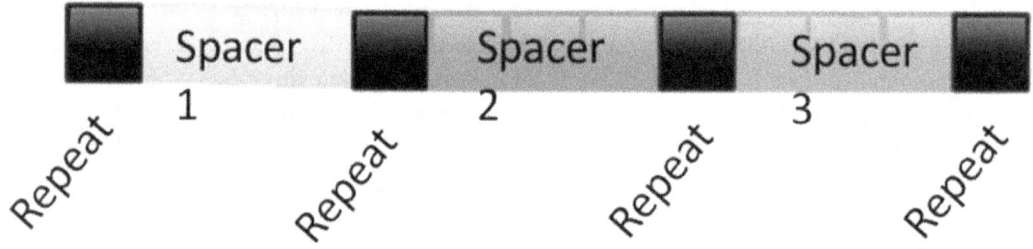

Image 34 CRISPR arrays. Assembled by Dr. Nancy Liu-Sullivan.

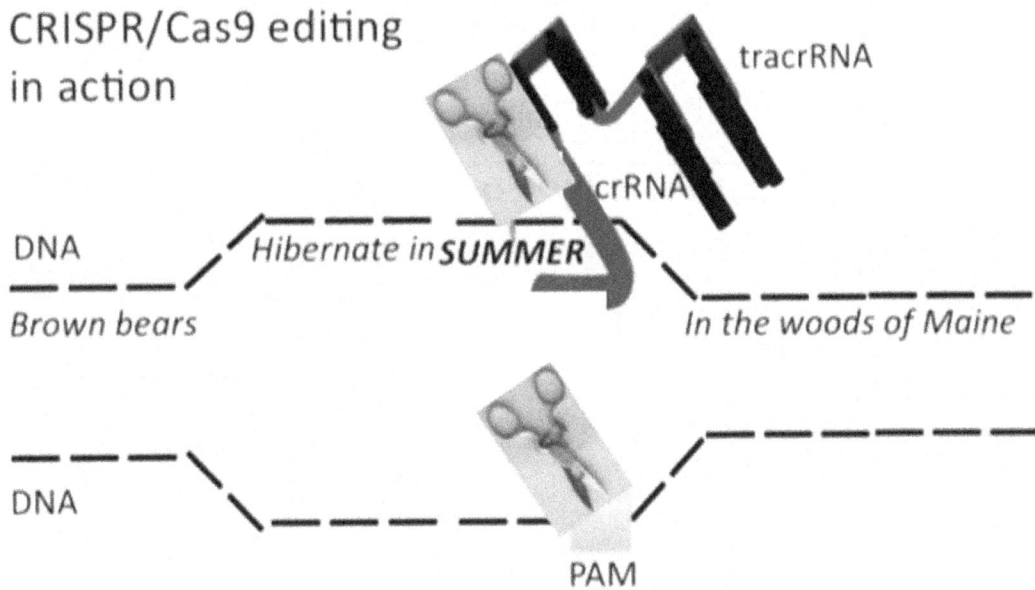

Image 35 PAM SCISSORS. Wilimedia Commons File: Forbici da occhielli.jpg and by Nancy Liu-Sullivan.

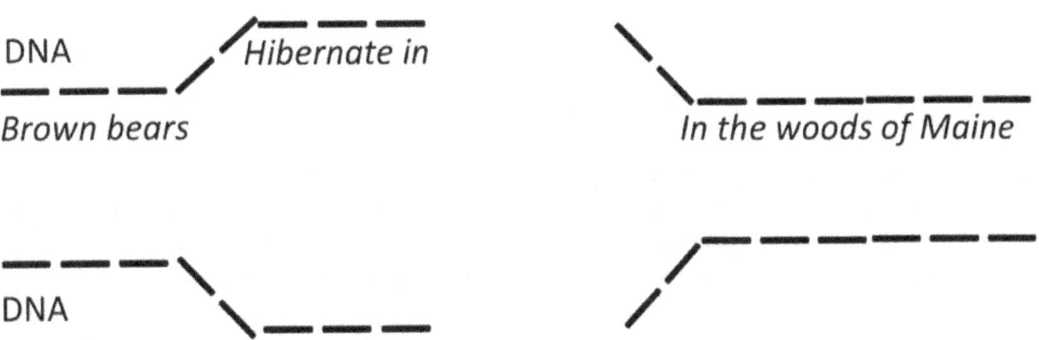

Image 36 DNA errors remove. Assembled by Dr. Nancy Liu-Sullivan.

CRISPR/Cas9 editing in action (3): ERROR CORRECTED

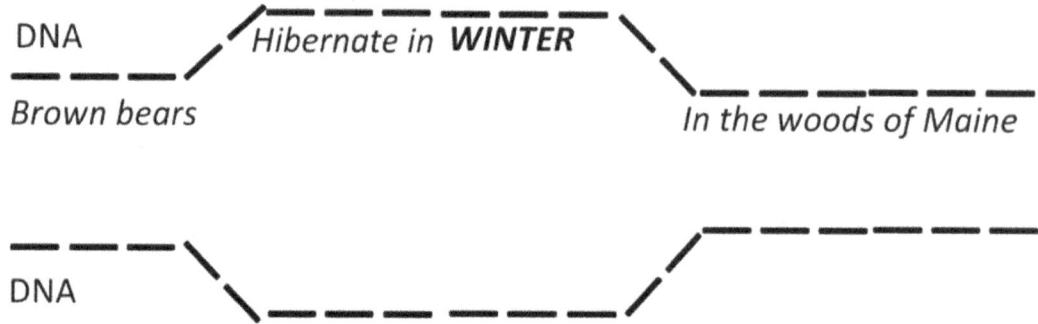

Image 37 CRISPR editing mission accomplished. Assembled by Dr. Nancy Liu-Sullivan.

Excitingly, CRISPR/Cas9 technology has successfully been translated in the clinics. The first FDA-approved therapy is Casgevy. More about it in our next essay.

Food for thought:

1. Phage is defined as a type of virus that specializes in infecting bacteria.
   A. True
   B. False

2. CRISPR is a remarkable molecular tool capable of editing DNA errors.
   A. True
   B. False

CRISPR/Cas9 QUARTET (2): SILENCING A CRITICAL GENE TO CURE SICKLE CELL ANEMIA

As the chief supplier of oxygen to every cell of the body, RBCs are our lifeline. A mutation drives RBCs out of shape, leading to a life-threatening medical condition called sickle cell anemia. Thanks to CRISPR/Cas9 gene-editing technology, we now have a genetic procedure capable of a cure. To understand how the drug works its miracles, let's first brush up on sickle cell anemia.

Mutant hemoglobin makes RBCs bent. Concave and flexible, normal RBCs are abundantly endowed with hemoglobin, an iron-rich molecule that binds to oxygen molecules to ensure oxygen distribution to every nook of the body as RBCs circulate. The iron portion also gives the red hue to RBCs. Perturbed by a genetic mutation, hemoglobin molecules crumble up inside RBCs, driving RBCs out of shape, rigid, and bent like the silhouette of a sickle. Bent RBCs malfunction with the tendency to clog up in blood vessels, causing tissue damage and interfering with normal blood flow, which can be life-threatening. The following figure illustrates normal RBCs in stark contrast to sickled RBCs.

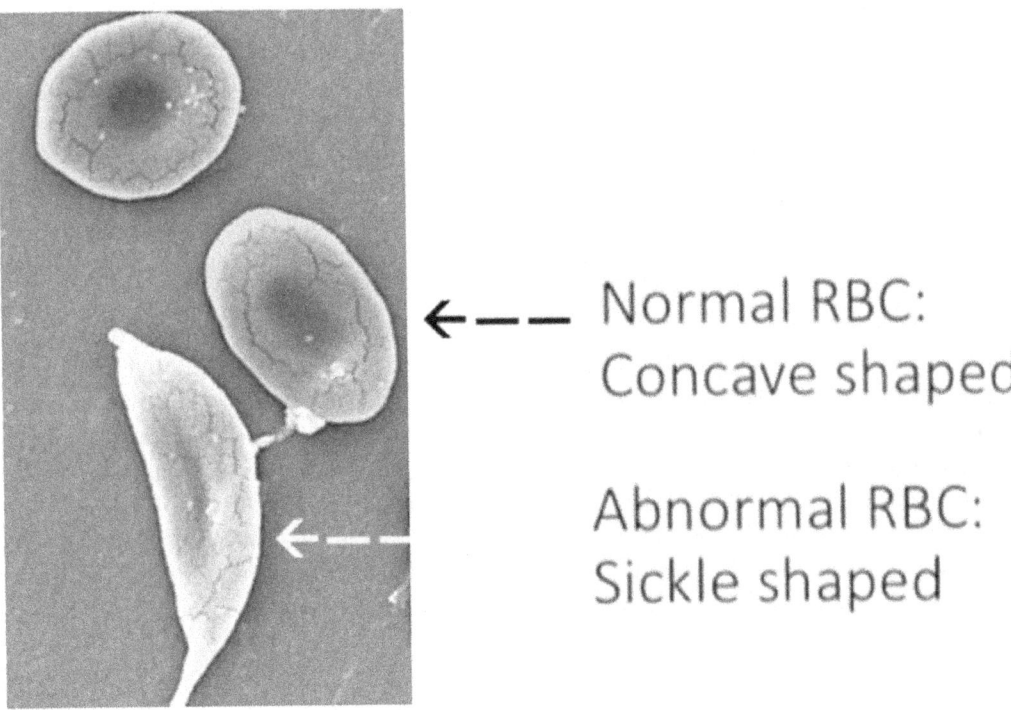

Image 38 Red blood cells: concave vs. sickle. Wikimedia Commons File: 1911 Sickle Cells.jpg.

CRISPR/Cas9 corrects the genetic typo. Symptoms of sickle cell anemia were first reported by an American physician in 1910. Besides being anemic (insufficiency of RBCs in circulation), patients also experience a lot of pain. Finally, in 1957, the causative factor was pinned down to a mutated gene. Fast forward to 2008, a gene termed *BCL11A* was identified by physician-scientists at Boston Children's Hospital as a suppressor gene that represses fetal hemoglobin gene (dubbed the *HBB* gene) responsible for making hemoglobin protein molecules that carry oxygen molecules inside RBCs. At the same time, CRISPR/Cas9 became a mature gene-editing tool. The combination of basic scientific discovery fused with cutting-edge genetic technology made it possible for a cure of sickle cell anemia. The name of the drug is Casgevy. How does Casgevy correct sickle cell anemia genetic typo? The steps are as follows:

Step 1: A medical specialist collects blood stem cells from sickle cell anemia patient. Since these cells are patient's self cells, they are also called "autologous" blood stem cells. By the way, all stem cells express a telltale trade marker protein called "CD34."

Step 2: CRISPR/Cas9 is then used to silence *BCL11A* gene with the goal of relieving suppression over fetal hemoglobin gene.

Step 3: The CRISPR/Cas9-edited stem cells that harbor silenced hemoglobin suppressor gene are then transplanted back to the patient. With the hemoglobin repressor yanked out, the fetal version of hemoglobin start to make correct copies of hemoglobin molecules that are happily housed in RBCs to carry out oxygen-transporting tasks.

Why is it a big deal to revitalize the fetal hemoglobin gene? Fetal hemoglobin gene is active after birth but gradually fades into the background and is replaced by the adult version of hemoglobin that occurs around 6 months of age. The "master mind" behind the switch of hemoglobin genes from fetal to adult version is a gene called *BCL11A*. Now, in patients with sickle cell anemia, the adult hemoglobin gene is the culprit of the disease due to a genetic typo. So, by silencing *BCL11A*, the error-free fetal hemoglobin gene gets a chance to be resurrected and start producing the correct version of the hemoglobin gene that fulfills the vital tasks of distributing healthy RBCs to the human body. The experimental design is genius!

How does CRISPR/Cas9 silence *BCL11A*? The silencing is a very straightforward process: After identifying the exact location of *BCL11A* gene aided by CRISPR guide RNA (gRNA), PAM raises a red flag at the cut site. Cas9, the molecular scissors, cuts both strands of DNA, leaving a broken gap. The cell's own DNA repair crew steps up to fix the broken DNA but makes an (inadvertent but intended) sloppy mistake. This mistake is exactly what scientists had hoped for, because the mistake triggers a mutation in the *BCL11A* gene. Our body cells, being the "perfectionist" that they are, make a swift decision of silencing the mutant gene in order to preserve DNA integrity. There! *BCL11A* gets silenced, which lifts repression over the fetal hemoglobin (*HBB*) gene. With the resurrected HBB, correct copies of hemoglobin proteins are made, which go on to supply robust RBCs vital for a functional human body.

With a long genetic name as "exagamglogene autotemcel" (also known as "exa-cel"), Casgevy is manufactured by CRISPR Therapeutics, a biotech company headquartered in Switzerland. A highly effective living drug, Casgevy also has a price tag *très cher*—$2.2 million for a single-dose, for a one-time treatment.

Following Casgevy, the FDA also gave approval to a second Sickle Cell Anemia therapy called "Lyfgenia" marketed by another US pharma called BlueBird Bio, using a different technological approach from CRISPR/Cas9. If you think Casgevy at $2.2 million is a sky-high price, think again. The asking price of Lyfgenia is $3.1 million. Hopefully, in time, the price will come down to allow greater accessibility to more needy patients not just in the United States but globally.

Food for thought:

1. Sickle-shaped RBCs in sickle cell anemia patients are unable to fulfill the task of distributing healthy hemoglobin throughout the human body.
   A. True
   B. False

2. Casgevy is a high-tech drug developed using stem cell transplantation combined with a CRISPR-edited gene that represses the adult hemoglobin gene. The repressive gene is called *BCL11A*. CRISPR-induced DNA errors lead to silencing of *BCL11A*. This allows the stem cell-resurrected fetal hemoglobin gene to take over.
   A. True
   B. False

CRISPR/Cas9 QUARTET (3): PIG DONOR HEART FOR HUMAN

September 20, 2023, marked another milestone of CRISPR/Cas9 gene-editing application in the clinic. On this day, at the University of Maryland Medical Center, an end-stage heart patient underwent transplantation of a CRISPR-edited donor pig heart encompassing a total of ten edited knocked-out and knocked-in genes critical for transplantation success.

Knock, knock! CRISPR technology moved very rapidly from bench (basic laboratory research) to the bedside (clinical applications). Compared to Casgevy, the CRISPR/Cas9 mutation-corrected drug, editing multiple pig genes in the donor pig heart entails a different level of complexity. The biggest challenge stems from how to optimally minimize immune rejections by the human recipient of the donor pig heart. As we know, our body is very particular about maintaining "selfness," and any entities that smell "alien" send immediate danger signals that prompt immune cells to rise up and pin down entities that are "non-self." This immune rejection, in turn, can also pose grave danger to the recipient as the rejection escalates to a "cytokine storm" that sweeps through cells, tissues, and organs in its path, wreaking systemic havoc. If not properly and timely treated, such violent immune over-reactions are life-threatening. To best keep the host immune system at bay, some critical genes in the donor pig heart need to be "knocked out," while certain other genes bear the necessity to be "knocked in." Let's look more closely.

Knocked-*out* genes. The sugar chemical groups on the surface of pig heart cells are a major culprit that triggers human host rejection. These sugar molecules are part of larger proteins found on pig heart surface and function as molecular antennas. The best way to yank out these dangerous sugar groups is to knock down or silence the entire antenna protein. Since proteins are the product of genes, to eliminate the protein, one must go to the root of the matter by eliminating the genes that encode the proteins. That was exactly what the Harvard CRISPR scientists did. One example of the sugar-bearing gene silenced by CRISPR/Cas9 is called "alpha-1,3-galactosyltranaferase" that writes the blueprint of a major sugar protein on the surface of pig heart cells. By the way, by convention, all gene names are italicized. Another cohort of genes knocked out by CRISPR/Cas9 involves a pig-specific gene called "*Swine Leukocyte Antigen*" (SLA), which are also known to trigger host rejection of xenotransplantation (cross-species organ transplantation such as pig heart to human). To prevent the donor pig's heart from outgrowing the human chest, a pig growth gene was also deleted using CRISPR/Cas9.

Knocked-*in* genes. In parallel to knocking out critical genes, CRISPR scientists also "knocked in" other critical genes that act as suppressors of cytokine monsoon in the host recipient. The target of repression is a protein called "Complement." By definition, this protein contributes to immune response by complementing or mediating other components. A family of more than thirty members, complement proteins reside in circulating blood. Of these, five stand out to form a "ring of fire" on the surface of body cells deemed "dangerous." The ring consists of Complement 5c subtype b, or *C5b*, joining hands with *C6*, *C7*, *C8*, and *C9*, collectively termed the "membrane attack complex" (MAC), as shown in the following figure:

A force of destruction, MAC pokes a giant hole on cell surface that triggers death of the targeted cell. To harness complement proteins, CRISPR scientists introduced or "knocked-in" genes that repress complements, officially called complement regulator genes. Key genes incorporated into the donor pig heart include a cluster of four: *CD46*, *CD47*, *CD55*, and *CD59*. The proteins made by these genes engage in diversified activities to tame the complement reaction pivotal for reducing host rejection.

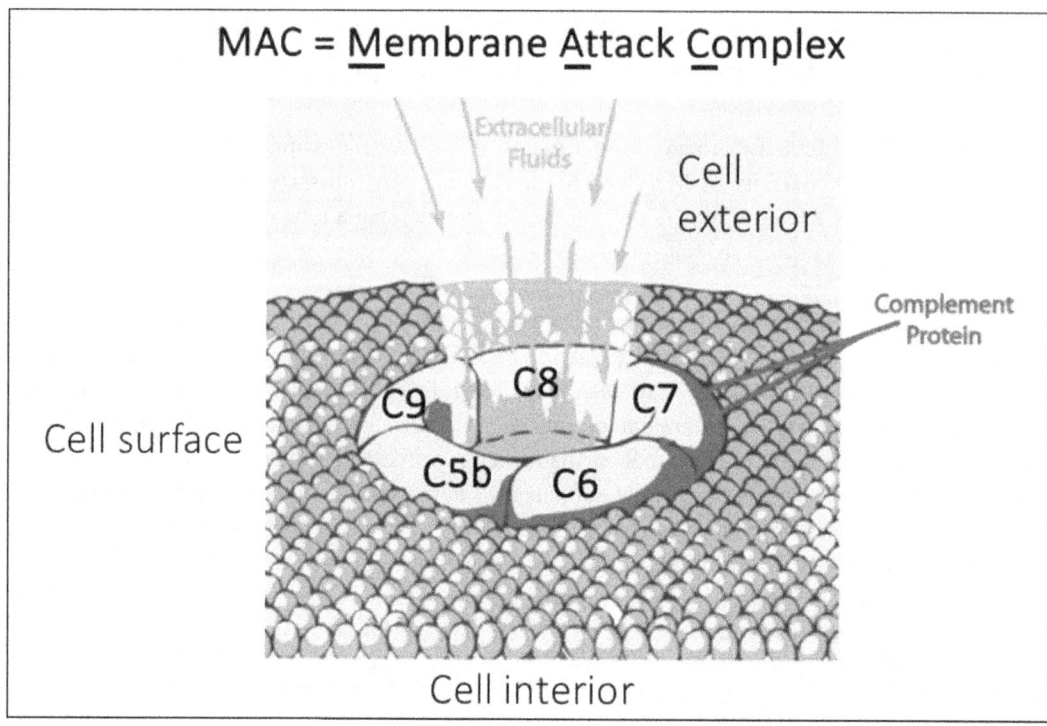

Image 39 Mac for membrane attack complex. Wikimedia Commons File: Complement death.PNG.

Room for improvement. Besides critical genes that were "knocked out" and "knocked in" to the donor pig heart prior to transplantation, the recipient patient was also administered medications that helped compensate for reduced immune strength. As for the outcome: the recipient had a positive post-surgery initial response, able to breathe on his own. But eight weeks after the pig sonar heart transplantation, the patient suddenly experienced an acute immune rejection reaction so severe that he did not survive the ordeal. There are many unanswered questions, one of which pertains to the adequacy of the genes selected for CRISPR/Cas9 removal. Clearly, there is ample room for improvement when it comes to CRISPR/Cas9 applications in the clinic.

CRISPR/Cas9 QUARTET (4): ENTERING THE ARENA OF GENE EDITING ETHICS

Patching up roof leaks, filling ceiling cracks, even remodeling the entire kitchen—these are typical home improvement projects that take care of anything above the ground level. Efforts to alter the foundation of the house, however, entail a completely different game plan. The same analogy can apply to CRISPR/Cas9 gene editing: Altering body cells, even stem cells, is akin to home improvement above the ground level. Tinkering with human embryos is wading into unknown, even perilous waters for the simple reason that genes programmed into human embryos represent the very being of the human species. To put it in a different way: Editing human embryonic genes would change the very genetic blueprint that has evolved to be uniquely human because the altered genes would be passed on to future generations. Not surprisingly, at a biomedical conference in Hong Kong, China, in 2018, a speaker shocked the world with a claim of having tinkered with the foundational human blueprint in embryos from an HIV-positive couple.

An outlandish claim. The astounding claim was made by a university professor from southern China: Using CRISPR/Cas9 technology, human embryos were edited to render them HIV-resistant. The two embryos were allowed to grow to full term, leading to the birth of twin girls. Which gene was edited? How does the disappearance of that gene resist HIV infection? Why was the scientific community so outraged?

A quick recap on HIV. The first case of AIDS (acquired immunodeficiency syndrome) was diagnosed in 1981 in New York City. AIDS is caused by HIV (human immunodeficiency virus). HIV preferentially attacks human CD4-T cells by binding to a surface protein complex made up of CD4 + a co-receptor of either "CCR5" or "CXCR4," as illustrated in the following figure adapted from *Clinicalinfo.HIV.org*.

The hook. For successful human T cell infection, a sugar spike protein called HP120 on the HIV viral surface hooks itself onto the human T cell receptor complex of CD4 + CCR5 or CD4 + CXCR4.

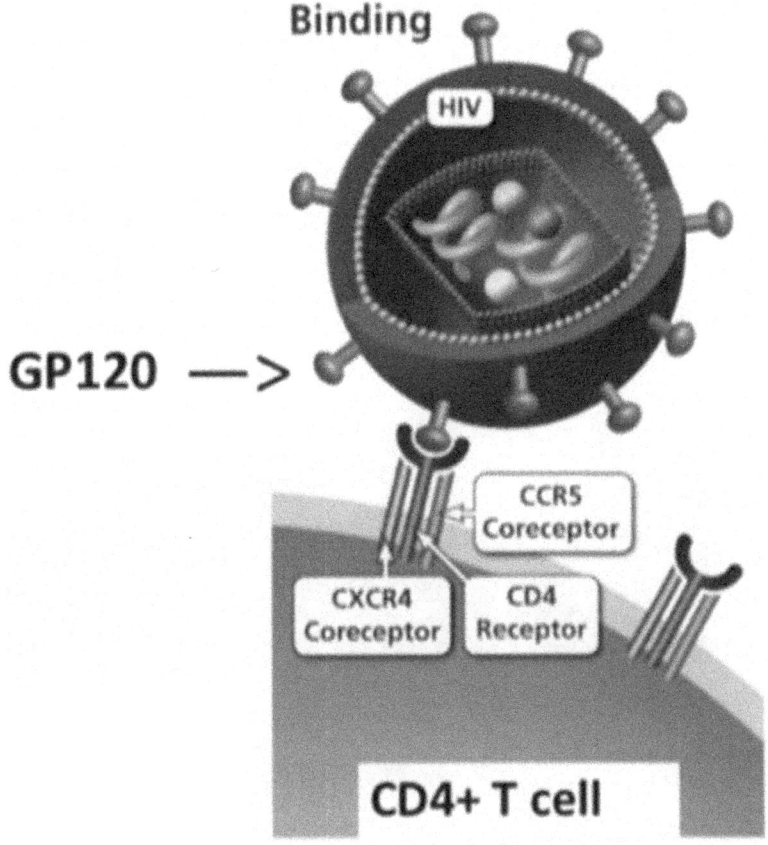

Image 40 HIV bites CD4-T cell. Clinical info.HIV.gov.

This hook allows HIV to enter human CD4-T cells, a step called "internalization." After that, the HIV RNA virus is reverse-transcribed back to DNA, which then gets sneaked into the human DNA. Once incorporated into the human genome (the collection of all genes), the virus hijacks the human protein assembly line to transcribe HIV DNA to HIV RNA, which then gets translated into HIV proteins, also called virions (HIV offspring). The virions then bud off the human host CD4-T cell outer membrane as free HIV agents for rampant next-round infections. The steps are illustrated in the following figure, adapted from Clinicalinfo.HIV.org.

The kill after the bite. After HIV successfully replicated itself by hijacking the human CD4-T machinery, it kills CD4-T cells by triggering the death button. Nearby uninfected CD4-T cells are not spared either by HIV as a result of cell debris from killed CD4-T cells. The debris is replete with toxins potent enough to kill uninfected CD4-T cells due to what is called the "bystander effect." Collectively the direct kill and indirect kill. HIV leads to quick reduction of CD4-T cell count in HIV patients. The normal range of CD4-T cell count in healthy individuals is 500—1,500 cells per microliter (cells/μL, also demarcated as cells/mm^3, pronounced as cells per millimeter cubed). If CD4-T count falls below 200 cells/μL, it indicates that the HIV patient has progressed to AIDS.

The Berlin patient. We have learned by now that successful HIV infection of human CD4-T cells requires two criteria: binding to CD4, the primary receptor, while simultaneously binding to the co-receptor CCR5 or CXCR4, which are distinct molecules. In particular, CCR5 is the entrance through which HIV-1 (one of the two subtypes of HIV) enters. Without a working CCR5 (which can happen

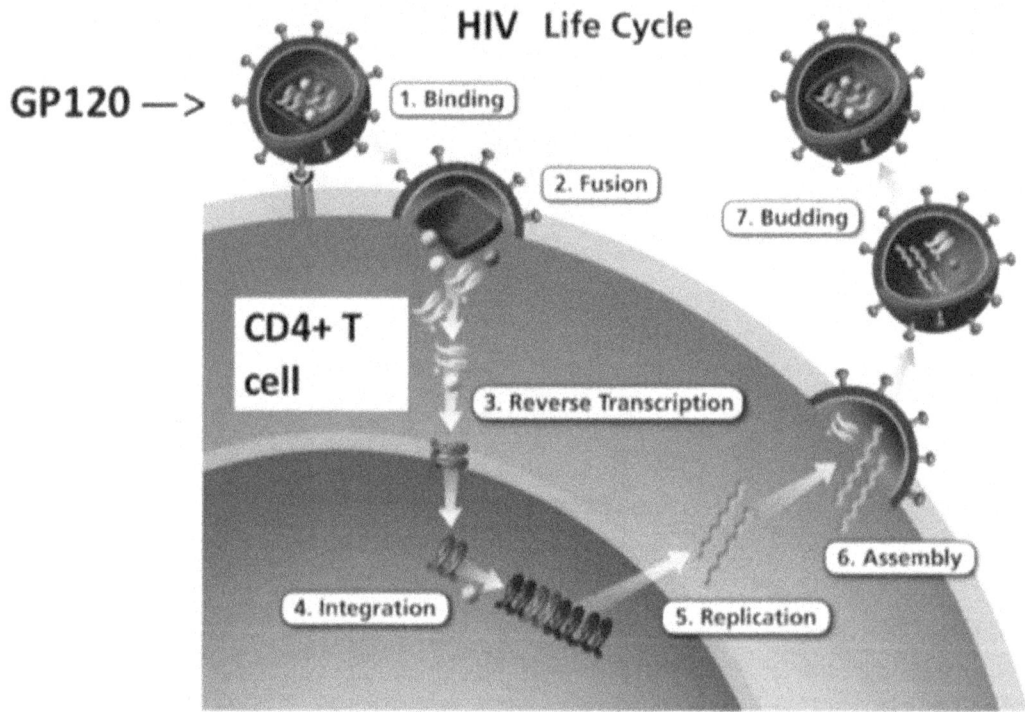

Image 41 HIV life cycle. Clinical info.HIV.gov.

by a naturally-occurring mutation in CCR5), HIV viruses are blocked out of human CD4-T cells. In 2007, an American residing in Berlin, hence the Berlin patient, received a stem cell transplant for the treatment of leukemia. By happenstance, the donor of the stem cells carries a non-functional CCR5. Since the Berlin patient's own bone marrow had to be cleared in order to receive the transplant, all his CD4-T cells that bear functional CD4 + CCR5 were also cleared. An HIV test indicated undetectable HIV viruses. To be sure, the patient was monitored for four years and was still HIV negative. So in 2011, it was announced that the Berlin patient was cured of HIV. A similar story happened in London with the same scenario: the London patient, positive for HIV, was diagnosed with leukemia and needed a stem cell transplant. The donor happened to carry a mutation that makes the CCR5 co-receptor protein dysfunctional. The London patient became the second person cured of HIV. Why not treat all HIV patients with transplantation? According to medical professionals, it is infeasible and the treatment is joy applied to HIV blood cancer patients in need of stem cell transplantation.

Molecular copycat. In an attempt to mimic the naturally occurring *CCR5* mutation, Prof. He, the Chinese scientist from Southern University, used the CRISPR/Cas9 gene editing tool and rendered an artificial mutation to the healthy original wild-type copy of the *CCR5* gene in two human embryos that subsequently gave rise to twins. Due to the claim that only one of the two copies of the *CCR5* gene carries the mutation, the twin girls have a mixture of *CCR5* genes: one is normal and the other is mutational. The very deed of making genetic alterations in human embryos breached the bioethical holy grail and triggered outrage from the international scientific community. A moratorium was initiated by Harvard molecular biology professor Dr. George Church. The moratorium was signed by several dozen leading scientists from all over the world and outright condemned the imprudent and irresponsible act by the rogue scientist. The scientist has since been out on trial and sentenced to three years.

A complex landscape. Is embryonic gene editing prohibited in the United States? The short answer: "It depends." Intriguingly, despite the fact the embryonic or germline editing is officially prohibited in the United States, if one reads the fine print of the guidelines, one would realize that prohibition of embryonic/germline gene editing is only prohibited in research supported by funding from government agencies. At this point, there is NO law that governs against CRISPR/Cas9-mediated gene editing in human embryos sponsored by private funding in the United States. As I was putting the finishing touches on this essay, news arrived that scientists at an American private university CRISPR-edited a faulty gene in human embryos that causes blindness. The research was made possible by a generous grant from a private foundation. There is, however, no plan to allow the edited embryo to grow to full term, according to the university. A responsible decision.

Food for thought:

1. CRISPR-editing embryonic genes (also called germline new) alter the foundational DNA blueprint in humans and are deemed unethical.
    A. True
    B. False

2. In the United States, editing human embryonic genes is strictly prohibited irrespective of finding sources.
    A. True
    B. False

D

DON QUIXOTE MOMENT OF THE IMMUNE SYSTEM

The protagonist in the epic Spanish novel by Miguel de Cervantes, *Don Quixote,* perceived dangers that were nonexistent. Consumed by delusions and steadfast about clearing dangers, *Don Quixote* famously charged at the giant windmills. Nothing was achieved except insanity and destruction.

Our immune system, too, can have its "Don Quixote moment" where immune cells confuse good old self body cells as "foreign" or "alien." The "character" in the immune context is "CD8 Killer T cells." To get to know our immune character, let's recap some basics.

T cell paranoia and autoimmune disorders. For unknown reasons, T cells that successfully passed the bite test can undergo molecular changes that make them mistake healthy self body cells for red flags of danger, with reasons not yet completely clarified. This immune paranoia ends up misguiding KT cells to start a molecular campaign of "slash and burn." The textbook definition of one's own immune cells attacking one's own healthy body cells is "autoimmune disorders." Rheumatoid arthritis (RA), Type I diabetes (T1D), lupus, and thyroiditis are common examples of autoimmune disorders. Nagging symptoms include general weakness, lethargy, pain, and fever. A vivid account of how an autoimmune condition can unmercifully shape one's everyday life is described by accomplished poet and literary editor Meghan O'Rourke in "What's wrong with me?" (https://www.newyorker.com/magazine/2013/08/26/whats-wrong-with-me). One indelible line in Ms. O'Rourke's insightful essay describes living with an energy-robbing autoimmune condition as *"You may always feel like you're 80%,"* that is, 80 percent on tolerable days!

Taming the autoimmune shrew. To clear "perceived enemies," killer T cells utilize a multitude of means, including poking holes in healthy body cells to trigger a form of cell death called "apoptosis." Fortunately, these out-of-control T cells can be tamed with immune suppressant drugs, a leading class of which includes corticosteroids that work by suppressing immune signaling cytokine molecules that promote inflammation. Below is a selective list of cytokines targeted by corticosteroids:

Corticosteroids Suppression Effects

—| Interleukin 1 beta (**IL-1β**): Situated at a critical junction of the inflammatory cascade, IL-1β induces fever and enhances blood vessel permeability (more porous), allowing blood content (such as fluids, proteins, and immune cells) to leak out of circulation to tissues that triggers classic inflammation symptoms of swelling, redness, warmth, even pain. What's more, IL-1β also attracts immune cells to travel near and afar to arrive and exacerbate the state of inflammation. Timely dampening of IL-1β action helps alleviate autoimmune flare ups.

—| Interleukin 4 (**IL-4**). A versatile cytokine, IL-4 drives CD4-T cells to differentiate to become pro-inflammatory Th2 cells in addition to promoting macrophages to develop into an inflam-

mation-prone subtype. Taming IL-4 with corticosteroids helps temper autoimmune episodes.
—| Interleukin 5 (**IL-5**). A specialty cytokine instrumental in enhancing activities of eosinophils, an inflammation-promoting immune cell type from the innate arm of immunity that is the culprit of a type of asthma. Toning down IL-5 tames autoimmune episodes.
—| Interleukin 6 (**IL-6**). Among a string of pro-inflammatory activities, IL-6 plays a pivotal role in the early phase of inflammation by stimulating the liver to secrete several acute-phase proteins, most notably C-Reactive Protein (**CRP**), which is a diagnostic marker of autoimmune conditions. Undoubtedly, striking down IL-6 activities with corticosteroids helps quiet autoimmune flare-ups.
—| Interleukin 8 (**IL-8**). A key cytokine that specializes in dispatching chemical signals to recruit immune cells and molecules, IL-8 is a *bona fide* chemokine that attracts neutrophils, an immune type from the innate arm of immunity. As the most abundant WBC at more than 65 percent, neutrophils are often the first WBC to arrive at sites of inflammation. No question that lessening autoimmune flare-ups with corticosteroids goes a long way.
—| Interleukin 13 (**IL-13**). During inflammation, pro-inflammatory immune cells roll out of blood vessels to migrate to inflammatory tissues. Instrumental to this process are a type of adhesion molecule called VCAM-1 that facilitates immune cells to anchor to blood vessel wall before migrating out of circulation. A designated role of IL-13 is to enhance potency of VCAM-1. Clearly, restraining IL-13 with corticosteroids helps keep autoimmune conditions at bay.
—| Interferon gamma (**INF-γ**). A complex cytokine, INF-γ has been traditionally recognized as a pro-inflammatory molecule, which, when interfered with corticosteroids, helps reduce severity of autoimmune conditions. In more recent years, however, a polar opposite of INF-γ has been observed as an anti-inflammatory cytokine; that is, this molecule is capable of quieting down inflammation flare-ups. To this end, caution ought to be taken when it comes to prescriptions.

Immune suppressant meds do have their double edge in that while helping with our autoimmune flare-ups, long-term use can severely weaken the immune system that renders patients more susceptible to opportunistic infections. Always a good idea to closely follow guidance of the doc.

Like *Don Quixote*, our immune system that goes after imaginary enemy cells ends up not a victor but "beaten and broken." Unlike hopeless *Don Quixote*, autoimmune conditions can be tamed down with meds, despite side effects. Hope AI expedites the process of identifying the genetic or epigenetic cause(s) of autoimmune disorders and sheds light on how to effectively rewire immune paranoid cascading pathways. Keep hopes up!

Food for thought:

1. Autoimmune conditions occur when individual's fighter T cells mistake healthy set cells for dangerous and launch friendly fire.
   A. True
   B. False

2. Prolonged use of corticosteroids or other classes of immune suppressants can lead to a weakened immune system that opens the door for opportunistic infections.
   A. True
   B. False

E

EXISTENTIAL THREAT TO GOOD ORAL BACTERIA BY RADIOTHERAPY

Root canal. Ouch! Cavities, swollen gums, decayed teeth, the list goes on. A sure pain for regular folks, but much worse for cancer patients, especially those who are undergoing radiation treatment for cancers of the head and neck. Special oral care can help. Let's find out how.

Radiation damage. Aiming at rapidly dividing cancer cells, radiation damages cancer cell DNA that results in tumor elimination, deterrence of tumor returning, or considerably slowed tumor growth rate, depending on cancer type, cancer stage, and treatment platform of choice. Radiotherapy can also cause unavoidable damage to normal cells, tissues, bone, and glands of the mouth in patients undergoing treatment for head and neck cancers, particularly oral cancers. Cells that line up the oral cavity are fast-growing, hence the most vulnerable for these patients. Even worse, the damaged cell lining is hard to heal since cells responsible for tissue repair, including immune cells, are also compromised by radiation treatment. At the microscopic level, radiation also upsets the balance of bacteria that reside in the mouth. Let's zero in.

Upsetting bacteria balance. Invited or uninvited, more than 700 different species of bacteria camp out in our mouth. Most of the bacteria that take residence in our mouths are good bacteria that help break down food or keep breath fresh. The bad oral bacteria, on the other hand, normally keep a low profile but seek every chance to come back to wreak oral havoc, the worst of which are painful cavities and nasty gingivitis. Radiation treatment, unfortunately, provides an environment that favors the bad bacteria. How come? Because radiation readily destroys oral enzymes responsible for keeping bad oral bacteria at bay. Lysozymes, for example, are potent antibacterial enzymes that kill bacteria by chewing away bacterial cell wall without which bacteria are unable to hang on to dear life, in a literal sense. Lysozymes are richly endowed in saliva which is produced by salivary glands that drain into the upper mouth, lower mouth, and under the tongue—the three major salivary glands respectively termed the *parotid gland, sublingual gland,* and *submandibular gland.* By damaging salivary glands, radiation zaps them out of commission in secreting saliva, creating an anarchical state for bad bacteria to run rampant. The deleterious effect of the surge of bad oral bacteria that cause oral infections is not confined only to the mouth but can affect the entire body because bad bacteria can easily breach through the already compromised oral lining and enter bloodstream.

Dental care is a must for cancer patients. In light of cancer treatment toxicities on oral health, the National Cancer Institute (NCI) recommends that dentists be an integral part of the cancer care team to monitor patients' oral immune systems along with good oral hygiene protocols *before*, *during*, and *post* cancer treatment. At the top of the dental care list is brushing twice a day with fluoride toothpaste. For patients who are intolerant to toothpaste, NCI recommends mouth rinsing using 0.9 percent saline solution. Chewing sugarless gum to stimulate saliva production is another recommendation.

Professional tips from experts at MSKCC are more specific: in addition to brushing teeth with a soft toothbrush using toothpaste containing fluoride or baking soda plus fluoride and within thirty to forty minutes after each meal. Mouth rinsing after meals is also highly encouraged. Interestingly, instead of using harsh mouth rinsing solutions available in drug stores, MSKCC recommends rinsing with water, although not just any water but *"A mouthwash with no alcohol or sugar, such as Biotene® PBF Oral Rinse or BetaCell™ Oral Rinse."* For a detailed description, please visit https://www.mskcc.org/cancer-care/patient-education/mouth-care-during-your-treatment. Why is sugar singled out in this recommendation?

Sugar, the usual suspect. Sugar sure has a very bad rep in the context of cancer: It fuels cancer's cellular energy production, encourages lactic acid accumulation within tumor micro environment (TME) that hampers immune Killer T cells and promotes activation of cancer-causing genes (***CANCER TRICKS AND TRAPS***, page 25–36). Sugar's bad rep also extends to our mouths. It turns out the sugar or carbohydrates we take from our meals or snacks end up feeding the bacteria in our mouths. Specifically, bacteria break down sugar by a biochemical process called *fermentation* that produces acid which can accumulate to erode enamel and cause cavities! What can counteract sugar remnants? *Fluoride.* It helps ameliorate tooth decay by filling tiny cavities with minerals in addition to interfering with bacterial acid-making processes. Tap water in almost all parts of the United States contains trace amounts of fluoride in light of the very reasoning that fluoride fights tooth cavities. Certain foods enriched with naturally occurring fluoride include tea, coffee, and potatoes. A delicious idea.

Food for thought:

1. Radiation treatment of cancer of the head and neck damages salivary glands in patients, leading to dry mouth which increases risks for oral infection.
    A. True
    B. False

2. Fluoride fills tooth crevices which prevents sugar remnants-associated acids from eroding tooth enamels.
    A. True
    B. False

F

FAMILY TREE OF BLOOD AND BLOOD CANCERS

The stem of a tree is the mother source of nutrients that sustains growth and maintains the very life of the tree. The "stem" in the human body is in the form of "stem cells" born out of the bone marrow, the cradle of all body cells.

Bone marrow is divided into two parts: "red marrow" and "yellow marrow." The red marrow is the source of all blood cells, whereas the yellow marrow takes care of "accessories" such as fat cells, cartilage, and tendons. The marrow of interest for this essay is red marrow.

Red marrow: Treasure trove for all blood cells. By virtue of its name, the red marrow is associated with the red spongy portion of the bone and is organized as a three-tier system.

Tier 1 harbors hematopoietic stem cells (HSC). Quick Word Anatomy: haimato = blood poietikos = to create, hematopoietic = blood-making; hematopoietic stem cells = stem cells that make blood.

Tier 2 consists of two branches: myeloid lineage of blood stem cells and lymphoid lineage of blood stem cells. Each lineage then branch off to the next tier.

Tier 3A is downstream of the myeloid line and contains four categories of cells:

1. *Megakaryocytes* that develop into thrombocytes, also called platelets (that clot/coagulate blood to repair wounds or injury)
2. *Erythrocyte*, also called RBCs (that supplies oxygen)
3. *Mast* cells (that liaison with allergies)
4. *Myeloblast*

Tier 3B is downstream of "lymphoid line" and consists of two types of cells:

1. Large *Natural Killer* (NK) cells
2. Small *lymphocytes*

Tier 4A is an extension to "Tier 3A" Category #4 of "Myeloblast" which further develops into three sub-categories as

1. "*BEN*" (my personal rendition of the acronym for my pre-med biology students) which consists of Basophils, Eosinophils, and Neutrophils;
2. *Monocytes* (that circulate in blood and are related to macrophages);
3. *Macrophages* (which are monocytes but, instead of roaming about in circulation, reside in tissues under the skin, in lungs, liver, or brain).

Tier 4B is an extension to "Tier 3B" Category #2, "Small lymphocytes" which further develop into "T cells" and "B cells." Upon activated in response to infection, both types of lymphocytes are ready to take immune defense action, with B cells becoming plasma cells that make antibody proteins to fight infection and T cells releasing toxic chemicals to bring down enemy cells.

The tree of blood cells from HSC to different sorts of mature blood cells is illustrated in the following figure.

Blood cancers. Harboring mutations that arise from either the lymphoid line (as in T cells, B cells, or plasma cells) or myeloid line (as in eosinophils or macrophages), blood cancers are classified into three types: (1) Leukemia, (2) Lymphoma, and (3) Multiple Myeloma, which can be subdivided into "acute" or "chronic."

Leukemia is a cancer of the blood or toe bone marrow manifested by rapidly proliferating mutant WBC that crowd out RBCs and platelets. Typical symptoms include extreme weakness and fatigue (even after adequate rest), unprovoked bruising or bleeding, unplanned weight loss, and a propensity for infections. Before the advent of T cell-based immunotherapy, chemotherapy or, on occasions, bone marrow transplantation were often first-line treatment choices. A summary of different types and subtypes of leukemias is provided in the following table:

Lymphoma often originates in lymph nodes but can also rise from anywhere in the body where lymph tissues reside, such as gastrointestinal tract. Unlike leukemia, which is "liquid blood cancer," lymphoma is a solid lump that is hard, immobile, and painless. While leukemia spreads from the bone marrow to the bloodstream, lymphoma spreads to the lymphatic system. Unlike leukemia, which can originate from blood cells of both myeloid and lymphoid lineages, lymphoma pertains to mutations in lymphocytes, namely B cells and T cells.

Lymphoma classification consists of "Hodgkin's lymphoma" (HL) and "Non-Hodgkin's lymphoma" (NHL). The hallmark of HL is the presence of *Reed-Sternberg cells* which are very large B cells consisting of a pair of sizable nuclei. NHL has two subtypes: (1) B cell lymphoma and (2) T cell lymphoma. Within B cell lymphoma, *Burkitt lymphoma* poses a considerable challenge

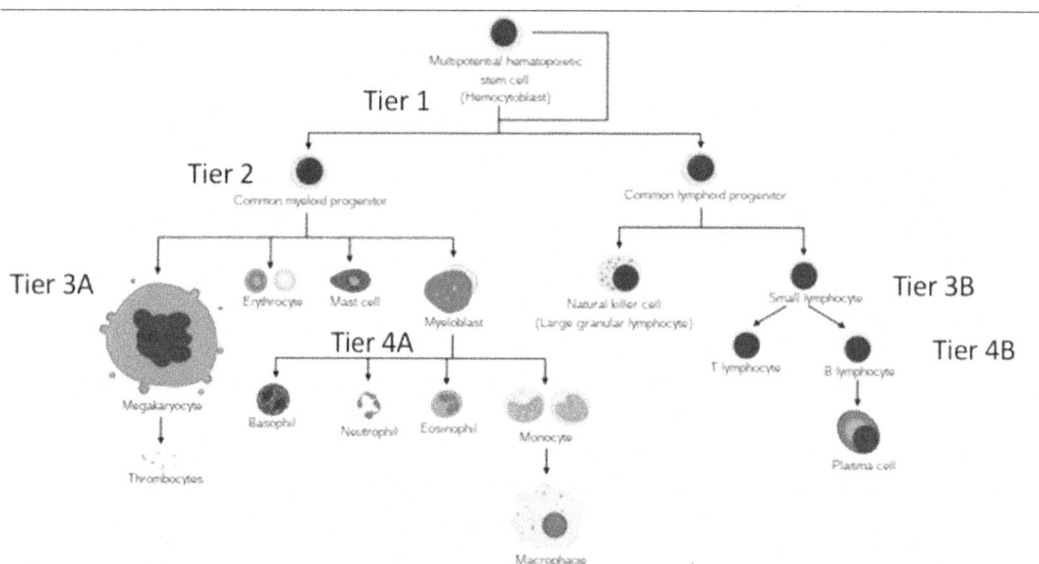

Image 42 Blood cell family tree. Wikimedia Commons File: Hematopoiesis simple.svg.

		Leukemia classification	
		Myeloid	Lymphoid
		Acute Myelogenous Leukemia (AML)	Acute Lymphocytic Leukemia (ALL)
		Chronic Myelogenous Leukemia (CML)	Chronic Lymphocytic Leukemia (CLL)
		Acute promyelocytic leukemia (APL)	
		Chronic Myelomonocytic Leukemia (CMML)	
Myeloproliferative Neoplasms (MPNs)		Chronic eosinophilic leukemia	
		Chronic myelogenous leukemia	
		Chronic neutrophilic leukemia	
		Essential thrombocythemia	
		Primary myelofibrosis	
		Polycythemia vera	

Image 43 Leukemia classification table. Assembled by Dr. Nancy Liu-Sullivan.

		Lymphoma		
	Hodgkin's lymphoma (HL)	Non-Hodgkin's lymphoma (NHL)		
Hallmark	Reed-Sternberg (B) cells	B-cell lymphoma	T-cell lymphoma	
		Large B-cell lymphoma	Adult T-cell lymphoma	
		Follicular B-cell lymphoma		
		Burkett lymphoma		
		Mantle cell lymphoma		
		Marginal zone lymphoma		

Image 44 Lymphoma classification table. Assembled by Dr. Nancy Liu-Sullivan.

for treatment due to the aggressiveness of tumor progression. Lymphoma classification summary is shown in the following table:

Similar to leukemia, symptoms of lymphoma also entail lack of energy, fatigue, weakness, easy bruising and bleeding, and being prone to infection. In terms of treatment, Non-Hodgkin's lymphoma (NHL) is hard to treat as a result of active metastasizing and spreading to lymph nodes in the vicinity of the original lymph node where primary lymphoma occurred. Hodgkin's lymphoma, on the other hand, is highly treatable chiefly due to the indolent nature of the tumor with only occasional or infrequent spread. T cell-based immunotherapy is also now available for the treatment of B cell mutation-derived lymphomas.

Multiple myeloma (MM). As the third type of blood cancer, MM arises in mutated plasma cells which are derived from activated B cells. Normal plasma cells produce antibody proteins to neutralize infectious bugs. Cancerous plasma cells produce a singular kind of antibody protein termed as M proteins that describes that the entire population of cancerous antibodies is from a single mutated B cell. M proteins are non-functional and incapable of playing the role of normal antibodies in assisting other immune cells during immune defense. Symptoms of MM consisted of unexplained fatigue, unprovoked bruising and bleeding, and elevated susceptibility to infection.

Knowing the what and the how. By now, you must have noticed that all three types of blood cancers share common symptomatic manifestations. While it is important to know what it is, it is of equal importance to know why it is. So let's scan through the symptoms and point out the corresponding contributing factors:

- ***Debilitating fatigue and weakness*** results from cancerous blood cells or cancerous antibodies' fast proliferation that takes over space of circulation, crowding our RBCs. In the absence of sufficient RBCs transporting oxygen up and down the human body, physiological functions of cells, tissue, and organs would be compromised, leading to overall weakness and fatigue.
- ***Easy bruising and bleeding*** results from expanding cancerous cells and antibodies overcrowding circulation, leaving limited space for platelets. A lack of timely blood clotting activities leads to bruising and bleeding not associated with physical injury.
- ***Heightened susceptibility to infection*** results from overwhelming numbers of muted Ella and antibodies taking over and squeezing out WBCs instrumental in fighting infections.

CAR-T immunotherapy answers the call. Cancer evades host immune surveillance by disabling immune cells, particularly T cells. Among an array of cancer tricks, keeping T cells in the molecular darkness or turning T cells into bystanders, or a combination of both, often cripples host immune system from putting up a good anti-cancer fight. Scientists strategized innovative ways to make molecular tweaks to patient T cells to revitalize them to be able to fight again. So far, six T cell therapy platforms have received FDA approval. For details, please visit the ***CAR-T THERAPY*** series (pages 48–67).

Food for thought:

1. All of our body cells come from the one marrow.
    A. True
    B. False

2. Blood cancers that harbor mutations in T cells, B cells, or plasma cells lead to leukemias, lymphomas, and multiple myeloma.
    A. True
    B. False

FEVER: TO SUPPRESS IT OR LET IT BE

Fever is no fun. The associated symptoms are even more unbearable. Who needs all the sweating, chills, shivering, headaches, and body aches, not to mention loss of appetite?! Some folks immediately fetch a Tylenol to suppress the fever. Others opt to tough it out. Should we suppress fever or let it run its full course? Let's examine it more closely.

Body temperature control center is in our brain. The normal body temperature is 98.6°F (37°C). A tiny gland in the brain, "hypothalamus" (shown below) is our body temperature sensor that is turned down when body temperature is elevated due to warm weather (*hyperthermia*) to allow our body to sweat to release excess heat. In the case of reduced body temperature (*hypothermia*), the hypothalamus sensor is turned up to retain body heat. The bottom line is to maintain a constant normal body temperature to sustain bodily functions at all levels. The following table summarizes different temperatures in Celsius and Fahrenheit

Fever is a necessary immune defense strategy. Is fever the same phenomenon as hyperthermia? Unequivocally not. Even though both involve elevated body temperature, hyperthermia results from hot weather; by contrast, fever is induced by our immune system in response to invading infectious

Body temperature	Celsius (°C)	Fahrenheit (°F)
Normal	37	98.6
Fever	38	100.4
High fever	39.5	103.1
Very high fever	41	105.8

Image 45 Body temperature and fever table. Assembled by Dr. Nancy Liu-Sullivan.

germs such as bacteria and viruses (collectively called "micro-organisms" because they are minuscule and invisible to the naked eye). The increased body temperature makes it tougher for invading microorganisms to survive. A family of molecules termed "prostaglandins" play chief mediating roles in fever production. Aspirin reduces fever by jamming up activities of prostaglandins. The details are in *ASPIRIN, WEEPING WILLOW, AND CREATIVE CHEMISTRY* (page 18).

Fever is hostile to infectious germs. Quite often, my immunology students ask if inflammation and infection one and the same. The answer is the two concepts are related but distinct. Inflammation is our body's immune cells in action in response to injury (such as a skin cut from stepping onto a broken seashell) or irritation (such as a nasty mosquito bite). Infection, on the other hand, indicates the involvement of infectious bugs (bacteria, viruses, or fungi). Inflammation typically occurs without infection, whereas all infections invariably set off inflammation. Fever is usually a sign of systemic response to infection. Fever creates a hostile living environment for agents of infection because elevated body temperature makes it difficult for bacteria and viruses to replicate. Fevers also speed up the movement of our body's immune cells to sites of infection. The sooner the immune cells arrive on site, the swifter they start releasing toxic chemicals against germs, and the faster battles against germs take action.

Fevers spike in the wee hours. As an added note, fever tends to spike at night as a result of reduced levels of cortisol, the stress hormone. Cortisol counteracts the immune system. So, with cortisol levels dwindling at night, the immune system is free to carry out defense battles against germs without cortisol disruptions. Produced by adrenals that reside on top of the two kidneys, cortisol keeps adrenaline (also produced by the two adrenal glands) action in check to ensure a balanced, homeostatic system.

When to see a doctor. As a mechanism to combat infectious germs, fever kickstarts when needed and subsides when combating mission is accomplished. Hence, the raised body temperature is a temporary phenomenon and typically lasts for three to four days. Prolonged high fevers exceeding a certain level can be harmful. Since this book does not intend to provide any medical advice, for fever and related questions, please consult your physicians. For further reading, please check out the Mayo Clinic recommendations, https://www.mayoclinic.org/diseases-conditions/fever/symptoms-causes/syc-20352759. As an added note, the folklore practice of poking fingertips to let out a small amount of blood as a means of reducing fevers does not carry any scientific basis. On the contrary, bloodletting can be of potential harm in that improper care of the poked fingertip can lead to infection.

Food for thought:

1. Fever helps fight infection because elevated body temperature makes it difficult for infectious agents to survive. Fever also promotes faster blood flow to facilitate speedy arrival of immune cells and pro-inflammatory cytokines to arrive at sites of infection.
    A. True
    B. False

2. Cortisol is an adrenal hormone that calms down heightened immune system activity. Cortisol activities are reduced at night, which explains why fever tends to reduce at night.
    A. True
    B. False

G

GINGER TALK

Ginger, nutmeg, cinnamon, and cloves form the four pillars of Christmas festivity. Gingerbread houses, in particular, have captured the hearts of so many, the young and the young at heart. Pungent with a hint of sweetness, ginger touches upon lots of aspects of our life, holidays and every day.

Ginger is a lauded herbal remedy. A root vegetable that originated in Southeast Asia, ginger has the reputation of being a flavorful spice with versatile and valuable medicinal properties. One property has an ocean connection. High winds in the high seas are a recipe for mighty waves, as vividly depicted in *Orphans of the Storm* and the BBC masterpiece *Brideshead Revisited*. The poor fellows on the transatlantic vessel succumbed to seasickness, their stomachs churning upside down, their guts wrenched. Well, ginger can rescue!

One small study reported prescribing 1 gram of ginger extract to a squad of naval cadets and found the remedy to be effective at preempting seasickness. Here, a mechanistic study alludes to ginger's anti-nauseant effect as a result of its capacity to break up intestinal gas, which acts as a form of intestinal disturbance. By reducing gas, ginger calms the digestive system and ameliorates nausea. That makes sense. Of course, additional and large-scale studies are needed. Ginger is also believed to alleviate nausea from chemotherapy as a short-term use. The operative phrase is "short-term use." As a general wise rule of thumb, the use of natural medicinal products and supplements that include ginger is best consulted with one's family physician.

Ginger's anti-inflammation properties. Ginger is said to contain salicylic acid (SA), the key ingredient in willow bark that tames inflammation. SA interferes with the making of a powerful family of inflammation molecules called "prostaglandins" that give us the sensation of pain. By eliminating this particular chemical, pain is eased and discomfort subsides. More on SA is discussed in *ASPIRIN, WEEPING WILLOW, AND CREATIVE CHEMISTRY* (page 18).

Ginger tames overactive immune cells. A recent study explored how ginger affects a major squadron of immune foot soldiers—"neutrophils," a major type of disease-fighting WBC abundantly found in our bodies. Among many strategies deployed by neutrophils against germs, one involves setting up a snare. As shown below, the trap pins bacteria down to facilitate elimination. Since the traps are set in the vicinity of neutrophils, these traps are called "Neutrophil Extra-Cellular Traps" or NETs. Now, NETs are essential in getting rid of unwanted bacteria, but prolonged NET activity can harm normal cells. So, it is important to make sure that neutrophil-mediated NET traps are regulated so as to avoid self harm.

Along this very line, the scientists who studied the effect of ginger on neutrophils made a surprise discovery. It turns out that ginger can effectively tame excess "Trap" activities exerted by neutrophils when they become overzealous in their germ-combating actions.

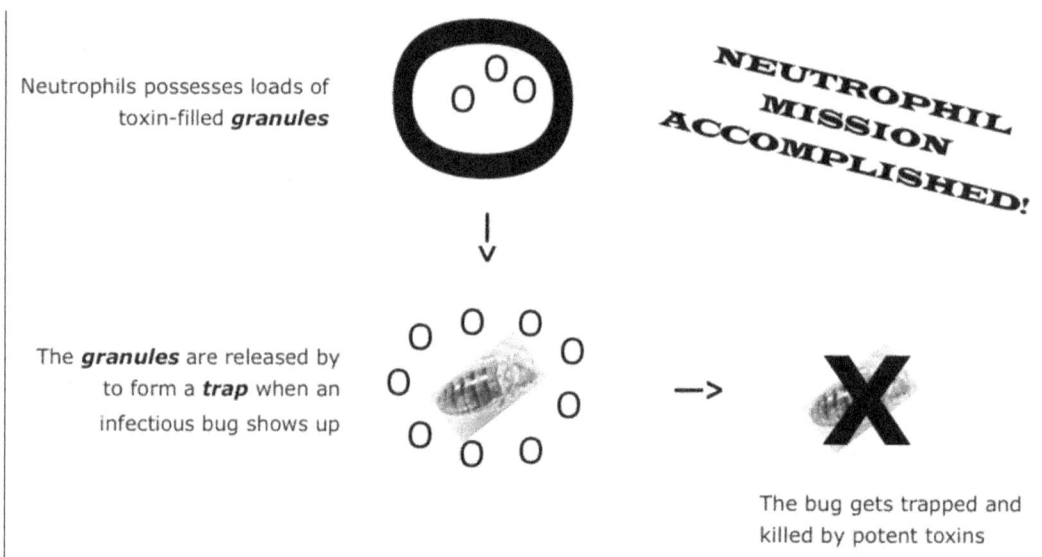

Image 46 Neutrophil immune traps. Assembled by Dr. Nancy Liu-Sullivan and combined with Wikimedia Commons File: Bed bug. Cimex lectularius.jpg.

Important to note that ginger supplements (as all medicinal food-derived supplements) contain much more concentrated key ingredients than the fresh ginger thin slices on Sashimi plates or the ginger sauce for potstickers. Hence, another gentle reminder to *always* consult your physician, however *ad nauseam* it may sound, and no pun intended.

Food for thought:

1. Ginger's anti-seasick properties come from its ability to relieve intestinal gas.
   A. True
   B. False

2. A recent discovery reveals ginger capable of calming down anti-germ activities by neutrophils which are from the myeloid lineage of hHSC.
   A. True
   B. False

H

HOUSTON, WE HAVE A PROBLEM!

Here is an unimaginable dilemma confronting a woman just diagnosed with breast cancer:

- **Choice A:** Lumpectomy—$3,750 to $9,722
- **Choice B:** Mastectomy—$13,000 + ($5,000—$15,000 per breast for reconstruction surgery)

Battle #1: Peer-to-peer appeals. Money is a means to an end or should be. The meaningful end for medical prescriptions is optimal treatment for the patient. Yet, the reality can be utterly cruel in that instead of a straightforward best medical treatment-based decision making by physicians and their patients, the decision can be dictated by restraining insurance company "policies" which can outrightly reject certain medical procedures out of monetary considerations.

Of course, to reject an expensive medical procedure purely on monetary grounds would send the insurance company to court. Hence, "medical necessity" becomes synonymous for "ground of rejection." Physicians who are trained to always look after patients' best health interests, irrespective of patient background—being wealthy or poor, educated or not being, ethnicity majority or minority. This sense of mission has prompted the practice of "peer-to-peer appeals," in which doctors reason, on behalf of the welfare of their patients, the need for certain, very often expensive, medical procedures. I wonder if forging battles to plead to insurance companies over rejected prescriptions is a required medical school training course! Likely, physicians learn on the job to strategize efficient courses of action against the maze of bureaucracies.

Battle #2: Out-of-pocket cost. In parallel to insurance coverage approval, cancer patients have an additional worry: How to pay out-of-pocket treatment costs? This could be a gross exaggeration, but most common folk households in America live from paycheck to paycheck. Who would ever imagine the need to set aside funds to cover exorbitant out-of-pocket expenses while battling the indescribable fear of a shocking diagnosis, not to mention concerns over job situations and a sense of guilt for having inflicted emotional tolls on the family?!

Duke University published a thought-provoking reality-check investigational study on medical costs and associated financial burdens weighed on breast cancer patients. The researchers presented very interesting findings obtained from an electronic survey study of 706 women over the age of eighteen who were diagnosed with breast cancer at different stages. Of these patients, 95 percent had medical insurance, 78 percent had received higher education, and 56 percent with more than $74,000 annual household income. All patients received surgical procedures ranging from breast-conserving surgery (43 percent), bilateral mastectomy (32 percent), to unilateral mastectomy (25 percent). The authors concluded that more than 1/3 of the patients (35 percent) experienced treatment-associated financial burdens. As we can easily imagine, not all medical costs are covered by insurance companies, not to mention co-pays. Below is a brief summary of out-of-pocket costs in four types of cancers based on a report provided by the US National Cancer Institute (NCI), under the National Institute of Health (NIH):

National Cancer Institute (NCI) 2019 data	
Cancer type	Patient out-of-pocket costs
Breast cancer	$3.14 billion
Prostate cancer	$2.26 billion
Colorectal cancer	$1.46 billion
Lung cancer	$1.35 billion

Image 47 Cancer out-of-pocket costs. Assembled by Dr. Nancy Liu-Sullivan.

CAR-T	Price	Pharma	Country
Tecartus	$533,500	Gilead/Kite	USA
Abecma	$524,833	BMS/Juno	USA
Carvykti	$504,300	Legend Biotech/Janssen	China
Kymriah	$475,000	Novartis	Switzerland
Yescartus	$424,000	Gilead/Kite	USA
Breyanzi	$410,300	BMS/Juno	USA

Image 48 CAR-T cost by country. Assembled by Dr. Nancy Liu-Sullivan.

The above table also reflects the prevalence of cancer in the United States, with breast cancer and prostate cancer continuing to be number one and the first runner-up. In light of cases of colon cancer among young people on the rise in recent years, it would be useful to find out how increased CRC incidence would shape the patient out-of-pocket map.

The table below is a summary of cancer immunotherapy, whose efficacy has taken blood cancer treatment by storm but also associated with a huge financial catch. The six CAR-T therapies approved by the FDA for the treatment of leukemia, lymphoma, and MM each marked with a hefty price tag. For patients whose tumors underwent CR after the therapy, the living drug based on engineered patients' own immune T cells is worth every penny. Still, a more patient-friendly price would allow access for more patients. Fortunately, CAR-T is covered by Medicare and Medicaid but only in select states. Private health insurance plans are a different story: many do provide coverage, but some completely reject it. A coordinated plan for cost reduction in CAR-T production and more sensible insurance coverage is in order and a tall one.

On a related topic, not all CAR-T therapies are created equal when it comes to price. Take "Yescarta" that treats multiple myeloma; for example, the international price range can carry quite a gap, as shown in the following table:

Allow me to add another thought-provoking table, which does not mean beyond what the table entails:

Shown above is the 2022 revenue data table that I assembled for our readers for ease of getting the full picture. "Impressively profitable" is the likely reaction. That said, pharmaceutical companies

CAR-T Yescarta comparative prices	
Country	**Price**
United States	$424,000
Canada	$358,000
France	$354,000
United Kingdom	$350,000
Germany	$306,000
Japan	$212,000
China	$188,000

Image 49 CAR-T Yescarta cost by country. Assembled by Dr. Nancy Liu-Sullivan.

BIG PHARMA IMMUNOTHERAPY REVENUE (2022)				
Checkpoint inhibitors	Keytruda	$20.9 billion	Merck	USA
	Opdivo	$8.2 billion	BMS	USA
	Tecentriq	$3.9 billion	Novartis	Switzerland
	Imfinzi	$2.8 billion	AZ	UK
	Yervoy	$2.1 billion	BMS	USA
	Libtayo	$448 million	Regeneron	USA
	Bavencio	$277 million	Pfizer	USA
CAR-T	Yescartus	$1.16 billion	Gilead/Kite	USA
	Abecma	$699 million	BMS/Juno	USA
	Kymriah	$536 million	Novartis	Switzerland
	Breyanzi	$182 million	BMS/Juno	USA
	Yecartus	$82 million	Gilead/Kite	USA
	Carvykti	$55 million	Legend Biotech	China

Image 50 Big pharma 2022 revenue. Assembled by Dr. Nancy Liu-Sullivan.

do have a bottom line to consider. They also support industry/academic collaborative projects, one of which I worked once as a lead scientist for a drug discovery endeavor that involved leading research universities including Harvard Medical School, Lawrence Berkeley National Laboratory, and Oxford University. All of the above said, a reasonable, happy median should be worked out to benefit patients more while sustaining company bottom line. Where there is a will, a way shouldn't be too far in the distance. Federal agencies can play instrumental roles.

Early detection holds the key. Back to the Duke study, the authors also drew another very important conclusion: costs patients must pay beyond insurance coverage are the lowest in cancers discovered at early stages when the tumor is confined within the primary tumor site without intruding into healthy cells, tissues, or organs nearby or distant—termed as "carcinoma *in-situ*." Yet another reason for routine screening in addition to leading a healthy lifestyle, especially for folks with a cancer family history. Preventive measures against cancer are discussed in the series of **RISK REDUCTION OF CANCER PENTALOGY** (page 166–176).

Food for thought:

1. Cancer care cost burden remains an elephant in the room.
    A. True
    B. False

2. Early detection and timely treatment continue to hold the key for patient welfare and for cost reduction.
    A. True
    B. False

I

IMAGINE! FRED'S TEAM, JOEY'S WINGS, BAILEY'S WARRIORS, AND EMILY WHITEHEAD FOUNDATION

"Think of giving not as a duty, but as a privilege." American entrepreneur and philanthropist, Mr. John D. Rockefeller, Jr. not only coined the very line but also lived by it. Extending a helping hand to the needy is a privilege, indeed, especially when it comes to raising funds for cancer research. This essay is dedicated to the brave cancer fighters and their kind supporters.

Fred's Team. The team was initiated by New York Road Runners, and the New York City (NYC) Marathon debuted in September 1970. Of the 127 registered runners, fewer than half made it to the finish line. Over subsequent decades, the NYC Marathon has expanded substantially in both participating runners and the extended route. The race in 1992 was indelible when a cancer patient in remission touched the finish line with an impressive record. The special runner was Fred Lebow, an avid runner, co-founder of the NYC Marathon, and a brave individual who had been undergoing brain cancer treatment at MSKCC. Thrilled by his cancer remission and determined to return the blessings, Fred encouraged participating runners to run with a glorious goal in mind: raising funds to support cancer research that is taking place 24/7/365 at MSKCC for nearly two centuries. Sadly, Fred's cancer relapsed, and he passed away in 1994. *Fred's Team* was organized in his memory the following year after Fred's passing, and runners continue to run to this day for a noble cause.

Joey's Wings. Gainesville, Florida, 2013. A precocious teenager named Joey Xu was diagnosed with a rare form of childhood kidney cancer known as "translocation renal cell carcinoma." Physicians exhausted all possible treatments but were unable to save Joey. Carried by the powerful wings of a legendary paper crane which symbolizes felicity and harmony in ancient Chinese culture, Joey bid farewell to his loving family the following year. *Joey's Wings*, a charity group, was established with the mission of raising awareness of childhood kidney cancers. In collaboration with MD Anderson Cancer Center headquartered in Houston, Texas, Joey's Wings has been coordinating efforts toward a tumor DNA sequencing database with the hope of shedding an edifying light for a more in-depth understanding of rare kidney cancers, with the goal of arriving at a cure one day!

Bailey's Worriers. Eight years old is a sweet age, having been a few years in formal schooling, proud to have mastered all twenty-six alphabetical letters, able to count up to 100 in math, after-school soccer or softball, piano or violin lessons—a thousand exciting ventures to explore and discover! Life, however, can be capricious and unpredictable. At the age of eight, Bailey was diagnosed with an extremely rare form of cancer of the skeletal muscle tissues called "rhabdomyosarcoma." At the time of the diagnosis, Bailey's cancer was already at a late stage. In fond memories, Bailey's mom recollects how Bailey fought a brave battle blessed with courage, grace, and a precious sense of humor, so much so that Bailey defied the odds of poor prognostics, lived to celebrate her ninth birthday, and carried on until one month shy of her tenth birthday. Today, through MSKCC's CYCLE FOR SURVIVAL campaign, Bailey's fight continues to shine an inspiring light on patients, physicians, and scientists.

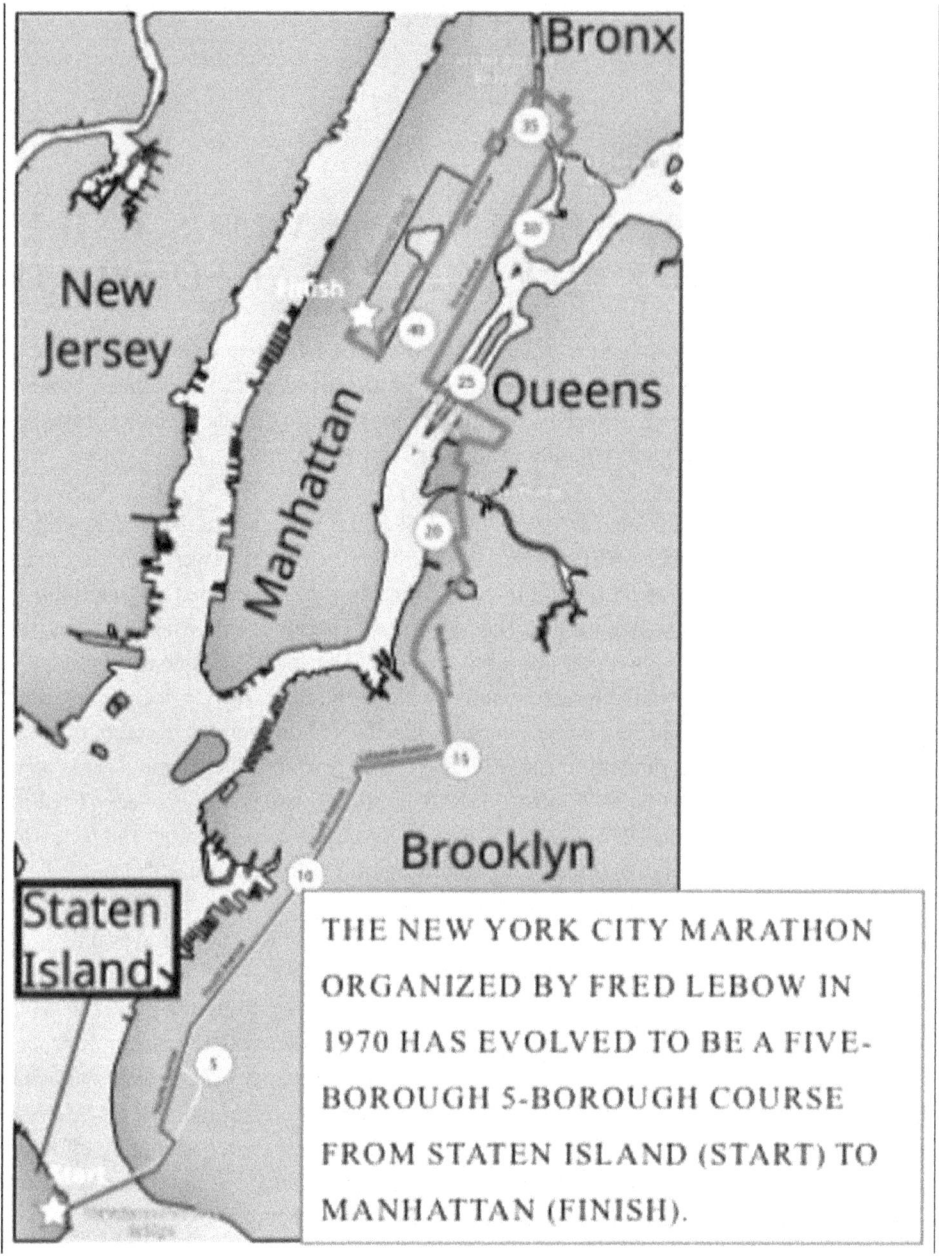

Image 51 New York marathon map. Wikimedia Commons File: Map of the ING New York City Marathon 2013.svg.

I joined many others in making an immediate donation to *Bailey's Warriors* after reading the heart-touching account by Bailey's mom. I completed this essay on September 4, 2024. The following day, literally less than twenty-four hours later, an article appeared in the journal Nature that described a major breakthrough discovery in "rhabdoid tumor" (different but related to "rhabdomyosarcoma"). Fasten your seatbelt for a molecular ride: as a hereditary genetic mutation, a defective protein called ***SmarCB1*** is crucial in organizing the formation of a protein complex dubbed "**Switch**" and "**Sniff**"

(SWI/SNF). Due to the genetic defect, the SWI/SNF complex is suppressed to dormancy, enabling an open season for tumor growth. For years, it had been a guessing game in how to wake up SWI/SNF until a consortium of scientists from St. Jude Children's Research Hospital, Memphis, Tennessee, and Harvard Dana-Farber Cancer Institute, Boston, Massachusetts, found the molecular "caffeine" to jazz up SWI/SNF. The name of the gene is, interestingly and by pure phonetic coincidence, ***DCAF5***. In a nutshell, when *DCAF5* is removed, SWI/SNF is liberated and swiftly swings back to action in swiping cancer cells in a clean yank! Of course, this observation has only been made in the laboratory at the moment. Translating the discovery into the real world of rhabdoid tumor patients is only a matter of time. Also, due to the relatedness of rhabdoid tumors to rhabdomyosarcoma that took Bailey away, discovery in rhabdoid may shed light on research for rhabdomyosarcoma.

Emily Whitehead Foundation. On the frontlines of the battle against cancer, some fought but had fallen, others fought and came through. The next story is about Emily Whitehead. At the age of five, Emily was diagnosed with an acute form of childhood leukemia. Despite treatment, Emily's cancer kept returning. Having tested all standard treatment regimens, the physicians literally ran out of options and gingerly hinted to Emily's parents ideas for hospice. Refusing to give up, Emily's parents kept searching. In 2012, two years after Emily's initial diagnosis, Emily and her parents found Children's Hospital of Philadelphia (CHOP). The right place at the right time. An ongoing experimental clinical trial was recruiting volunteer patients next door at the University of Pennsylvania School of Medicine. A brand new cancer therapy that leverages patients' own immune fighting T cells to fight their own cancer cells. Emily became the first pediatric patient for the trial. After an entire month including overcoming a severe case of cytokine storms, Emily became cancer-free and has remained free for more than a decade. The experimental drug developed by team Carl June received FDA approval in 2017 and has since saved many more lives. For a detailed description, please refer to ***CAR-T THERAPY (2): A PHILADELPHIA STORY*** (page 51).

Imagine! John Lennon envisioned a pristine world with only blue skies. Imagine a world without cancer—not necessarily a world without cancer *incidence* since our cells do tend to divide imperfectly, particularly as we age, but to imagine a world with powerful vaccines that preempt cancer, with sensitive tools that detect cancer early, and with robust personalized therapeutics that unleash immune prowess to cure or keep cancer at bay—Actually part of our imagination has already come true, exemplified by the UK success story of cervical cancer prevention through vaccines against HPV infections. Combating cancer takes a village. Just imagine!

"-*ITIS*" AND INFLAMMATION

A revered Harvard professor once remarked on his esteemed colleagues so engrossed in their narcissistic academic dwellings that they were suffering from "*Harvard-itis*." In good humor, of course; tongue in cheek over a martini dinner, most likely. Don't get me wrong. Harvard continues to be a scholastic beacon. My very first translation assignment took place on the hallowed Harvard campus.

"*-itis*" **in a medical context.** It is a suffix that describes a medical condition of inflammation. To name a few examples:

- Bronchitis → inflammation of the windpipes or bronchi.
- Colitis → inflamed guts.
- Dermatitis → inflamed skin.
- Meningitis → inflamed shielding membrane of the brain and the spinal cord.
- Rhinitis → inflamed nasal membrane.

Of course, a different contributing factor is associated with each form of "-itis," ranging from physical injuries to allergens and bacterial/viral infections.

Immune in active defense mode. Inflammation is a sure sign that our immune system is working hard to remove unwanted substances from our body. A splinter, a paper cut, even a mosquito bite all trigger an inflammatory response in the injured area with the cardinal manifestations of turning red, getting swollen, feeling warm, and sensing pain. Our immune first responders arrive at sites of injury to put up a formidable fight. Immune cells at defense forefronts are typically neutrophils, macrophages, and dendritic cells.

Immune cells also secrete powerful molecules that further enhance inflammation. One such molecule—interleukin-1 (IL-1)—is responsible for fever. Hence, IL-1 is also a pyrogen defined as a fever-causing substance. Other molecules, such as prostaglandins that signal aches and pains, are also released by immune cells that serve to inflame the inflammatory response. We discussed the function of aspirin in suppressing prostaglandins and alleviating pain (see *ASPIRIN, WEEPING WILLOW, AND CREATIVE CHEMISTRY,* page 18). There are also growth factors, molecules that promote cell growth, found at sites of inflammation to help repair and rebuild damaged tissues. Inflammation can be classified into two categories, shown below:

Acute inflammation is typically caused by cuts, allergens (substances that trigger an allergic reaction such as peanuts, shellfish, pet dander, and pollen), chemical irritants (such as detergent, coal tar, tobacco smoking, alcohol, and food additives), and, believe it or not, emotional stress. The classic symptoms of acute inflammation are characterized by redness, warmth, swelling, pain, and temporary loss of function of the inflamed area. Acute inflammation typically lasts no more than three days.

Sub-acute inflammation is sandwiched between acute and chronic inflammation. If the acute inflammation does not clear after three days and lasts anywhere from two to six weeks, it is called "sub-acute inflammation." Sub-acute inflammation is the transition from acute to chronic inflammation.

Chronic inflammation. If sub-acute inflammation persists beyond 6 weeks, it then enters the territory of "chronic inflammation." Chronic inflammation occurs when the causative agent of acute inflammation (such as infectious bacteria or viruses) fails to be eliminated after 6 weeks. Chronic conditions can persist for months, several years, even decades. Hepatitis B and Hepatitis C, for example, each starts as an acute form of liver inflammation and often can deteriorate to "chronic hepatitis B" or "chronic hepatitis C." Both forms of chronic hepatitis are known to develop into liver cancer, although the transformation can take up to several decades.

Food for thought:

1. Acute inflammation typically lasts for three days.
    A. True
    B. False

2. Chronic inflammation usually results from acute inflammation and sub-acute inflammation that fails to clear beyond six weeks and can linger for years, even decades.
    A. True
    B. False

	ACUTE INFLAMMATION INFECTION	CHRONIC INFLAMMATION
CAUSAL FACTORS	Physical injuries (cuts or burns), Microbial infections (viral or bacterial)	Long-term exposure to irritants (tobacco), Prolonged illnesses, Autoimmune conditions
CLINICAL MANIFESTATIONS	Localized redness, swelling, pain, warmth/heat	Systemic effects involving persistent pain, prolonged fatigue, frequent infections
ONSET	Rapid/sudden	Gradual
DURATION	Short term (days — weeks)	Long term (months — years — decades)

Image 52 Acute vs. chronic infection. Assembled by Dr. Nancy Liu-Sullivan.

J

JAMES ALLISON: AN INDEFATIGABLE TRAVELER

Growing up in Alice, Texas, James developed an incredible sense of curiosity. Not satisfied with the mere *What*, he always dug deeper to explore the *Why*. That intellectual curiosity followed his entire research career path from Alice, Texas, to Berkeley, California, to Manhattan, New York, then in full circle back to his home state of Texas, over the span of close to half a century, accompanied James the undergraduate to Dr. James Allison holding a PhD in biology to Director Allison, the immunology expert with a laser-sharp focus on a type of fighter immune cells called T lymphocytes.

October 1, 2018, an ordinary day turned indelible: Dr. Alison received a surprise long-distance telephone call from Sweden that he and Dr. Tasuku Honjo had been awarded the 2018 Nobel Prize in Physiology or Medicine. What's more remarkable is that this was the very first Nobel Prize granted for therapeutic accomplishments in cancer. The therapy that aims at harnessing patients' inner immune power to combat cancer has demonstrated a game changer in cancer treatment.

It all started with curiosity over why confronting cancer cells, the host T cells act as if they are in a state of malaise. What is stopping the T cell engine from charging forward? Dr. Allison was determined to search until all possible stones were turned. Dedication, inspiration, and lots of perspiration led to the discovery of a molecular "wedge" on cancer cells that jam the locomotives on the T cell machinery. The "wedge" is designated as *CTLA-4,* which stands for "cytotoxic T-lymphocyte associated protein 4," also known as "CD152." Without intervention, CTLA-4 on immune T cells is bound by another protein on a different type of immune cell called "B7." This binding bogs down T cells and renders them immobilized. Elucidating this intricate mechanism of action by Dr. Allison laid the foundation for producing an antibody drug that "jumps" in front of B7 to occupy the binding pocket on CTLA-4 to jam it up. Jammed-up CTLA-4 leaves no room for B7 to bind, hence freeing up T cells to tackle cancer cells. The experimental drug was first tested at MSKCC. The unexpected result awed everyone. Here is what happened:

Ipi, the miracle drug! In 2006, a small investigator-initiated clinical trial was organized by Dr. Jedd Wolchok, a leading expert in cancer immunotherapy at MSKCC. The patient diagnosed with late-stage melanoma had very bleak prospects in prognostics. As a last resort, Dr. Alison's anti-CTLA-4 antibody drug was tested on the patient. A miracle happened! The drug enabled elite trooper Killer T (KT) cells in the patient to be liberated to fight back cancer cells. At the end of a series of immune battles, the patient experienced complete tumor remission. Dr. Alison has kept personal communications with the cancer-free patient over the years. One day, a piece of mail addressed to Dr. Alison arrived. Inside the mail was a photo of the recovered patient's first child. A second piece of mail followed a few years later announcing the arrival of the second child. Tears streamed down Dr. Alison's cheeks as he recalled the occasions. The miracle drug is *Ipilimumab*, abbreviated as "Ipi" with the trade name of Yervoy and received approval from the FDA in 2011. The same drug also worked wonders for our former President Jimmy Carter, whose severe melanoma had metastasized to the brain but was reverted by Ipi.

Today, like any day, is a routine day of work for Dr. James Allison, except for a new hat: as the executive director of the Immunotherapy Platform at MD Anderson in Houston, Texas, he leads a group of dedicated scientists to chart new waters in cancer immunotherapy.

JILL O'DONNELL-TORMEY: THE CHOICE THAT MADE A TRANSFORMATIONAL DIFFERENCE

Two roads diverged in the field of cancer research: To remain a bench investigator or to shine a resplendent beacon on new terrains of cancer therapy? Having chosen the latter, Dr. Jill O'Donnell-Tormey has made all the difference.

Captain with a mission. A native of Staten Island, the "Borough of Parks" of New York City, precocious Jill attended Notre Dame Academy, an elite local school that instills in its pupils an ardent passion for knowledge and an honorable mission for life. Guided by both principles, Jill excelled in science, graduated with honors in chemistry from Fairleigh Dickinson University, New Jersey, and pursued doctoral studies at the State University of New York (SUNY) Downstate Medical School, Brooklyn, New York. The strong passion and sense of mission to pursue knowledge to save lives continued to propel Dr. Jill O'Donnell-Tormey forward, first at Rockefeller University and then at Cornell University Medical Center. By happenstance, Dr. O'Donnell-Tormey noticed a recruitment post by the famed CRI. Established by Dr. Helen Coley Naut, the daughter of Dr. William Coley, the founding father of cancer immunotherapy, CRI is the very first research institute in the world dedicated solely to exploring novel immune-powered cancer treatment platforms. Dr. O'Donnell-Tormey echoed! The rest of the story is well known: Dr. O'Donnell-Tormey became CRI's Public Relations Officer, and six years of excellence later, she was entrusted to helm the entire CRI flagship for the following four plus decades.

Remarkable fruition. Forty years of able leadership with utmost dedication and impeccable vision, trips to Washington, DC, meetings with the nation's lawmakers, reviewing research grant applications, and dedicating educational essays to readers at large about the brilliance of cancer immunotherapy—a magnificent trail of fruition tells tall orders and taller tales instrumental in translating basic research discoveries into life-saving meds by cancer patients' bedside. The summary below is a microcosm of the enormity of leadership by CRI in cancer immunotherapy research:

The scientists awarded for their endeavors in cutting-edge cancer immunotherapy research represent the best, the brightest, and the hardest-working in the field of cancer translational studies. It also serves as a scientific gauge of how leading cancer centers all over the world have steadily shifted resources and talent to exploring new paths of unleashing immune power to annihilate cancer! Of note, awardees associated with Harvard University, Harvard Medical School, and Harvard-affiliated hospitals and research institutes are grouped together under Harvard University. The three research programs supported annually by the Cancer Research Institute, led by Dr. Jill O'Donnell-Tormey, include (1) Technology Impact Award, (2) Lloyd J. Old Star Program, and (3) Clinical Innovator. For detailed descriptions of projects and scientists, please visit https://www.cancerresearch.org/cri-funded-scientists. Among the three programs, the Lloyd J Old Star awards scientists who engage in "high-risk, high-reward" cutting-edge cancer immunotherapy projects. The 2024 class consists of five innovative scientists from Australia, Israel, and the United States, each awarded "$1.25 million over five years." Information about their respective exciting projects can be found at https://www.cancerresearch.org/media-room/2024/cancer-research-institute-announces-new-lloyd-j-old-stars-class.

CRI-FUNDED CANCER IMMUNOTHERAPY PROJECTS	
UNIVERSITIES/RESEARCH INSTITUTES	# PROJECTS
Harvard University/Harvard Medical School/Dana Faber Cancer Institute/Brigham & Women's Hospital/Massachusetts General Hospital/Boston Children's Hospital	28
Memorial Sloan Kettering Cancer Center	14
Icahn School of Medicine Mount Sinai	7
MD Anderson	6
University of Pennsylvania/Abramson Cancer Center	6
Yale University	6
Stanford University	5
University of Washington	5
Moffitt Cancer Center	4
The Rockefeller University	4
Columbia University Medical Center	3
Duke University	3
Emory University	3
John's Hopkins University School of Medicine	3
New York University Medical Center	3
Salk Institute for Biological Studies	3
University of Minnesota	3
University of Pittsburgh School of Medicine	3
Washington University School of Medicine	3
Weill Cornell Medicine	3
Baylor College of Medicine	2
Oregon Health and Science University	2
The University of Texas Southwestern Medical Center	2
University Health Network (Canada)	2
University of California, San Diego	2
University of Wisconsin-Madison	2
Vancouver Cancer Centre	2
Weizmann Institute of Science (Israel)	2
Albert Einstein College of Medicine	1
Cancer Research Institute-Irvington	1
Centre Leon BERARD (France)	1
Champalimaud Foundation (Portugal)	1
Fondazione Humanitas per la Ricerca	1
Fred Hutchinson Cancer Research Center	1
Fundacio Institute D'investigacio Biomedica de Bellvitga L'Hospitalet del Llobregat	1
Georgetown University	1
Hefei Comprehensive National Science Center (China)	1
Huashan Hospital Fudan University (China)	1
Institut Curie (France)	1
La Jolla Institute for Immunology	1
Leiden University Medical Center (Netherlands)	1
Ludwig Institute for Cancer Research/University of Lausanne	1
Lund University (Sweden)	1
Massachusetts Institute of Technology	1
National Cancer Institute	1
National Institute of Allergy and Infectious Diseases, NIH	1
Northwestern University	1

Image 53 CRI-funded projects, I. https://www.cancerresearch.org/cri-funded-scientists tabulated by Nancy Liu-Sullivan.

CRI-FUNDED CANCER IMMUNOTHERAPY PROJECTS (Continued)	
UNIVERSITIES/RESEARCH INSTITUTES	# PROJECTS
Odette Cancer Centre Health Sciences Centre	1
Sage Bionetworks & Institute for Systems Biology	1
St. Vincent Hospital Applied Medical Research Institute	1
The J. David Gladstone Institutes	1
The Scripps Research Institute	1
University College London	1
University Hospital of Lausanne, Switzerland	1
University of Alabama at Birmingham	1
University of Calgary (Canada)	1
University of California, Berkeley	1
University of California, Los Angeles	1
University of Chicago	1
University of Colorado at Boulder	1
University of Connecticut	1
University of Massachusetts Medical School	1,
University of Oxford	1
University of Virginia Health System	1
University of Western Australia (Australia)	1
Vita-Salute San Raffaele University	1
TOTAL # CRI-FUNDED CANCER IMMUNOTHERAPY PROJRCTS = 165	

Image 54 CRI-funded projects, II. https://www.cancerresearch.org/cri-funded-scientists tabulated by Nancy Liu-Sullivan.

Granddaughter of a milkman, daughter of a construction worker and a homemaker, excelling as the first-generation college graduate, doctoral researcher, and President and CEO of CRI in charge of $400+ million research operations and, most importantly, offering visionary guidance on unearthing new paths and strategizing novel platforms that strive to mobilize patients' inner immune power to combat cancer, Dr. O'Donnell-Tormey is an indefatigable living legend of the timeless American success story. Hats off to Dr. Jill O'Donnell-Tormey!

K

KATALIN KARIKÓ: LOST FUNDING, GOT CANCER, BUT BEAT BOTH

She left her home country Hungary in 1985 for the United States to continue her pursuit of molecular biology. Constant worrying about lab funding and health scares is a vivid depiction of the constant downs of her life then. Yet, she remained unwaveringly focused on her treasured research project and used it as a great buffer against life's vicissitudes. Today, she is standing tall to receive the coveted 2023 Nobel Prize in Physiology or Medicine.

From Budapest to Philadelphia. Her name is Katelin Karikó. Some three plus decades ago, Dr. Karikó, a PhD scientist from Budapest, Hungary, arrived in the United States to expand the horizons of her research endeavors. At the University of Pennsylvania (UPenn), she became a "contract" scientist, meaning that as long as she continued to secure grants to support her research, she would be allowed to continue to have a lab on campus. At a critical juncture in her research journey, she failed at grant renewal and was told either to pack up and go or stay but at a demoted post with less pay. When it rains, it pours: As if losing a critical grant wasn't crushing enough, Dr. Karikó was also informed of a cancer diagnosis. A doubly cruel trouble fell on the same person at the same time! Well, how Dr. Karikó prevailed redefined the adage that reads, "You are the only one that can change your fate."

Undeterred by the setbacks, Dr. Karikó started a "lobbying" campaign to see which top lab at UPenn was willing to "adopt" her to continue to pursue her mRNA research. Dr. Drew Weissman, a physician-scientist, was immediately drawn to the idea of applying mRNA technology to medicine. The two scientists began to work collaboratively on overcoming mRNA bottlenecks.

A cold welcome! The ultimate aim of the joint project was to turn mRNA into a molecular dispatcher to distribute reagents or meds as needed to the human body. A quick recap: mRNA is the centerpiece of the central dogma coined by Dr. Francis Crick, who co-discovered the double-helical structure of DNA with Dr. James D. Watson. The dogma: DNA is transcribed to mRNA and mRNA gets translated into a long chain of amino acids called "polypeptides," followed by elegant three-dimensional folding into a protein. In short: **DNA → mRNA → Protein**.

Since mRNA is a bridge that propagates DNA to protein, to introduce any protein of interest, just present the mRNA to the body and the cell's protein machinery will process the mRNA into the target protein. It sounds like a straightforward step, but the reality turned out to be extremely complicated. Three major molecular "brouhahas" emerged between the external mRNA and the hawkish host immune surveillance system:

1. The mRNA is unstable and ephemeral, with a very short shelf life.
2. The mRNA triggers an immune response acute enough to kill the messenger.
3. The mRNA-associated immune response can deteriorate to a molecular gale termed "cytokine storm," manifested by immune "slash and burn," as described in the ***DON QUIXOTE MOMENT OF THE IMMUNE SYSTEM*** (page 87).

Clearly, these mRNA self-defeating caveats must be corrected in order to make the technology viable. After several years of many long hours of conducting experiments, confronting abject failures, and going back to the drawing board, there was finally light of hope at the end of the dark and dank tunnel: The two scientists identified the crux of the mRNA problem concerning mRNA building blocks called "bases," as described below.

Molecular "make-over" did the trick! As shown in the following figure, the naturally occurring building blocks of RNA consist of two complementary pairs of "G—C" and "A—U," where G = guanine; C = cytosine; A = adenine; U = uracil. Like salt and pepper, G is always paired with C and A with U, as shown in the following table:

Substituting "U" with "Ψ." Can't beat you, get around you. This was exactly what the dynamic research duo of Dr. Karikó and Dr. Weiss strategized. Instead of beating up on stubborn "U" (Uracil) that caused all the problems when mRNA was released into the human body, the two scientists brainstormed and settled on the idea of a Ψ (pronounced as *sigh*) modification, and it worked! The modified Ψ (that replaced U) renders mRNA stable, invites no cytokine storms, and is also nicely tolerated by our hawkish immune system with no fuss. Bingo! A *sigh* was finally let out.

mRNA technology applies to life-saving vaccines. Thus far, Ψ-modified mRNA technology has transformed biomedical science, as exemplified by Covid-19 mRNA vaccines and mRNA therapeutic cancer vaccines as described in ***CANCER VACCINES (6): IMMUNE WRITING STENTORIAN FROM THE MESSENGER.*** (page 46). Deservedly, Dr. Karikó and Dr. Weissman stood high as the co-laureates for the 2023 Nobel Prize for Physiology or Medicine. And as the role portrayed by Queen Latifah in *The Last Holiday*, the cancer diagnosis in Dr. Karikó also turned out to be a medical error. Today, Dr. Karikó has returned to her *alma mater* university in Hungary, teaching, mentoring, and conducting experiments to tackle more biomedical questions.

	BUILDING BLOCKS		STABILITY
DNA	A—T	G—C	Stable
mRNA	U—A	C—G	Very unstable
Modified mRNA	Ψ—A	C—G	Improved stability

Image 55 RNA modified. Assembled by Dr. Nancy Liu-Sullivan.

L

LES TROIS PIONEERS OF MODERN CANCER IMMUNOTHERAPY (1): MICHEL SADELAIN

Having completed medical school at the University of Paris, Dr. Michel Sadelain moved to Canada to pursue doctoral studies followed by postdoctoral research at the Massachusetts Institute of Technology (MIT). In 1994, Dr. Michel Sadelain, MD/PhD, became the leader of a research laboratory at the MSKCC. Three decades of unwavering dedication to uncharted terrains in cancer immunotherapy have carved out a meaningful life-saving path for patients.

First-Generation CAR-T: Brilliant but ephemeral. As Dr. Sadelain kick-started introducing genes to T cells using a viral carrier on the East Coast of the United States, first at MIT (1992) then at MSKCC (1994), a group headed by Dr. Zelig Eshhar at the Weizmann Institute of Israel was working on engineering T cells with part of an antibody molecule—a CAR. In 1993, the Eshhar group unraveled the alpha product of CAR-decorated T cells that aimed to kill cancer cells. This first-generation CAR-T model worked but lamentably lacked durability; that is, the engineered T cells failed to last in cancer patients long enough and powerful enough to unleash T cells' formidable 1–2 punch to wipe out cancer cells. This first-generation CAR-T was appropriately equipped with CD3z, the T cell activator, but was apparently inadequate. What was missing?

CD28 co-pilot to turbocharge CAR-T! Formidable fighters against unwanted cells in the host body, T cell activation is a carefully choreographed platform where a triple set of signaling must all be in shipshape for T cell launching. These include (1) Primary signaling (T cell receptor recognizes enemy antigen displayed on HLA), (2) Secondary signaling (also called co-stimulators, which consist of several candidates), and (3) Tertiary signaling (the involvement of immune signaling molecules called cytokines). Why has T cell evolved to be under such draconian regulation when it comes to T cell activation? The answer is to make sure that T cells are *exclusively* activated in response to stimulus from non-self cell antigens to prevent accidental or random T cell activation and action against self body cells—conditions collectively called autoimmune diseases.

Upon careful examination of the T cell landscape and lots of rounds of experimentation and returning to the drawing board, team Sadelain selected CD28 as the CAR-T booster. *And* it worked like a charm! The action by CD28 greatly turbocharged CAR-T with sustainable power while also boosting secretion of cytokines which promote CAR-T cell proliferation and expansion. This milestone accomplishment fundamentally placed CAR-T on the right path to success. Still, there was something else missing: How to ensure that the powerful and long-lasting CAR-T drives toward the desired cancer cells for destruction?

CD19: A GPS that guides CAR-T to leukemia with precision! To escape immune attack, one cunning cancer trick is to conceal its surface "antigens" or HLA designated to display the cancer antigen to keep T cells in the dark. Indeed, as Dr. Sadelain poignantly points out that cancer cells are poor antigen presentation entities. Can we cut to the chase and install a *GPS* on CAR-T to guide it directly and unmistakably to cancer cells?! Would it be possible to get around this cancer trick?! The

GPS imagination then is the CAR-T reality now: four of the six CAR-T drugs approved by the FDA carry the CD19 molecular GPS that targets particular types of leukemia and lymphoma.

What's so special about CD19? It turns out CD19 is a universal ID antigen on all B lymphocytes (or simply B cells). By *all,* we mean cancerous B cells as well as normal B cells. CD19-guided CAR-T kills a lot of cancerous B cells than normal cells because of the sheer fact that cancerous B cells proliferate multiple orders of magnitude faster than normal B cells. You might ask: If a patient's normal B cells are also wiped out by CD19-CAR-T, wouldn't it also deprive those patients of any chance of producing their own antibodies since antibodies are made by plasma cells that differentiate from activated B cells? Fair question. And the answer is affirmative. However, science has figured out a way to help CD19-CAR-T recipients acquire precious antibodies. For details, please refer to *CAR-T THERAPY (2): A PHILADELPHIA STORY* (page 51). Since the inspiring light has shone onto CAR-T by CD19, additional molecular GPS apparatuses have been visited, one of which is a reality in the clinics, manifested by the two MM-targeting CAR-T drugs approved also by the FDA. Several work-in-progress GPS candidates are in the making for solid cancerous tumor types.

Three decades ago, molecular tinkering with T cells was met with a polite but cold welcome by the immunology circle. Now, thirty years later, after a long and circuitous journey through many troughs, everyone is a convert to CAR-T. The two engineering marvels innovated by Dr. Sadelain—CD28 and CD19—have instilled sharp cancer target recognition and durability power, as manifested on the clinical scoreboard: upto 50 percent of blood cancer patients undergoing CAR-T treatment have experienced complete or partial tumor remission. Word has it that Dr. Sadelain has moved to Columbia University Medical Center (CUMC) to lead the cancer research center. CUMC's gain!

LES TROIS PIONEERS OF MODERN CANCER IMMUNOTHERAPY (2): CARL JUNE

A proud graduate of the US Naval Academy, Annapolis, Maryland, followed by vigorous training at Baylor College of Medicine, Houston, Texas, and subsequent extended stints at the World Health Organization (WHO) headquarters in Geneva, Switzerland, at Fred Hutchinson Cancer Center, Seattle, Washington, at the US National Naval Medical Center in Bethesda, Maryland, then back to Bethesda, Maryland, until joining the faculty at the University of Pennsylvania School of Medicine, Philadelphia, Pennsylvania, in 1999. Drawing on an eclectic array of research expertise, Dr. June has made milestones in bringing laboratory findings to the cancer patients' bedside.

Survival tales of Bill and Doug. Leukemia brought them together, and both were fortunate to have been accepted into the clinical trial of experimental CAR-T therapy led by Dr. Carl June. Immune T cells were drawn from Bill and Doug, respectively, engineered in the laboratory with intricately designed gene constructs that guide T cells to leukemia cells, followed by returning the special T cells back to the bodies of Bill and Doug. A single dose of this CAR-T managed to annihilate leukemia cells in one swift scoop: both patients had complete remission; that is, their leukemia cells were all gone! This milestone event took place in 2010. Bill was the first-ever adult patient in the CAR-T clinical trial, and Doug was the first runner-up. Both remained cancer-free post-treatment. Bill had a severe case of Covid-19 infection and passed away in 2021. Doug is still cancer-free according to the University of Pennsylvania School of Medicine newsletter in 2022 and continues to devote his time, heart, and mind to funding and raising cancer awareness.

The story of Emily. Also under the care of Dr. Carl June, Emily became the first pediatric patient in a CAR-T clinical trial. The treatment was successful, and Emily has been leukemia-free since 2012 when she was a six-year-old. For a more detailed story of Emily, please refer to *CAR-T THERAPY (2): A PHILADELPHIA STORY* (page 51). As for which prototype of CAR-T approved by the FDA saved Emily's life, the answer is Kymriah—the very first CAR-T granted the green light by the FDA in 2017, five years after the successful clinical trial initiated by Dr. Carl June at UPenn School of Medicine in 2012. This second-generation CAR-T was designed to be equipped with a T cell enhancer different from the one designed by Dr. Michel Sadelain, which is whipped with CD28. Dr. June elected to enhance the prototype of Kymriah with another enhancer termed 4-1BB (also called CD137) with equally robust enhancing capacity to ensure sustainability as well as T cell expansion. On an important note, the use of 4-1BB for CAR-T was the result of joint efforts by research groups at St. Jude Children's Research Hospital (Memphis, TN), UPenn School of Medicine/Children's Hospital of Philadelphia (Philadelphia, PA), Moffitt Cancer Center (Tampa, FL), and the National Institutes of Health (NIH, Bethesda, MD). It takes a village!

LES TROIS PIONEERS OF MODERN CANCER IMMUNOTHERAPY (3): STEVEN A. ROSENBERG

Growing up in the Bronx, NY, in the dark shadows of the deaths of relatives in concentration camps in Poland, young Steven cemented the ideal of using medicine to heal and comfort. Two decades later, Steven became a physician-scientist and began service at the National Cancer Institute (NCI, Bethesda, MD)—the fruition of the National Cancer Act in 1937 (as shown in the following Image).

Image 56 National Cancer Institute, NCI. Wikimedia Commons File: National Cancer Institute logo.svg.

This year, 2025, the NCI celebrates its eighty-eighth birthday, and Dr. Steven A. Rosenberg celebrates his eighty-fifth year of humility as he soldiers on as NCI Chief of the Surgery Branch while continuing to ponder over the profound yet at once befuddling question that has prompted him to devote his entire research career: How exactly is cancer shaped by the immune system?

Some tumors cryptically self-clear. It all began at a Harvard Medical School affiliated hospital where Dr. Rosenberg worked as a resident. Reviewing the chart of a patient suffering from an acute gallbladder case, Dr. Rosenberg noticed a stomach cancer diagnosis made twelve years ago, and no other treatment procedures were administered to the patient except for a failed attempt to surgically remove the metastasized tumor. Twelve years later, the patient was back at the hospital with an acute case of gallbladder attack in need of surgery. To everyone's surprise, no tumors were present. The patient had somehow mysteriously undergone an apparent spontaneous tumor remission! Even though there had been prior literature describing similar events, for Dr. Rosenberg, nothing is as powerful as witnessing a real case in front of his very eyes as an attending physician!

Seizing the forest through telltale trees. If the first patient case described above sparked a hunch, the subsequent second patient case served up an ample dose of evidence of an intimate connection between cancer and the host immune system for Dr. Rosenberg. Here is what happened. A patient received a kidney transplant and was put on standard suppressant drugs to prevent the recipient's immune system from rejecting the donor kidney. Unexpectedly, the kidney recipient started manifesting full-blown metastatic cancer and was taken off immune suppressants. Where did cancer come from? It turned out that the donor kidney had a speck of a cancerous nodule likely so microscopic that it was overlooked by the transplant team. What transpired next stunned everyone: after the removal of drugs that tamed the immune system, the patient's immune system rejected both the donor kidney and all cancer cells! Another case of spontaneous cancer clearance in front of the very eyes of Dr. Rosenberg! No chemo, no radiotherapy, no surgery. The simple act of liberating the patient's own immune system did the trick. The role of the immune system played a decisive role here, in no uncertain terms. How did the immune system drive the spontaneous disappearance of all cancer cells? Dr. Rosenberg spent the next fifty years decoding that enigma, making milestone discoveries, and most meaningfully, translating them into patient care and saving lives.

Patient #67. As immune elite troopers, Killer T (KT) cells are at the forefront against unwanted cells, including cancer cells. Like a high jump athlete who relies on a flexible pole to assist jumping over the bar, KT cells too need assistance in growth and expansion from a cytokine molecule called "interleukin 2" (IL-2). Dr. Rosenberg had an epiphany: Why not infuse cancer patients with IL-2 to add more steam to KT?! Wasting no time, Dr. Rosenberg initiated an experimental trial. A total of 283 volunteer patients diagnosed with treatment-resistant melanoma and kidney cancers visited Dr. Rosenberg's trial clinic to receive "high-dose IL-2 therapy" followed by meticulous post-treatment observations on the effect of IL-2 on patients' cancerous tumors. Patient #1, #2, #3, . . . #66, showed unremarkable effects. Next was the turn of Patient #67, Ms. Linda Taylor, and the effect was remarkable: IL-2 therapy led to the complete disappearance of Ms. Taylor's melanoma, the most aggressive form of skin cancer. Ms. Taylor is the very first melanoma patient who has shown high sensitivity to Dr. Rosenberg's innovative IL-2 therapy that made her hard-to-tackle melanoma disappear. The indelible moment was captured in a photo of Ms. Taylor side by side with Dr. Rosenberg, who saved her life (https://nihrecord.nih.gov/2023/10/13/rosenberg-s-research-spans-half-century-and-counting).

By the time the seven-year (1985–1992) clinical trial had completed, eighteen additional cancer patients joined Ms. Taylor in achieving CR, that is, all cancer cells disappeared as a result of IL-2 treatment. More importantly, the majority of the nineteen patients' cancer remissions were sustained for multiple years, which indicates durability of the IL-2 therapy. This line of therapy received FDA approval in 1992 for the treatment of metastatic kidney cancer and in 1998 for the treatment of metastatic melanoma. In both circumstances, IL-2 serves to boost cancer patients' immune systems to combat cancer cells.

New grounds to tackle melanoma. Another milestone in cancer immunotherapy developed by Dr. Rosenberg involves taking advantage of immune cells that have migrated to the tumor village, or "tumor micro environment" (TME), but instead of acting like fighters, these cells are found to be cancer onlookers. The mechanistic details of this phenomenon are described in ***CANCER TRICKS AND TRAPS (3): THRIVING IN LOW OXYGEN*** (page 28). In parallel to developing IL-2 therapy, Dr. Rosenberg also ventured into "tumor-infiltrating lymphocytes" (TIL) that aimed to re-energize immune cells that have entered the TME. The intricate experimental steps are as follows:

Step 1: Tumor tissues are surgically removed from which immune cells (TILs) are extracted.
Step 2: To increase cell population, the TIL cells are grown in the laboratory in the presence of IL-2 to boost T cell expansion (up to 15 billion cells!)
Step 3: The prepared TIL cells are frozen down to maintain stability and stored until use at the patient's bedside.
Step 4: Prior to TIL therapy administration, the cancer patient receives medication to deplete "regulatory T cells" (Tregs) to prevent them from weakening TIL.
Step 5: Upon completion of depleting Tregs using chemotherapy drugs, the patient is all set for a two-week treatment regimen in which TIL cells are thawed and fused back to the patient intravenously.

LET THEM EAT CAKE: ON CANCER CARE DISPARITY

"Qu'ils mangent de la brioche!" was supposedly exclaimed by an eighteenth-century French princess when poor peasants were unable to afford bread for their families. It is said that brioche, a gourmet pastry, would be even more out of reach for the destitute! Embedded in the senseless utterance was a hopelessly troubling gap between the rich and the poor. Sadly, now, some three hundred years later, societal disparity remains a thorny issue in many walks of life, particularly in cancer care. Delightfully, a guiding national policy to ameliorate the gaps is underway as overviewed below.

Scope and measures. Defined as "differences in cancer measures" by the National Cancer Institute (NCI), cancer disparities pertain to the following measures:

The gaps. The data table below speaks softly of very loud lines of evidence of cancer care-associated cancer inequitable outcomes. Despite progress made, inequities persist in several types of cancers associated with various groups of Americans, including African Americans, Hispanic Americans, American Indians, and Pacific Islanders. As for contributing factors, the NCI study cited a range of components that shape cancer disparity outcomes as stand-alone factors or, most plausibly as combinatorial factors.

CANCER DISPARITY MEASURES	
MEASURES	NOTES
Incidence	Newly diagnosed cases
Prevalence	All existing cases
Mortality	Cancer deaths
Survival	Length survived after diagnosis
Survivorship	Quality of life after cancer treatment
Morbidity	Medical complications associated with cancer
Financial burden of cancer	Cost expenditures on cancer treatment and related medical conditions
Screening rates	Percentage of cancer screening
Stage of diagnosis	Stage of cancer at the time of diagnosis
Adapted from http://www.cancer.gov/about-cancer/understanding/disparities	

Image 57 Cancer disparity measures table. Tabulated by Nancy Liu-Sullivan based on http://www.cancer.gov/about-cancer/understanding/disparities

CANCER DISPARITY MANIFESTATIONS			
CANCER TYPES	GROUP/REGION AFFECTED	DISPARITY MEASURE	CONTRIBUTING FACTORS
Cancers in general	African American	Cancer mortality	• Low incomes • Low health literary • Inadequate accesibiiity to screening. • Lack of access to treatment facilities • Lack of of health insurance • Lack of paid medical leave • Harsh living environment such as lack of clean water or exposure to carcinogens • poor diet • Obesity • Chronic stress
Breast cancer	African American Women	Cancer mortality	
Prostate cancer	African American Men	Cancer mortality	
Colorectal, lung, & cervical cancers	Rural Appalachia	Cancer incidence	
Colorectal cancer	Less educated Americans	Premature cancer death (before 65)	
Kidney cancer	American Indianans	Cancer mortality	
Cervical cancer	Hispanic, African American, & American Indian Women	Cancer incidence	
Cancer risks from smoking & alcohol	LGB youths	Cancer risks	
Liver cancer & intrahepatic bile duct cancer	American Indians followed by Hispanics, Asians/Pacific Islanders	Cancer incidence & mortality	
Adapted from http://www.cancer.gov/about-cancer/understanding/disparities			

Image 58 Cancer disparity manifestations table. Tabulated by Nancy Liu-Sullivan based on http://www.cancer.gov/about-cancer/understanding/disparities

A vision to change. The comprehensive NCI cancer disparity report serves as an informative roadmap for the missions of the various councils and work groups. Good to see that the National Cancer Institute (NCI) has established an Equity Council and Working Groups to address the high-need issues. Various task force committees have been set up to focus on multiple dimensional aspects, particularly on inequities in cancer risk factor education, cancer screenings, and clinical trial participation.

My two cents with all sincerity. It is not at all my place to say, but immediate efforts can be carried out to address some of the immediate gaps such as

- *Dispatching "Cancer Screening Across America Caravans" to rural and remote regions;*
- *Building online cancer consultation service stations to allow folks from all corners and walks of life to get opinions from oncologists at world-class cancer centers;*

- *Providing tuition free medical education to those willing to serve rural/remote areas upon obtaining medical license;*
- *Providing on-the-job training fellowship opportunities for rural/remote hospital physicians to shadow oncologists from NCI-designated cancer centers;*
- *Supporting liaisons between cancer patients and suitable clinical trials. More on this: The NCI does offer guided steps (*https://www.cancer.gov/research/participate/clinical-trials-search/steps*); however, it would be more rational for professionals who are conversant with how to best match patients with the most suitable clinical trials to devote their expertise on the matter;*
- *Allocating $$$ to help ease hardships of long-distance transportation to folks from underprivileged areas for access to cancer radiation treatment with heightened precision and reduced side effects such as "proton beam therapy." HEIC leads to our next topic below.*

Radiation: Photon versus Proton. As a major pillar of cancer treatment, radiation therapy works by knocking cancer DNA out of whack to kill cancer cells. But not all radiotherapy platforms are created equal. Conventional cancer radiation therapy delivers to tumor site powerful X-rays, also called **photon beam therapy**. X-ray photon beams are generated by a powerful machine called "linear particle accelerator" (LINAC). How powerful are the X-ray beams from LINAC? Powerful enough to break tumor DNA and destroy tumor cells. There is, however, a major drawback: The energy scatters and damages healthy cells in the vicinity of the tumor. What's more, the X-ray also travels through the body to exit at the other side, meaning that all healthy cells along the X-ray path become collateral molecular damage. Is there a source of radiotherapy that is more focused on cancer targets while sparing healthy cells? Yes, the answer is ***Proton*** **beam therapy**. In contrast to "photon" particles which carry zero mass, "proton" particles do carry mass and are quite heavy, with the advantage of precisely targeting tumor tissues with 60 percent less damage to healthy tissues compared to X-ray radiotherapy. The reduced damage stems from the fact that once hitting the designated target, proton beam deposits all its high energy in the tumor *without* exiting, hence sparing healthy tissues along the would-be exit path. Another advantage of proton beam therapy is its capacity to access tumors located in inoperable locations, such as soft-tissue sarcomas and pediatric brain cancers. For the latter, proton beam therapy can best help preserve healthy brain tissues of the developing brain. Despite unparalleled advantages over conventional X-ray beam machines for cancer radiotherapy, proton beam therapy technology does have a catch: a very dear price to set up, to operate, and to maintain, as shown in the following table:

Shown above, linear particle accelerators (LINAC) offer conventional X-ray therapy (at considerably high doses and frequencies compared to X-ray diagnostic imaging such as chest X-rays or mammograms) at a steep price of more than one million dollars, but only a fraction compared to cyclotron centers that generate proton beams: more than $200 million per center! Shown below is the Proton Beam Center at Mayo Clinic, Rochester, MN.

Currently, there are forty-five proton beam centers in the United States, and six new ones are under construction. That said, the center locations appear to be concentrated in the southeastern and northeastern regions, based on information provided by the National Association for Proton Therapy (https://proton-therapy.org/findacenter/). To put this in a worldwide perspective, the United States has 45+, Japan 12, Germany 6, China 5, France 3, and the United Kingdom 2.

Less toxic IMRT. Back to the United States, necessity is the mother of invention—a tried-and-true formula that also applies here. Radiation experts at MSKCC developed an innovative platform to maximally reduce regulator radiotherapy toxicity while enhancing cancer-killing efficacy. The

LET THEM EAT CAKE: ON CANCER CARE DISPARITY

RADIATION TREATMENT MACHINES IN US		
Machine type	Utility	Cost
LINEAR accelerator	X ray radiotherapy	$750,000 - $1.5 million
Cyclotrons	Proton beam therapy	$200 million+

Image 59 Radiation treatment machines in the United States table. Assembled by Dr. Nancy Liu-Sullivan.

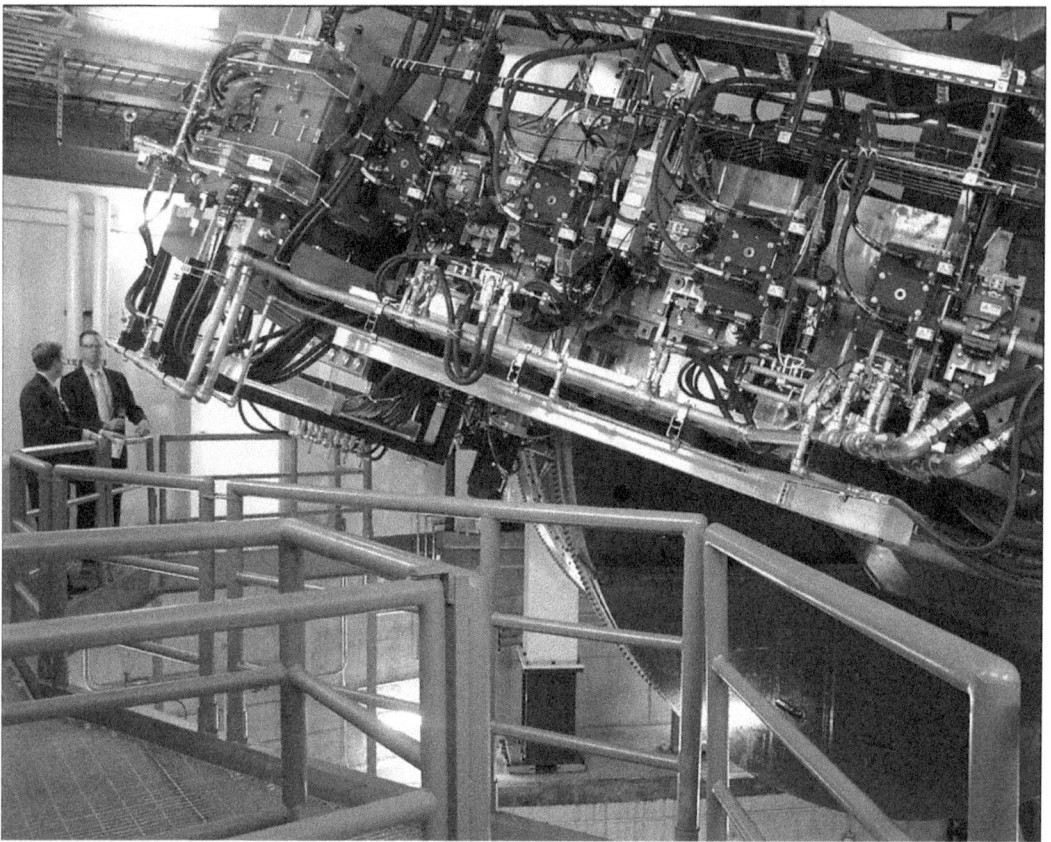

Image 60 Proton beam centers, Mayo Clinic. Wikipedia Commons File: MayoProton.jpg.

procedure is called led IMRT or Intensity-Modulated Radiation Therapy in which the tumor of interest is demarcated in three-dimensions (3-D) using a CT (computed tomography) scan. This allows radiotherapy rays to be delivered to the tumor from multiple angles using higher doses (but in smaller beams of multiples and in different shapes mapped to the tumor contours). The sharper precision that pinpoints the tumor helps avoid healthy tissues and organs in the vicinity of the tumor. The radiation beams used in IMRT are generated by photon beams from LINAC machines. Of course, the high-energy photon beams must exit the patient's body, which unavoidably causes damage to healthy tissues in the exit path. Well, IMRT is not perfect but leaves considerably less damage when compared to conventional high-energy photon beam treatment. That said, until proton beam therapy becomes more widely available, IMRT offers a good alternative to conventional photon beam therapy for cancer patients. For details of MAKCC IMRT, please visit https://www.mskcc.org/cancer-care/diagnosis-treatment/cancer-treatments/radiation-therapy/what-imrt

Food for thought:

1. Proton beam therapy does less damage to patient's normal tissues due to its direct focus on the tumor without exiting the patient's body, unlike conventional high-energy X-ray photon beam therapy that tends to scatter around the tumor and exit the patient's body on the other side, leaving a trail of normal tissue destruction.
   A. True
   B. False

2. IMRT stands for intensity-modulated radiation therapy. By mapping the tumor contour using computer topology, this therapy is capable of directing the high-energy photon radiation path to the tumor contour using multiple smaller beams, hence minimizing radiation scattering to normal tissues surrounding the tumor.
   A. True
   B. False

LURKING CARCINOGENS IN CIABATTA AND RYE

I ventured into amateur bread-making a few years ago. My first try failed miserably. The bread turned out to be a shapeless, mushy mess. Something was missing in the mix. It turned out to be potassium bromate.

What gives texture in bread? Let's rewind a bit and talk about flour. Flour turns into a tough mass after kneading with water. That is the result of adjacent molecules of gluten, a type of protein, forming bridges to create a tangled network. These bridges consist of two sulfur atoms and their formation requires a process known as "oxidation." The slow way to achieve oxidation is to unhurriedly mix flour with water in the presence of oxygen from the air in your kitchen. Industry cannot afford to take the leisure of hours of bread kneading, for time is money. To this end, a fast and efficient method of using a simple chemical called potassium bromate ($KBrO_3$) was invented. Instead of waiting for hours to allow connective molecular bridges with the help of slow oxygen from the air, $KBrO_3$ does the oxidizing trick almost instantaneously.

But wait, there is a catch! Potassium bromate is a "carcinogen," a substance known to cause cancer in laboratory mice. It is banned in the EU, the United Kingdom, Canada, Brazil, India, Japan, and China, but not in the United States. At least not yet. The reassuring reasoning is that by the end of the baking process, there is only an infinitesimal amount present in the finished product. But is there really a safe level of exposure? Is there a threshold below which potassium bromate poses no problem? Should US consumers be concerned?

DNA errors and genetic mutation. It is a long and circuitous road from initial exposure to a carcinogen (or carcinogens) to the final formation of a malignant tumor. It all starts with damage to DNA, the molecule that is commonly referred to as the "blueprint for life." There are three possible outcomes: (1) Our cellular DNA repair system is able to fix the damage so that the cell can continue to divide and multiply, faithfully reproducing the repaired DNA; (2) The DNA damage is too far gone to be fixed, and our DNA repair system directs the cell that harbors the faulty DNA to be destroyed (thank goodness!); (3) DNA repair fails, and the cell containing the error slips through the cell cycle with the defective DNA, and over time, cumulative mutations in growth-regulatory genes drive uncontrolled cell growth while at the same time mutations in tumor suppressor genes disable the DNA repair apparatus. The combination of faulty genes that drive growth and prohibit DNA repair is the worst mutational scenario.

Potassium bromate, cancer, and the hidden link. Let's cut through the chase: Potassium bromate produces *free radicals* which are electron stealers. Electrons are the "glue" holding molecules together. A theft of electrons can result in bond breakage. We have learned that DNA is formed by nucleotides which consist of three parts: (1) A nitrogen base (A, T, G, or C), (2) a sugar group (pentose), and (3) a phosphate group. Stringing nucleotides together (in pre-programmed sequences) forms the two-stranded double helix. Base A is paired with T and C to G. Linking A↔T and G↔C are chemical bonds called hydrogen bonds. When DNA becomes the target of potassium bromate, the chemical bonds that hold the bases or between the base and the sugar group are subject to free radical attack. If DNA damage is fixed in time, DNA order can be restored. If repair fails, the error is passed on, leading to genetic mutation and resultant cancer. There is evidence in support of a link between potassium bromate and kidney cancer and thyroid cancer.

The dose makes the poison, but why chance it? Now back to potassium bromate in baked goods. Occasional consumption of bread that contains potassium bromate is unlikely to pose any serious health danger. On the other hand, trace amounts of potassium bromate, a tiny amount of food dye, a little sprinkle of artificial sugar, an iota of forever chemicals, a whiff of radon gas leaked out of the basement, or benzene from car exhaust... Before you know it, you are collecting a plate of chemicals that are known, probable, or possible carcinogens. While it is impossible for anyone to stay in a totally sealed cocoon, it wouldn't hurt to shy away from undesirable toxic substances, where possible, however mild.

Given that bread can certainly be made without potassium bromate, why take the unnecessary risk? Good bread can be baked the old-fashioned way. After all, the French would not put up with mushy bread. Nutty and savory baguette needs no unwanted additives of any kind. The exact composition of the dough, believe it or not, is written in French law.

Special note: The original version of this essay was published in McGill University Office of Science and Society weekly digest.

Food for thought:

1. Potassium bromate helps bread speed up rising in baking. Potassium bromate is also a carcinogen.
    A. True
    B. False

2. One way carcinogens cause cancer is by compromising DNA integrity and disrupting normal cell division.
    A. True
    B. False

M

MILANO, OSSO BUCO, AND IMMUNE POWER

Milan is famous for many feats, from Roman ruins to the fashion center of the world. There is one more deliciously defined feast of Milan of lesser notoriety: a gourmet dish called *Osso Buco*.

A bowl of delicacy. Imagine special cut veal nested in a harvest of bright veggies braised in a sacred sauce of white wine and bovine bone marrow. Understandably, to vegetarians and "veganarians," the mere mentioning of veal triggers grossly emetic sensations. With you! Here, the focus is on bone marrow, a vital organ that defines and defends our very life.

Bone marrow is a blood cell cradle. Bone marrow comes in two flavors: red bone marrow and yellow bone marrow. Harboring blood stem cells, the red bone marrow is the mother source of all blood cells, including RBCs, WBCs, and platelets. Yellow bone marrow harbors different sets of stem cells that specialize in becoming our body's supportive cells, including bone cells, cartilage, tendons, ligaments, and fat cells. To sustain various biological and physiological needs of our body, the bone marrow judiciously makes a wobbly 500 billion assorted cells each day, rain or shine! In ***CRISPR/Cas9 QUARTET (2): SILENCING A CRITICAL GENE TO CURE SICKLE CELL ANEMIA*** (page 78), we described how a faulty gene that causes sickle cell anemia can be corrected with gene therapy by introducing the correct copy of the gene into stem cells which when returned to the patient's bone marrow matures as RBCs that express the correct hemoglobin gene to alleviate the patient of sickle cell anemia.

Stem cells are easy targets of radiation. Stem cells are versatile foundations capable of becoming specialty cells. The process of a "general stem cell" branching off as a "speciality cell" is called "differentiation." Examples of differentiated cell types include (1) "epithelial cells" (e.g., the cells that form the protective lining of our guts), (2) "endothelial cells" (that form the lining of our blood vessels), (3) "keratinocytes" (cells that form the protective outer layer of our skin, also called *epidermis*), and many more.

DNA damage and radiation sickness. Differentiated cells are sturdier as if they were veiled with an invisible guarding shield. Therefore, it is no surprise that "opportunistic" radiation generally stays away from differentiated cells. Which types of cells are easy targets of harmful radiation? The *undifferentiated* cells, most notably stem cells from the bone marrow. How exactly? By damaging the DNA harbored in those cells. When a cell's DNA is broken and stays broken without a quick fix, one fate of the cell is to die off. The same fate confronts stem blood cells—a condition called *radiation sickness,* which can be acute or chronic, and depending on the severity, the sickness could be transient or permanent. Drastic reductions in WBCs unquestionably dampen the overall immune system. With immune defense guard down, radiation sickness patients are extremely vulnerable to infections, and to this end, the prescription of antibiotics is one of the treatment measures. The admirable Madam

Curie, who spent decades working with potent radioactive materials, eventually developed pernicious aplastic anemia, a form of blood cancer, where irreversibly damaged bone marrow stops making blood cells. The destructive nature of radioactive rays to human health was not fully elucidated in Madam Curie's time. Blood cancer took Madam Curie's life when she was only sixty-two. Hailed as a national hero in France, Madam Curie's body is preserved at the Panthéon, and due to strong radioactivity emitted from her body, her casket is shielded with 1-inch thick lead to block off radioactivity for the safety of visitors. Lead is known to block radiation rays due to its high density. Despite this protective measure, even today, nearly one century since Madam Curie's passing, visitors are still required to put their signatures on a liability waiver form in addition to wearing protective gear.

Back to *osso buco, which* originated in Lombardy, Italy, the stew is said to be rich in two types of amino acids, proline and glycine, which help strengthen the immune system. Of course, there are many other ways to boost the immune boosting: a balanced diet, some physical exercise, adequate sleep, and be happy—just to name a few.

Food for thought:

1. High-energy (ionizing) radiation seeks after vulnerable undifferentiated human cells such as blood cells from the bone marrow.
   A. True
   B. False

2. Consuming bone marrow broth is the only way to keep a strong immune system.
   A. True
   B. False

N

NODES THAT CHANNEL LYMPH: STRONGHOLDS OF TRUSTED IMMUNE RADARS

Shaped like a bean the size of a pea, lymph nodes play a vital defense role in our health.

Location and function. Found abundantly in armpits, neck, chest, abdomen, and groins of approximately 600 in our body, each lymph node is replete with fluid of bodily waste such as dead cells and molecules shed by bacteria, viruses, and even cancer cells. This clear fluid is put under the radar screen for scrutiny by the immune cells. As soon as a "danger" molecule is spotted, the immune cells are on high alert, quickly multiply, and mount an immune response to eliminate danger.

Not all swollen lymph nodes are the same. The response to imminent "danger" by immune cells is not only swift but also palpable: lymph nodes swell up due to the large numbers of immune cells undergoing expansion and gathering needed immune arsenals to fight back against the danger. The average diameter of a lymph node in an adult person is ~12 millimeters (12 mm, or 1/2 an inch). By contrast, when a lymph node swells up to become a lump, its diameter reaches 25 mm—doubled!

While both infection and cancer give rise to enlarged lymph nodes, there is a distinct difference. Simply put: a swollen lymph node in response to infection is enlarged but feels tender and painful. A swollen lymph node driven by cancer, on the other hand, is also enlarged but rock-hard and painless. Another gauge to distinguish the two contexts is the time factor: an infection-enlarged lymph node usually goes away within seven weeks, whereas cancer-associated lymph node lump is persistent, lingering beyond seven weeks. Here is a helpful tip from MD Anderson Cancer Center: a swollen lymph node from infection feels like touching the soft tip of your nose, whereas a lymphoma blood cancer-related swollen lymph node feels like touching the hard tip of your chin. Moreover, early-stage lymphoma has skin manifestations such as itchiness and rashes, while more progressive lymphomas are associated with symptoms of fever, fatigue, night sweats, and unplanned weight loss, among others. More detailed info can be found by visiting https://www.mdanderson.org/cancerwise/swollen-lymph-nodes-and-other-symptoms-of-lymphoma. It's always a wise idea to consult your family physician.

Shown above is the anatomic structure of a lymph node. Lymph enters and exits the lymph node via intricately designated routes. The pine nut-shaped pockets inside the lymph node represent compartments that house different types of immune cells. Lymphatic vessels run alongside blood vessels of artery and vein.

A slice of entomology trivia. Lymph is transparent and cloudless, resembling the Latin semi-goddess of pulchritude "lympha," seen by clear and pristine water. Beauty and purity aside, lymph nodes are barometers of health and illness.

Lymph nodes and lymphoma. A true story: During the lockdown of the Covid-19 pandemic, a mother from one city and her son working in another city were having their usual video chats. The mother noticed a visible lump on her son's front neck. Intuitively, the mother felt something unusual and

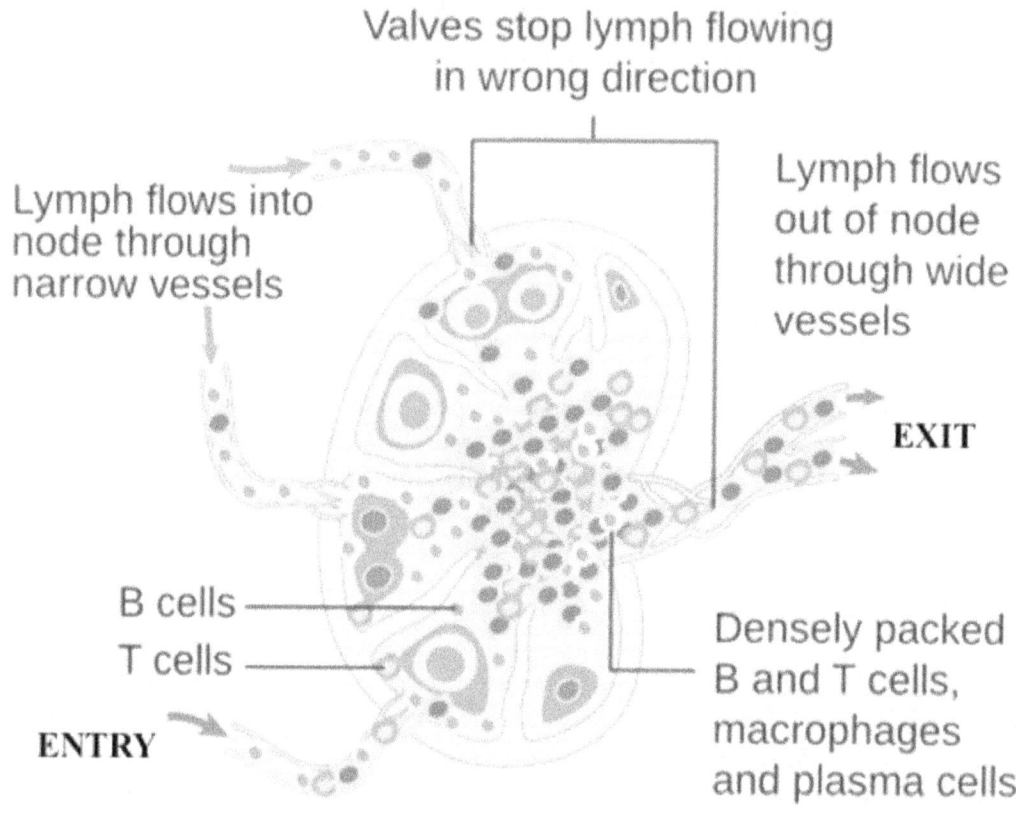

Image 61 The lymph node. Wikimedia Commons File: Diagram of a lymph node CRUK 022.svg.

urged her son to have it checked. The swollen lymph node turned out to be an early-stage lymphoma. Timely detection and treatment saved the son's life. Catching cancer early is always a swell idea!

How to pump up lymph? The lymphatic system has no analogue to the heart, which is the "pump" that circulates blood. Without the "luxury" of a working pump, our lymphatic system has to rely on the activities of surrounding muscles to push lymph circulation. This is where exercise comes into the picture! The more muscular movement, the faster the lymph moves, and the more continuously immune cells are delivered to where they are needed for immune battles. The old adage "*You rest, you rust*" makes a lot of immunological sense.

Food for thought:

1. A swollen lymph node due to infection typically lasts for no more than seven weeks, soft and painful. By contrast, cancer-related swollen lymph nodes persist beyond seven weeks, hard but painless.
    A. True
    B. False

2. Physical movement is a great way to get the lymph going and to stay healthy.
    A. True
    B. False

O

"OPEN SESAME" AND THE IMMUNE SECRET CODE

Legend has it that *Alibaba* heard a hum of "Open Sesame." Soon after, the door to the thousand-year-old cave opened and hidden treasures were revealed. What does the fable have to do with immunity? Odd, indeed! But the link is actually plain to see.

Naturally endowed immune power. Our immune system houses two branches, namely "innate immunity" and "adaptive immunity." Think about the movie *Good Will Hunting*: the precocious young lad who tried to make a living by working as a janitor at a leading engineering school solved a difficult math problem by eavesdropping outside the lecture hall. When the professor noticed the solution to the math problem on the hallway writing board, he immediately recognized the talent in the young lad—talent he was born with, talent not obtained from formal schooling. Back to innate immunity: the designated immune cells for the *innate immunity* branch are capable of snapping into action to eliminate infectious bugs on their own with no need for special training or tutorials. For a long while, though, scientists had no idea how the awesome innate immune cells spot and recognize immune danger until a group of German biologists uncovered the secret "*Sesame Open*" molecular code of how innate immune cells crack open infected cells. What are the equivalents of "sesame doors" on cells?

Hints from fruit flies! Perusing through any residential street in America, one notices arrays of houses with colorful doors, some white, others brown, and Dr. Albert Einstein had the door of his Princeton, New Jersey, residence painted bright red. No matter what the color of the door, all doors are equipped with a lock, and clicking the block with the matching key allows one to enter the house. Most houses possess a front door, a back door, and a side door. Our cells, immune cells included, also have different molecular doors, each with an associated key. Instead of humming the magic words of "Sesame Open," the first clue to innate immune cells was identified by a group of German scientists at the Max Planck Institute. The organismic model they were using was *Drosophila* (fruit flies). We discussed in an earlier essay here in this book that scientists knock down a gene of unknown function to determine which function of the organism would be affected—the famous loss-of-function studies. The German scientists, too, were investigating the genetic basis of fruit fly body pattern formation using the same methodology. They knocked out individual genes in fruit flies and followed up on what alterations were produced, one gene at a time. One particular gene yielded an extremely unusual change in fruit fly offspring with an incompletely sealed abdominal cavity, although the flies were very much alive. One scientist exclaimed in German, "*Das ist toll*," which translates as "*That's amazing*" in English. The word "amazing" in this context does not carry the same connotation as "positively wonderful"; rather, it denotes "unusually peculiar" or "weird." The two lead scientists, Dr. Christiane Nüsslein-Volhard and Dr. Eric Wieschaus from the Max Planck Institute, were awarded the Nobel Prize in 1995 for their discovery of the *toll* gene. Is there a connection between a body pattern-formation gene found in fruit flies and innate immunity in humans? Sounds oceans apart, but the answer is *yes*, although it took two decades and several groups of scientists to have finally figured it out.

Immune connection. Subsequent observations on fruit fly offspring that failed to carry the *toll* gene revealed that those deformed species were also extremely vulnerable to fungal infection—the first and crucial hint to the gene's role in immune response. Several research groups in the United States carried out parallel investigations exemplified by Dr. Charles Janeway, based at Yale School of Medicine. What was unraveled was not just the human equivalent of *toll* but a family of proteins termed toll-like receptors (TLRs). Dr. Janeway's particular contribution was the discovery of TLR4, which is ubiquitously expressed on the surface of innate immune cells, most notably macrophages and dendritic cells (DCs). If TLR4 is the "key," which "lock" does it open on infectious bacteria such as *E. coli*? The answer is LPS, which stands for lipo-poly-saccharide, a complex sugar group. Using the TLR key, macrophage cells interact with the LPS lock on *E. coli*, followed by swiftly engulfing, chewing up, and literally splitting out the defunct *E. coli* pieces. The process described above is classic phagocytosis—a common but powerful weapon of bug destruction, as shown in the following Image:

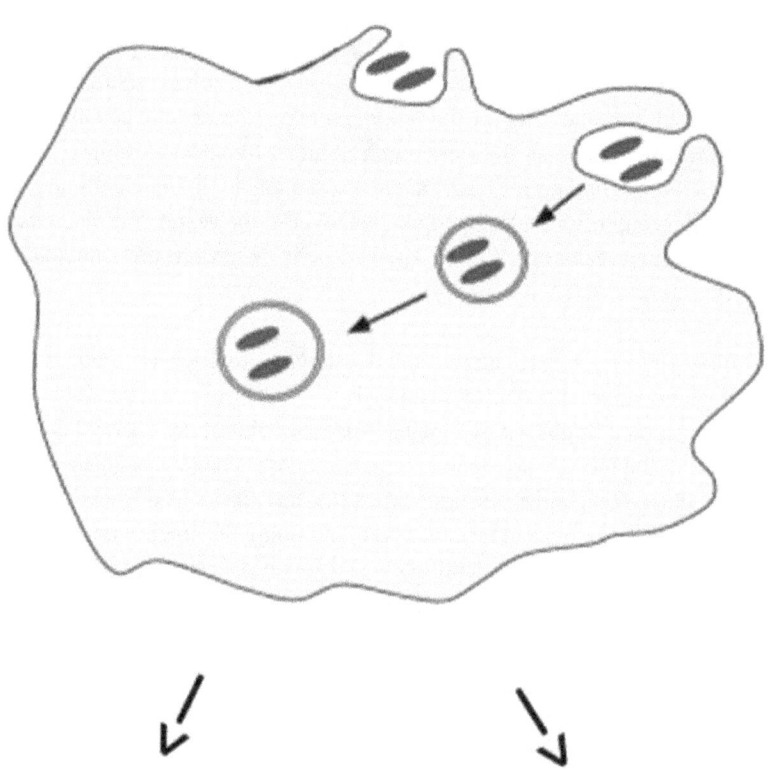

Image 62 *E. coli* is engulfed by an immune cell. Wikipedia Commons File: Phagocytosis and Exocytosis.svg modified by Nancy Liu-Sullivan.

As shown above, the fateful "key-lock" interaction leads to engulfment and destruction of the bacterium to complete the immune battle. If, however, the bacterial population gets too overwhelming for innate immune cells to handle, elite troopers from the adaptive immunity would be called upon to continue the battle. This process starts with macrophages (or dendritic cells) carrying a slice of enemy antigen "intel" and traveling to local lymph nodes to meet up with T cells, leading to the activation of Killer T (KT) cells which are equipped with the famous "1-2 punch" secret weapon against tough invaders. In parallel, B cells would be activated, undergo a differentiation process to become plasma cells that secrete *E. coli*-specific antibodies which, in turn, facilitate and enhance phagocytosis. Immune teamwork, indeed! An in-depth description is in ***AN ATLAS OF IMMUNE BIG PICTURE*** (pages 5–6).

The innate arm of immune cells is said to be "promiscuous" in a molecular sense, meaning it is not a faithful 1:1 pairing of "key" to the one-and-only "lock." On the contrary, TLR4 alone can interact with LPS and a host of other "locks." And of course, LPS is not the only "prize possession" of *E. coli*, all gram-negative bacteria express LPS. This also expands TLR4's versatility as one "master key" for "multiple locks." A family of great variety, TLRs consist TLR1, TLR2, TLR3, TLR4, and numerous others, as depicted in the following figure:

As shown above, innate immune cells are in possession of several members of the TLR family that bind to corresponding antigens found on infectious bugs, where LPS = Lipopolysaccharides, ssRNA = Single-stranded RNA, dsRNA = Double-stranded RNA. Additional antigens include Pam3, CSK4, and Flagellin. These are but the tip of the iceberg of the large pool of antigens that are displayed on the radar of innate immune cells.

Kudos and twists. Groundbreaking work on how innate immune cells recognize immune danger was awarded the 2011 Nobel Prize for Physiology or Medicine to Dr. Bruce Beutler and Dr. Jules

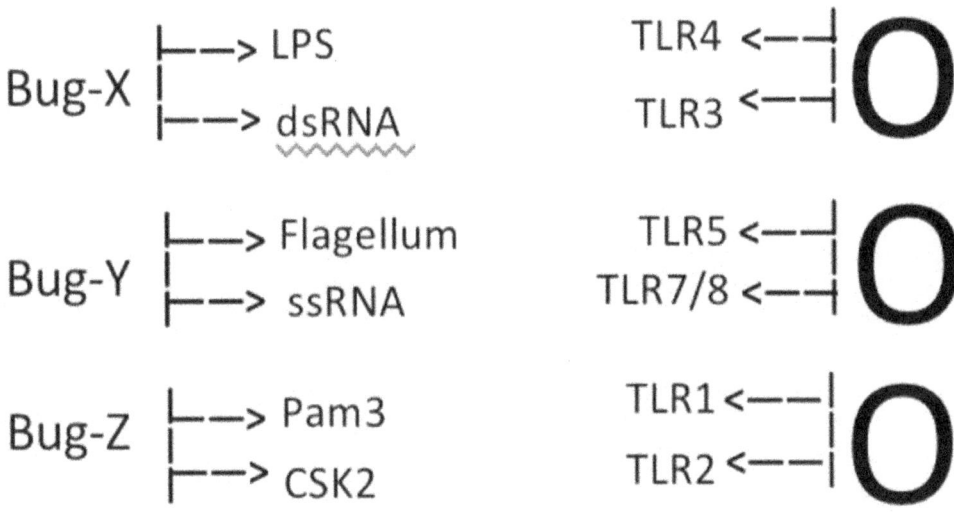

Lock on infectious bug   **Key** on innate immune cell

Image 63 Molecular tango between immune cells and infectious bugs. By Nancy Liu-Sullivan.

Hoffman, both from Yale University School of Medicine. The third scientist was Dr. Ralph Steinman who discovered dendritic cells (DC). Since the Nobel Prize is not awarded to worthy scientists promiscuously, Dr. Charles Janeway did not live to see his breakthrough discovery recognized by the Nobel Prize Committee. The second twist has a happier ending: Dr. Ralph Steinman had passed away three days prior to the public announcement made by the Nobel Prize committee without knowledge of Dr. Steinman's passing. The committee decided on keeping the award as is (*ZENITH OF SUCCESS NOT DEFINED BY A PRIZE,* page 221).

Food for thought:

1. Innate immune cells, by definition, battle infectious microorganisms with no need for training or prepping.
   A. True
   B. False

2. For innate immune cells to engage infectious microorganisms, a key (such as TLR4) is to open the lock (such as LPS on *E. coli* bacterium).
   A. True
   B. False

P

P53 PENTALOGY (1): ELEPHANT'S GUARDIAN ANGEL

Very low cancer in elephants Giant but gentle, poised yet playful and equipped with a remarkable memory capacity, elephants are popular creatures among humans. Unlike humans, however, elephants are rarely afflicted with cancer. As shown in the table above, cancer incidence among elephants is less than 1 percent, in stark contrast to humans of a wobbly 25 percent, that is, 25 percent of the human population gets diagnosed with cancer in their lifetime. What is elephants' secret recipe for cancer resistance? Before delving into this question, let's recap some cell biology basics.

DNA blueprint. According to the most updated calibration of human cells, on average, an adult male has 36 trillion, an adult female 28 trillion, and a ten-year-old 17 trillion. To sustain bodily functions, 500 million blood cells are made in a person every minute! Cells grow by dividing; that is, one mother

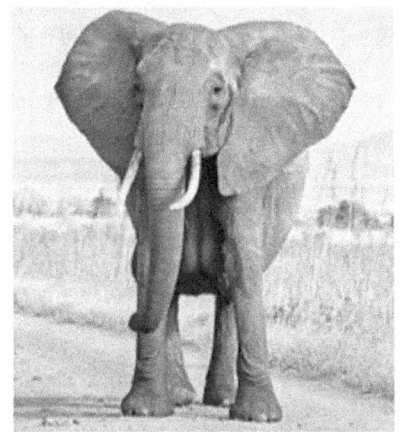

Genetic features	Elephants	Humans
Life span	65 years	72 years
# of chromosomes	56	46
# of cells	3,500 trillion	100 trillion
Cancer incidence	Less than 1%	25%
p53 tumor suppressor gene	20	1

Image 64 Facts of elephants table. Wikimedia Commons File: African Bush Elephant.jpg modified by Nancy Liu-Sullivan.

cell divides into 2, 2 become 4, 4 to 8, 8 to 16, and so on and so forth, all offspring cells carrying the same exact DNA blueprint as the ancestral mother cell. Consisting of a pair of complementary strands, DNA winds up like a flexible ladder. To replicate DNA, the two strands must separate, followed by each strand serving as a template to make carbon copies at the end of the DNA replication event. The two original complementary strands become two pairs of 2-stranded species, each serving as the genetic makeup for each of the two offspring cells. There is also a team of enzymes assisting the DNA replication process. In short, DNA replication is extremely prone to errors, some minor, others egregious. DNA errors ought to be fixed and fixed in a timely fashion; otherwise, if erroneous DNA is allowed to be carried on to offspring cells, it would alter the original DNA blueprint, which is defined as a mutation. It is estimated that it takes five or more incidents of genetic mutations to arrive at a malignant tumor in humans. Fortunately, DNA repair genes and tumor suppressor genes are in charge of spotting DNA errors, halting the cell cycle machinery to fix the errors, and maintaining DNA integrity. The molecular protagonist here is p53 (also called TP53). We humans can be hubristic about how superior we are to other species but not when it comes to p53. More to be discussed next.

Elephants are richly endowed with *p53*: As shown in the table above, each human cell carries a single *p53* gene. Since we inherit one copy from each parent, we possess two alleles (versions) of the single *p53* gene. By stark contrast, elephants possess **twenty *p53* genes** (or forty alleles). The sheer richness in the number of *p53* in elephants allows an ample supply of primary troopers and backup troopers to spot and fix erroneous DNA in these large but gentle mammals. Elephant cells are also found to be twice as efficient in signaling DNA damage compared to their human cell counterparts, providing further supporting evidence of elephants' remarkable capacity for efficient troubleshooting for the maintenance of genome integrity. It is, therefore, no surprise that elephants have an extremely low cancer incidence of less than 1 percent as opposed to 25 percent in humans.

Genome's guardian angel. Inspired by p53-rich genome-aided deterrence of cancer in elephants, scientists are expanding the repertoire of p53 studies with the goal of developing p53 gene therapy to treat cancers that harbor p53 aberrations. Recent observations (made by MSKCC's lab helmed by Dr. Scott Lowe) have shed new light on the intricate interplay between *p53* (the genome guardian angel) and *Kras* (the potent cancer gene): Loss of *p53* and presence of *kras* drives aggressive cancer, whereas the absence of *Kras*, accompanied by the presence of *p53*, confers tepid benign tumor, indicating that (1) when *p53* is intact, activities by the potent cancer gene *Kras* can be curtailed and (2) the double whammy of loss of *p53* combined with *Kras* is a sure recipe for full-blown cancer. By breaking cancer into its component parts in temporal and spatial dimensions for an in-depth understanding of how selective pressures drive the transformation from normal cells to a benign transition and finally degrading to full metastatic cancer, anti-cancer medications can be strategized. Go Team Lowe! For a detailed description of work by Dr. Lowe's lab, please visit https://www.mskcc.org/news/scientists-solve-30-year-old-mystery-about-p53-protein-dubbed-guardian-genome.

Food for thought:

1. Elephants owe their low cancer rate to a valuable set of twenty tumor suppressor genes called *p53*.
   A. True
   B. False

2. The combined loss of *p53* with dominance of cancer-causing gene *Kras* spells full-fledged cancer development.
   A. True
   B. False

P53 PENTALOGY (2): A GENE OF MANY HATS

We described in the previous essay that *p53* is a critical tumor suppressor gene (TSG). Mutations in *p53* are found in more than 50 percent of all human cancers. Besides TSG, *p53* has two additional molecular hats.

The tumor-suppressor gene "hat." Instead of becoming taller, wider, or bigger, our cells grow by making carbon copies of themselves, and they do so by going through cell cycle progressions. Imagine the cell cycle as an Olympian-scale track and field stadium. To pass the qualification to run the tracks, runners must go through a checkpoint station where their physical fitness is examined. Occasionally, certain runners commit moral mistakes by using banned stimulants to boost performance. Those individuals are given warnings and are invited out if the same problem persists. A similar process also takes place at our cell cycle checkpoints. Each cell's DNA is methodically scrutinized: if all is good, a green pass is issued. If an error is spotted, the DNA "sheriff," p53, steps in to take care of business. A terrific team player, p53 has a partner called "p21" that relays p53's decree to a key cell cycle gatekeeper molecule called "CDK4." The signaling cascade can be summed up as: **p53** —> (stimulates) **p21** —| (halts) **CDK4** —| (blocks) **Cell cycle machine**. This delicately orchestrated platform makes sure of no faulty cells with erroneous DNA get a chance to pass on DNA mistakes to offspring cells in order to nip potential cancer in the bud.

The DNA repair gene "hat." Despite acting as the draconian "czar" of cell cycle quality control, *p53* does have a forgiving side. Specifically, *p53* gives cells that harbor faulty DNA a chance to repair. Certain DNA blunders can be fixed easily and become good as new. What exactly does p53 do as a molecular fixer? Traditionally, it is thought that p53 works as a DNA correction coordinator that sends SOS signals to recruit professional DNA repair molecules to arrive at injured sites to patch things up. That being said, new studies have described p53 as also playing a direct role in righting the wrongs of erroneous DNA. The water is deep in p53 biology. More awaits to be uncovered to piece together a panoramic view of this versatile molecule.

The cell-suicide gene "hat." For thornier errors that have gone beyond repair, p53 acts like a no-nonsense molecular executor by shuffling cells that harbor irreversible DNA damage to cell suicide machine. Again, instead of being the actual hand that carries out the killing of dangerous cells detrimental to genomic wholesomeness, p53 simply presses a cell-death button on cells destined for elimination. This triggers a cascade of events that quickly relays the death signal to a molecule called Caspase 3(Casp3). High levels of active Casp3 in a cell are a sure sign of cell death work-in-progress. This special cell death program initiated by p53 is the famous *apoptosis*. **Quick Word Anatomy**: *apo* = away, *ptosis* = falling. Combining apo + ptosis = falling off. In the context of cancer biology, apoptosis vividly portrays a scene of rogue cells being teased away from a body of good cells.

What happens when p53 goes haywire? A mutation is manifested by a change in DNA that deviates from the DNA norm. Since a specific DNA segment encodes a gene, when the code is erroneous, the resultant gene becomes a variation of the original gene. The landscape of *p53 mutation* is a complex one which can lead to loss of p53 protein normal tumor-suppressor function or degrade p53 to a cancer-causing gene! Between p53 loss-of-function (LOF) and gain-of-function (GOF), LOF is more commonly observed in human cancers. The National Institutes of Health (NIH) presents a comprehensive list of cancers associated with p53 mutations identified thus far. These include breast cancer, bladder cancer, lung cancer, melanoma, and many more. For details, please refer to *https://medlineplus.gov/genetics/gene/tp53/*.

Food for thought:

1. Suppressing tumor, fixing DNA errors, and promoting death of cells that carry faulty DNA sum up the three molecular hats of *p53*.
   A. True
   B. False

2. Mutations in *p53* that induce loss of normal p53 protein tumor suppression functions are more commonly found in human cancers.
   A. True
   B. False

P53 PENTALOGY (3): INTIMATE IMMUNE CONNECTIONS

The discovery of p53 entails an interesting behind-the-scenes story in that four research groups simultaneously reached the same milestone in 1979—speaking of *like minds thinking alike!* Confronting the new kid on the block of molecular genetics some forty years ago, scientists initially surmised p53 as a tumor-promoting gene, also called an "oncogene." It was not until 1989 that the true nature of p53 surfaced as a confirmed tumor suppressor gene (TSG), not just any TSG but a master TSG. As Hollywood elects the best picture every year, so too does the field of biological sciences. The "Molecule of the Year" in 1993 was awarded to p53 by the *Science* Magazine, which itself is a crown jewel professional journal, together with *Nature* and *Cell*. The work on p53 continues to advance. Here, let's go over a feature of p53 mutation related to immune response.

Dancing an immune tango. More than 50 percent of cancers are inflicted with p53 mutations, which renders p53 non-functional in suppressing tumors, correcting DNA mistakes, or promoting the death of dangerous cells, thus creating a molecular open season for cancer cells to become rampant. For years, attempts to develop drugs that target p53 have failed due to mounting challenges. One major challenge involves the reversal of drug development in that typically inhibitor drugs are developed to tackle cancer cells that grow wildly and need to be curbed. It is a different story with p53: As a tumor suppressor molecule, its normal functions need to be enhanced instead of being blocked. New observations have revealed a mutant p53 *Achilles' heel* in cancer.

It turns out that the tumor antigen ID on mutant p53 proteins is unique enough to alert the host immune system. Through an immune tango between the p53 mutant antigen and dendritic cells (DCs), tumor "Intel" gets displayed on the molecular silver platter called HLA. Once in possession of precious tumor Intel, DCs interact with B cells and CD8 Killer T cells. The consequence of this pair of interactions is of significant utility by producing antibodies that can bog down p53 mutant cancer cells on the one hand,

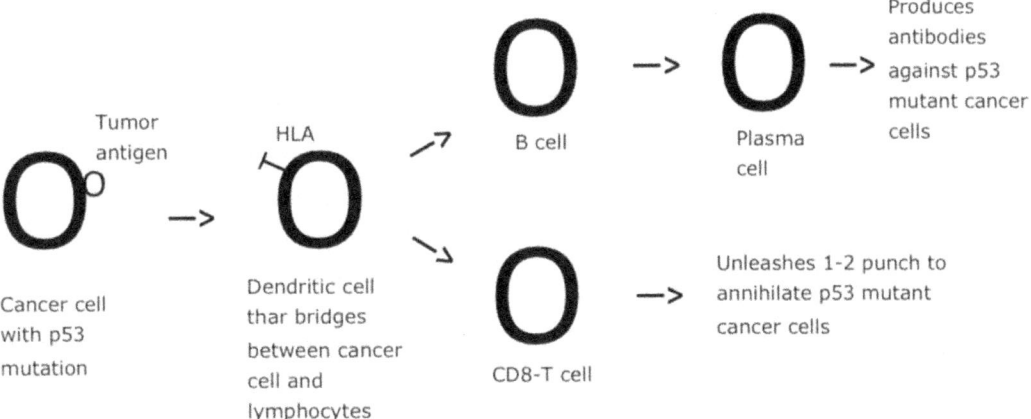

Image 65 Cancer cell under immune fire. By Nancy Liu-Sullivan.

and on the other hand, by energizing KT cells to launch a "1-2 punch" to proactively reject and destroy cancer cells that harbor p53 mutations. The details are delineated in the following figure:

The scenarios described above are being investigated with the hope of translating them into cancer immunotherapy one day. However, considering the multi-dimensional nature of p53 in health and in cancer, tackling p53 mutants by taking advantage of unique tumor antigens takes time to be hashed out. Where there is a will, there is a way.

Cancers in which p53 undergoes mutations are tough to treat, understandably. However, a particular type of skin cancer does harbor intact p53; yet patients have very poor treatment responses and bleak prognoses. Let's find out how this p53 molecular puzzle was solved in the next essay.

P53 PENTALOGY (4): DECODING THE *APAF1* ENIGMA IN MELANOMA

Almighty p53 becomes feeble in both gene and protein forms in many types of cancer. Patients do not respond to treatment, and their survival rates dwindle. All logical: when the body's chief tumor suppressor is dysfunctional and the DNA repair apparatus is down, early tumors no longer bear any checks and become anarchical. There is, however, a befuddling exception: in a subtype of melanoma, p53 bears no mutation and is fully functional, yet patients do not fare well in their expected treatment responses. Let's find out how a research group at Cold Spring Harbor Laboratory (CSHL) solved the puzzle.

Popping the "death" question. How does p53 suppress tumor cells? A single-word answer is "death," as also described in ***P53 PENTALOGY (2): A GENE OF MANY HATS*** (page 135). P53 initiates, before a problematic cell turns cancerous due to irreversible DNA damage, a programmed cell death termed *apoptosis*. I can still remember vividly my graduate school biochemistry professor, from the land of Shelly, Yeats, and Barron, dictating with all sincerity to the class how the second consonant "p" in apoptosis is silent! Coming from an English literature background from a few moons ago but always a biologist-want-to-be, I readily echoed!

P53 and company. Not at all a one-molecule island, p53 mobilizes a cascade of proteins to coordinate apoptosis, as shown in the following figure:

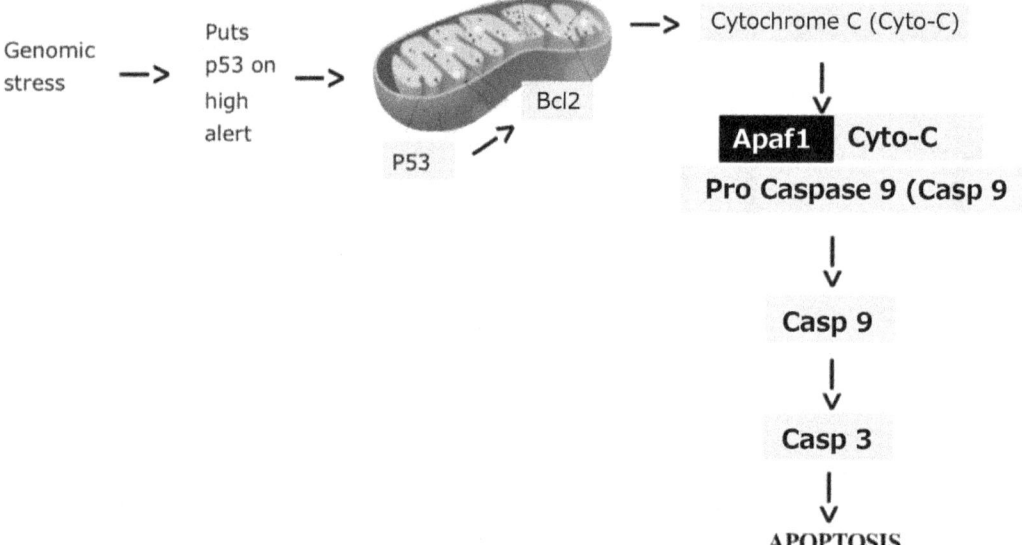

Image 66 P53 in action. Wikimedia Commons File: Mitochondrion structure.svg modified by Nancy Liu-Sullivan.

A simplified version, the figure illustrates the cascading events of apoptosis initiated by p53. It starts with microscopic-level stresses exerted on DNA from exposure to UV, radon gas, or benzene from tobacco smoking, among a long list of risk factors. Yes, a common denominator of all of the above is "carcinogen," defined as substances that either directly cause cancer or increase cancer risks. Of course, transitioning from toxic exposure to cancer takes years. Why so long? The answer resides in p53!

p53 rescues genomic stress. Going back to the figure above: thanks to p53's apoptotic prowess, certain cells are timely eliminated before they could turn cancerous.

Step 1: Following genomic stress event,
Step 2: p53 is activated
Step 3: and enters mitochondria,
Step 4: followed by Bcl2 activation in the mitochondria followed by
Step 5: the release of "Cytochrome C" (CytoC); Note: CytoC comes from a family of "cytochromes" proteins and plays an essential role in mediating the making of ATP, the cellular fuel. Now, CytoC release is like the sound of the starting gun; it only starts the race, the relay mission will have to be carried out by the runners, as delivered below:
Step 6 to Step 9: CytoC release triggers a partnership between CytoC with Apaf1, which sequentially brings Casp9 and Caps3 to the race all the way to the finish line: APOPTOSIS—the destruction and demise of problematic cells in danger of becoming cancerous.

Melanoma *Apaf1* enigma decoded. Instilled with extreme recalcitrantly rogue traits, cancer cells do everything to defy cellular rules and regulations, as manifested in a subtype of melanoma cells observed by scientists at Cold Spring Harbor Laboratories (CSHL) back in the early 1990s. Discerning patterns to determine trends is an essential step in the long journeys of scientific discovery. Typically, cancers that bear p53 mutations are apoptosis-resistant and hard to treat. Melanoma stands out as an *outlier*: Its p53 is present and in good form; yet, melanoma is just as resistant as cancers with faulty p53. How odd! Leaving no stone unturned, the CSHL scientists kept on and made a key discovery: An important relay station downstream of p53 turns out to be defective! The name of the gene is *Apaf1*. One runner out, the entire apoptotic cascading race is out, allowing, unfortunately, melanoma cells to gleefully grow and defy death without any restraints. It is important to mention that Dr. Xiaodong Wang from Emory University led a team of scientists in mapping out the apoptosis signal transduction pathway. An onerous task, but done AMD done well! Dr. Wang now heads the Beijing Biological Research Institute.

Reinstating Apaf1 to resume apoptosis. Back to CSHL: No time to rest on the laurels of detecting a glitch downstream of p53, the CSHL scientists also elucidated what brought down *Apaf1*, a molecular event termed "methylation," where the chemical "methyl" group is added to the *Apaf1* gene that turned Apaf1 silent; that is, Apaf1 becomes dysfunctional, unable to relay apoptosis signaling initiated by p53. Knowing where the problem resides solves half of the problem. Indeed, the addition of an anti-methylation chemical agent effectively lifted Apaf1 suppression. The resurrection of Apaf1 resumed smooth sailing along the p53 apoptosis pathway, which brought about total destruction of melanoma. Amazing!

The head of the CSHL research laboratory that ironed out the melanoma apoptosis wrinkle is Dr. Scott Lowe, an accomplished molecular biologist who now helms the cancer biology flagship at MSKCC. MSKCC's gain.

Food for thought:

1. P53 initiates tumor cell apoptosis.
    A. True
    B. False

2. Team Lowe uncovered a faulty relay station downstream of p53 that blocked the apoptotic pathway. Resuming Apaf1 function cleared the block and successfully sent melanoma cells to their demise.
    A. True
    B. False

P53 PENTALOGY (5): MEETING THE NEMESIS

Commonly known as the culprit for cervical cancer, HPV also increases the risks of several other cancer types in the head and neck regions. A recently uncovered role of HPV puts the virus in a new light of its cancer-enabling schemes.

HPV and cancer. How does HPV cause cancer? A good but loaded question. A quick answer of "*HPV causing gene mutation that eventually leads to cancer*" is an oversimplified response, as there are multiple HOWs beneath the tip of the mutation iceberg. Let's sort it out.

All viruses grow and expand by hijacking the host genetic system. HPV is no exception. Worse, the two-stranded DNA virus can also surreptitiously blend its DNA to that of the human host. This uninvited DNA mingling changes the human DNA composition. Any deviation from the original DNA sequence is, by definition, a mutation. HPV-induced mutations serve to produce two vicious cancer-causing oncoproteins termed as "E6" and "E7." Akin to "onco-genes" being genes that cause cancer, "onco-proteins" are the gene products that cause cancer. "E" in the series of HPV proteins stands for "element." Indeed, E6 and its wicked partner E7 have turned out to be extremely "elemental" in cancer-causing deeds.

HPV: Arch nemesis of p53. In parallel with integrating into the human cell genome, E6 and E7 team up to molecularly gang up on p53! As we are now quite conversant with the crucial roles p53 plays in maintaining genome soundness and the dire ramifications of disabled p53 on the genome, it should come as no surprise that disabling p53 by HPV serves as a key link between chronic HPV infection and several types of cancer. How exactly does the wicked HPV E6-E7 evil duo disable p53?

Shuffling p53 to the shredder. Life and death are the norm of proteins—a process called degradation. Discarding the old and welcoming the new, protein degradation is a major mechanism by which our body maintains its molecular and cellular fitness. Protein degradation is carried out by a shredding process called "ubiquitination" which tags proteins destined for destruction with a molecule called "ubiquitin." The tagged proteins are subsequently sent to a protein shredder called "proteasome." This is precisely how HPV E6 and E7 team up to destroy p53. With genome guardian p53 out of the way, HPV is now able to wreak havoc on human host cells with no molecular qualms. This process is illustrated in the following figure:

As shown above, **Step 1:** Stress activates p53; **Step 2 and 3:** Activated p53 goes on performing tasks of stopping normal cells from becoming cancerous in the nick of time; **Step 4, 5a, and 5b:** HPV releases two ring leaders, E6 and E7 to degrade and subdue p53.

The arch nemesis finally meets its match! Yes, the "V" word comes to mind: Vaccines against HPV. The small family of vaccines serves as a training platform to mentor the host immune system in the way, shape, and form of the HPV virus to enable the production of HPV-combating antibodies.

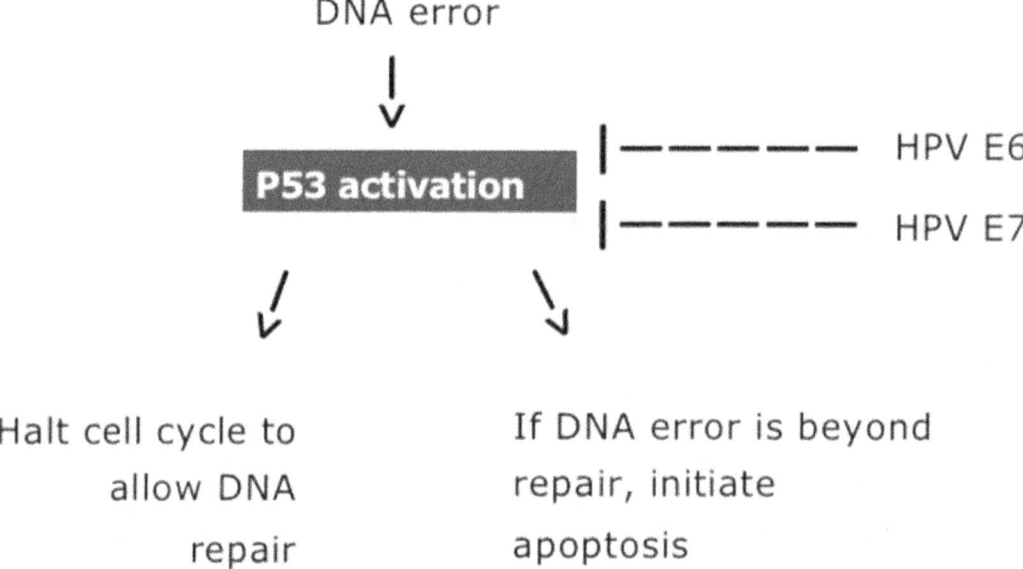

Image 67 P53 subdued by HPV. By Nancy Liu-Sullivan.

Clearance of HPV viruses cleanses the host body's chance of infection, leaving no opportunity for HPV infection-driven cancer to develop. The decades-long vaccination campaign has yielded impressive fruitions: In Scotland in the UK, health officials have announced absence of diagnoses of cervical cancer caused by HPV. A great start! More in-depth descriptions of HPV vaccines combating human cancers can be found in *CANCER VACCINES (2): PREEMPTING CERVICAL CANCER WITH HPV VACCINES* (pages 39–41).

Food for thought:

1. HPV evil duo consisting of E6 and E7 shuffles p53 to a molecular shredder to clear the way for HPV infection-induced cancer cells.
   A. True
   B. False

2. HPV vaccination has demonstrated proof of preempting cervical cancer 100% in the United States.
   A. True
   B. False

Q

QUIRKY SILHOUETTE ON THE WALL AND MUCH MORE

It all started in Bavaria, southern Germany, at a nuclear physics laboratory, in 1895. Dr. Wilhelm Röentgen had been working round the clock for a few weeks on fluorescence production in vacuum tubes. One day, he noticed a spooky greenish ray permeating through the seamlessly sealed test tube and projecting onto the screen wall. What on earth?!

When Dr. Röentgen placed an object between the mysterious energy source and the wall, the ray shone through the object, creating a vivid silhouette on the wall. Magical! Dr. Röentgen coined the electromagnetic wave "X" ray to reflect the first encounter with the unknown ray. In reverence to the discoverer, X-ray is also termed Röentgen ray. Shown in the figure below is the X-ray film of the right hand of Dr. Röentgen's wife. Note the vivid capture of the ring on the finger. Note also that the fingers appeared whitish on the film because bones are high-density tissues that absorb high levels of X-ray.

Radiation creates free radicals. X-ray joins gamma ray as electromagnetic waves; both are ionizing radiation (IR). Two additional types of IR are alpha particle rays and beta particle rays. IR is widely acknowledged for its powerful DNA damage capacity via a direct attack on DNA strands or indirectly via free radicals generated by breaking water molecules in cells. The following figure explains types of IR and means for shielding.

As presented in the above table, IR can take the form of waves or particles. Alpha particles are bigger but lighter than beta particles. Alpha particles can be blocked by a piece of paper or by intact skin. Beta particles are smaller but heavier than alpha particles and can penetrate intact human skin by 0.8 centimeters (cm) but can be shielded by aluminum. Gamma and X-rays, by astounding contrast, are much more powerful and can only be stopped by lead or thick concrete.

Free radicals break DNA. DNA is housed in the nucleus of cells. Up to 70 percent of cell content is water, the good old H_2O, where "H" stands for hydrogen and "O" for oxygen. Water is vulnerable to ionizing radiation (IR). When IR shines through water, it bumps one H out of H_2O, resulting in "-OH," pronounced as "hydroxyl." This newly created species is very unstable because by losing one hydrogen (H), the balance of electrons is disrupted; hence, it turns into "free radicals."

To strive for balance, free radicals resort to "stealing" electrons from neighboring atoms. The victims of such molecular theft could be DNA stored in the cell nucleus. The loss of electrons on DNA strands renders the DNA broken. When too many breaks occur, DNA repair crew becomes overwhelmed, unable to fix all, and before long, DNA mutations arise. Typically, when mutations accumulate in three types of critical genes, namely, cancer-causing genes (or oncogenes), tumor suppressor genes, and DNA repair genes, the affected cell is spellbound for mutation-induced cancer formation in the long run. The IR —> Free Radical —> DNA damage connections are illustrated in the following figure:

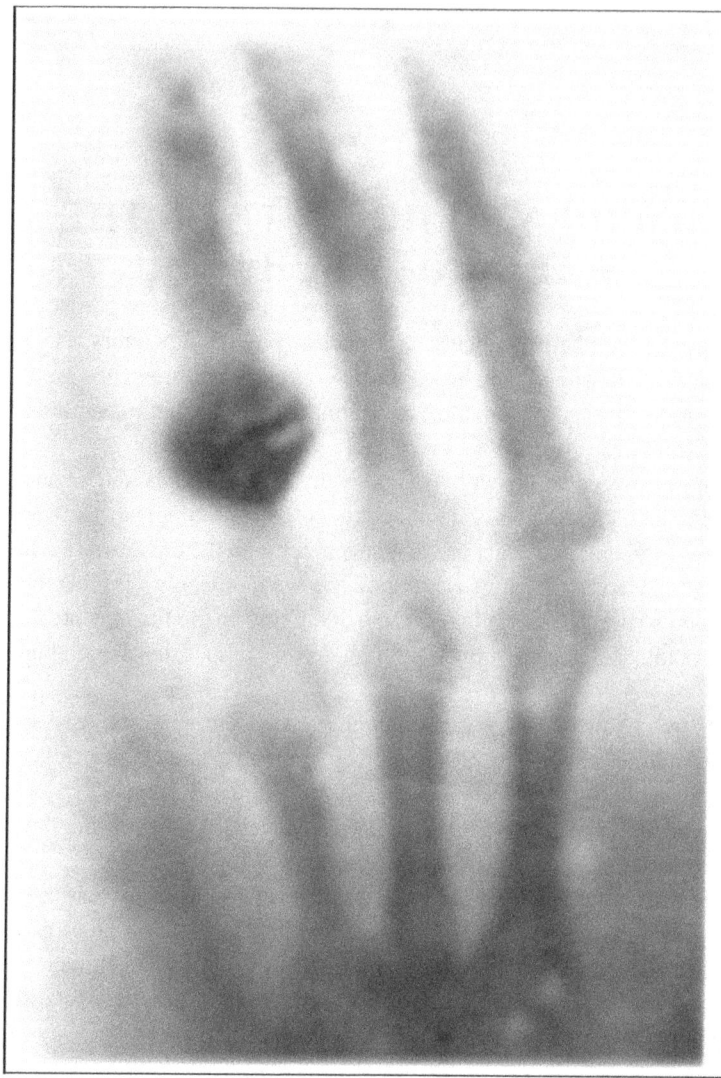

Image 68 Hand with wedding ring: the first-ever medical X-ray. Wikimedia Commons file: First medical X-ray by Wilhelm Röntgen of his wife Anna Bertha Ludwig's hand—18951222.jpg.

Of the four types of ionizing radiation described above, X-rays are the most relevant to our everyday life as a medical imaging platform for broken or fractured bones as well as a tool for cancer diagnostics and radiation therapy. Thanks to scientific advancement, today we are fully aware of how X-ray radiation is effective at treating cancer but also potent enough to cause cancer. That wasn't the case at the turn of the twentieth century, in the glorious days of ingenious inventor Thomas Edison, described in the next essay.

Special note: The original version of this essay was published in the McGill University Office of Science and Society weekly digest.

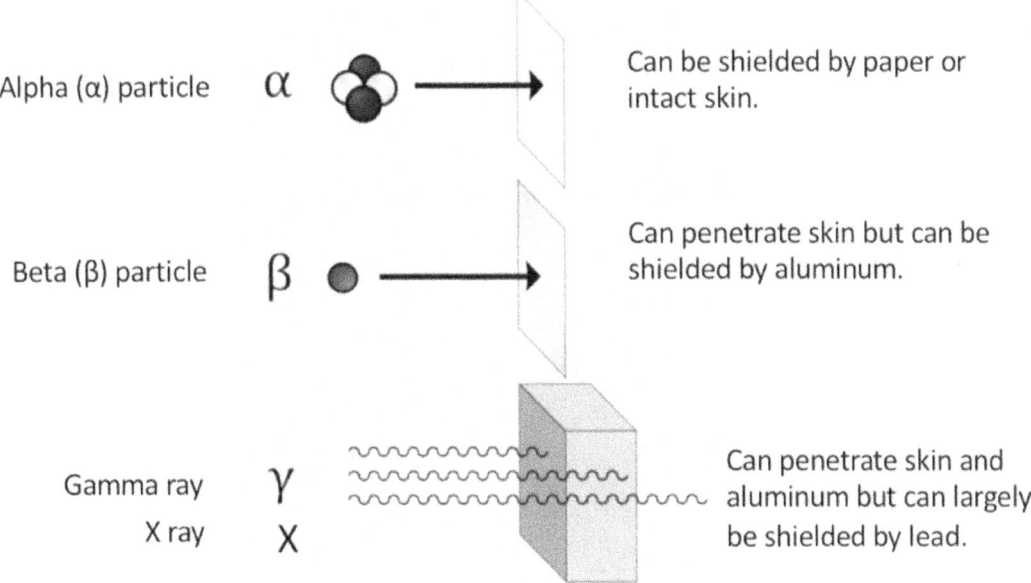

Image 69 Ionizing radiation blockers. Wikimedia Commons File: Alfa beta gamma neutron radiation .svg.

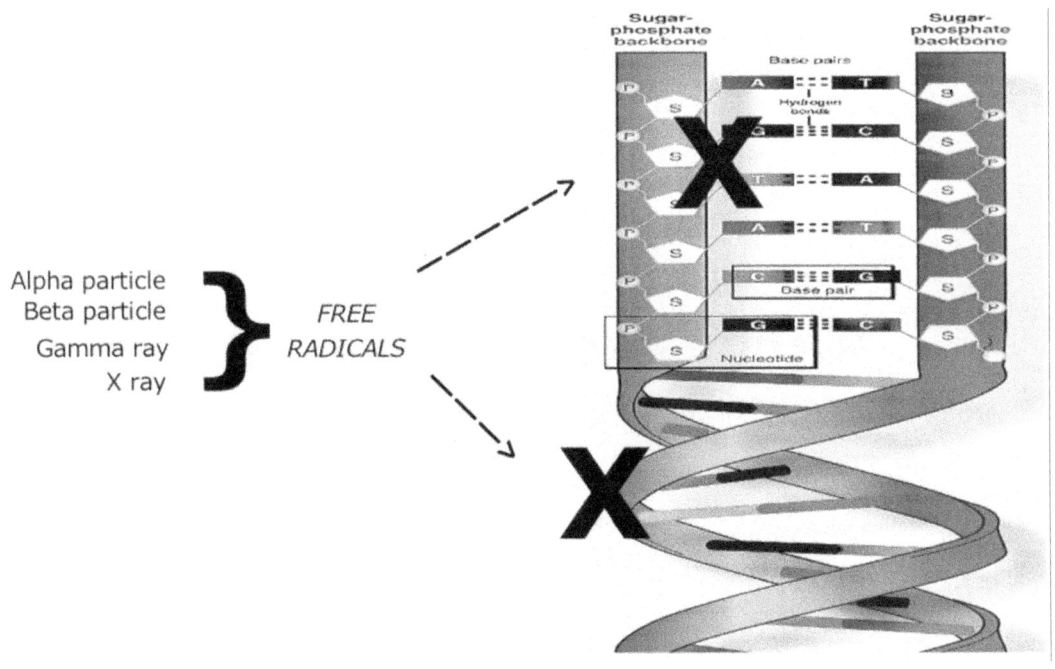

Image 70 IR and free radicals. Wikimedia Commons File: Phosphate backbone.jpg.

Food for thought:

1. X-ray can turn water molecules within cells into free radicals which cause DNA breakage.
   A. True
   B. False

2. X-ray is a double-edged sword in that it can detect and treat cancer but can also cause cancer.
   A. True
   B. False

R

RADIATION AND CANCER (1): EDISON'S NAIVETY AND MANKIND'S LESSON

Despite so many claim-of-fame inventions, Thomas Edison got one thing woefully wrong.

X-ray took the world by storm. Capable of shining through humans to reflect unadulterated inner workings of tissues and bones on a sheet of radiographic film, X-ray fascinated all walks of life. Engineers and inventors lost no time exploring the enormous potential of this enigmatic energy with the goal of improving the quality of life in various facets. Team Thomas Edison excelled. Edison and his research assistant Clarence Dally developed a prototype "fluoroscope" that literally endowed doctors with "X-ray vision." Broken bones, fractured bones, deformed bones, metal nails or pins—nothing could hide away. To optimize the instrument, Edison and Dally worked into the wee hours experimenting with different X-ray tubes.

Edison erred. X-ray's penetrating power made it an excellent medical imaging apparatus. Madam Curie, the discoverer of uranium and polonium, drove X-ray trucks to the battlefields of the First World War around 1916 to help take X-ray images for medical diagnostics of injured allied soldiers. Many quickly learned about the usefulness of X-ray as a tool but none were aware of the ray's devastating harm. Not Madam Curie nor Thomas Edison.

Back in Edison's laboratory, Edison and Clarence Dally were working on two parallel research projects. Dally opted to work with high-energy tubes on fluoroscopes. Long hours every day for eight plus straight years spent in close proximity to intense X-ray tubes without any protection took its terrible toll, to Dally's horror and Edison's astonishment. It began with a burning sensation on Dally's hand, followed by swelling and skin peeling. The inflammation turned into aggressive skin cancer that spread, first to his upper arms and then to his lower limbs so extensively that amputation was carried out to preserve his life. Astounded and extremely guilt-ridden, Edison halted all research on X-rays in his laboratory, footed all Dally's medical bills, and continued to keep Dally on the payroll until his passing.

Dally's sacrifice not in vain. Having worked on the same X-ray research topic, Edison himself did not come out unscathed either: his vision was severely compromised. How come that Edison's condition did not deteriorate to the gory stage of cancer like Dally's? The answer stemmed from the particular caliber of X-ray tube: Edison survived owing to working with low-energy tubes; he also steered clear of any radiation-related research for the rest of his life. Edison even openly declared to the exacting press that he was stupefied by X-ray. The sacrifice by Dally and Edison were not in vain. Mankind managed to learn three precious lessons in the X-ray playbook: (1) high-frequency X-rays are associated with acute physical damage; (2) longer exposure to X-rays exacerbates bodily harm; and (3) X-ray machine handlers ought to be shielded with protective gear.

Ignorance is no bliss. X-ray did not scare everyone away. Unlike Edison, other folks, either unaware of the danger or so fascinated by the awesome imaging power of X-ray that they threw caution to the wind, continued to play with X-ray. Dally passed away in 1904. Yet from the 1920s through the 1950s, a form of foot X-ray became popular in the United States, Canada, the United Kingdom, and Switzerland. Shoe stores boasted X-ray as the new toy in town. Enticed, people, young and old, rushed to lay their feet on the X-ray box for a perfectly fitting pair of shoes. Exposure during a twenty-second X-ray imaging exposed the individual to **0.13 Sv**. To put this in context, let's crunch some numbers:

- 0.13 Sv = 130 mSv = 13,000 mrem
- 620 mrem = Annual average exposure to high-energy radiation in the United States
- 100 mrem = Dose limit of annual public exposure to high-energy radiation, meaning beyond 100 mrem harms kicks in.

So, a single trip to the shoe store for a cool foot X-ray exposed a customer to more than twenty-one times (21×) the annual average radiation exposure and 130 times (130×) above the limit of annual public exposure dose. Dangerously alarming! Due to a lack of record keeping, demographic data on radiation poisoning or radiation-related cancer would be kept in the darkness forever. Finally, in 1957, the state of Pennsylvania banned the use of foot X-ray. By the 1970s, thirty-three states in the United States also banned the machine. Live and learn.

A silver-lining sequel. A single foot X-ray several decades ago exposed an individual to 13,000 mrem which was dangerously high. Since then, X-ray machine design has gone through several rounds of revisiting the drawing board for a much-reduced and hence safer exposure with enhanced efficacy. Below is a list of common medical procedures and associated radiation exposure. "mSv" stands for *milliSievert*, a unit common in Europe, whereas "mrem" stands for *milli rem*, a unit common in America.

As shown above, even a whole body combined PET/CT cancer screening amounts to an exposure of 2,270 mrem, which is very high still with respect to the annual exposure limit of 100 mrem as the comprehensive scan involves three-dimensional imaging. Still, compared to the 13,000 mrem exposure from a single shoe store visit, tremendous progress has been made with modern X-ray machines. Progress is a good thing!

Food for thought:

1. The story of Dally taught us that exposure to high-caliber X-ray tubes without shielding leads to severe skin damage that progresses to skin cancer.
   A. True
   B. False

2. The annual safe limit of radiation exposure is 620 mrem.
   A. True
   B. False

RADIATION AND CANCER (2): SPLENDID RAYS AND SKIN CANCER

Helios, the sun god in Greek mythology, rode a chariot across the sky, east to west, sunrise to sundown, year-round, as dusk gleams silvery moonlight accompanied by stars that extend to infinity followed by

Medical procedure	Radiation exposure (mrem)
Single dental X ray	0.1
Single chest X ray	10
Single mammogram	40
Single CT head scan	200
Single CT chest scan	600-800
Single CT abdomen scan	500-1,000
Single CT/PET whole body scan	800-3,000
Reference values	
Exposure that causes acute radiation sickness	100,000-200,000
Whole body exposure that leads to mortality	1,000,000

Image 71 Radiation types and exposure. By Nancy Liu-Sullivan.

dawn that welcomes renewing sunlight. The sun is not always gentle and rosy in mythological senses but instead can get stupendously stormy and frightfully tempestuous, a phenomenon called a "solar storm." Fortunately, planet Earth is protected from powerful solar rays by invisible but humongous "bubbles" around the Earth. Termed the *magnetosphere*, these giant bubbles form a magnetic shield that blocks off many harmful rays from the sun including, thank goodness, extremely detrimental X-rays and gamma rays. There is, however, one exception: ultraviolet (UV).

Ultraviolet (UV) rays from the sun cast harmful rays on Earth unannounced, undramatically, with no visible fanfare. Abbreviated as UV, ultraviolet rays are a form of electromagnetic (EM) radiation. Radiation is classified by wavelength and frequency on the EM spectrum. A clear trend shown in the figure below indicates that the shorter the wavelength, the higher the frequency (busier cycles), and the higher the energy (more severe harm). Examples of high-energy radiation include alpha, beta, gamma, and X-rays. Conversely, the longer the wavelength, the lower the frequency, and the lower the energy level; hence, the less the level of harm, one example of which is *microwave* although it is recommended to stay two feet away from a microwave apparatus heating a cup of lentil soup in action! UV is a "middle-of-the-roader" that resides between high- and low-energy radiation. However, make no mistake: UV can harm! Let's look closer.

UV's three forms: Ultraviolet rays are classified into three types: UVA (95 percent), UVB (5 percent), and UVC. Both UVA and UVB rays can penetrate the outermost layer of skin called the epidermis, and both are linked to skin damage and increased risks of skin cancer, in addition to compromising the human immune response. UVC is the most energetic; hence, potentially the most damaging. Fortunately, UVC gets filtered by the ozone (O3) layer of our Earth's atmosphere. Where the ozone layer is damaged, however, UVC will readily cast rays on Earth and affect living organisms, including humans. By the way, byproducts termed "CFCs" (chloro-fluoro-carbons) spewed from a long list of everyday items ranging from air conditioners to blowing substances in foam insulation, packaging materials, propellants in aerosol cans, and ubiquitous refrigerators

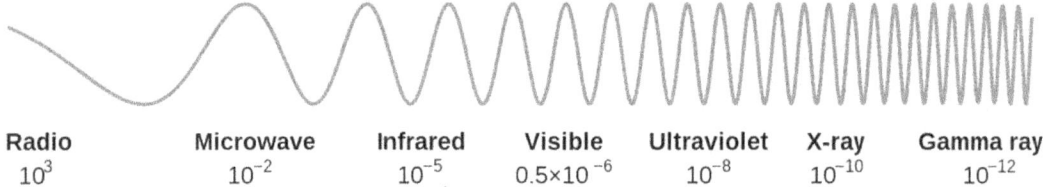

Image 72 Radiation: wavelength, frequency, and power. Wikimedia Commons File: EM Spectrum Properties edit.svg.

are all capable of weakening ozone's capacity of filtering out UVC. Adding to this environmental woe is CO_2—carbon dioxide (CO_2)—another infamous ozone-depleting greenhouse gas. Speaking of CO_2, Columbia University Climate School had an intriguing Q and A posting. The question is here paraphrased: *CO_2 only accounts for 0.04% of the atmosphere. How can such as a minute amount drive outlandish global warming*?! The answer, also paraphrased here: the Earth absorbs solar energy and in turn emits heat (as infrared radiation). Despite the fact that CO_2 makes up less than 0.1 percent of Earth's atmosphere, the other 99 percent consists of nitrogen (78 percent) and oxygen (21 percent), the atoms harbored in CO_2 dance to the same rhythm as the heat emitted by the Earth—the technical term being that the atoms of CO_2 vibrate in such a way best suited to absorb heat. Neither nitrogen nor oxygen are capable of such atomic minute steps. What happens after CO_2 gases absorb the heat given off by Earth? The heat gets evenly split with half returning to Earth and the other half being released into the atmosphere; the latter is none other than the infamous *greenhouse*! To be fair, greenhouse gases are not always bad in that they form a blanket that traps heat to generate a temperature on planet Earth livable for humans. In the absence of the gaseous blanket, the Earth would be too frigid for organisms to survive. The problem arises when excess greenhouse gases gather in the atmospheric blanket, driving Earth's temperature up, driving global warming. By the way, CO_2 has an abettor in exacerbating the greenhouse effect: water vapor. For a detailed description, please visit https://news.climate.columbia.edu/2019/07/30/co2-drives-global-warming/. While much could be done about water vapor, we can and should effectively minimize our carbon footprint as a no-choice choice! Back to UV, how does it put human health in harm's way?

UV and skin cancer. UV, especially UVB, is associated with *thymine dimers*—a type of DNA damage where two adjacent thymine bases are cross-linked to one another instead of being paired with adenine on the DNA double-helical spiral, as shown in the following figure. Any alteration of the DNA sequence is by definition a deviation from the original masterpiece; hence, a mutation. UV-caused thymine dimers are usually timely corrected by our DNA repair crew. If the damage is profound and beyond repair, the cells that bear the damage gets expelled via apoptosis (programmed cell death). If both above mechanisms of damage control fail, a mutation happens that can eventually progress to skin cancer—non-melanoma skin cancer.

There are three distinct types of skin cancer: Basal cell carcinoma (BCC), squamous cell carcinoma (SCC), and melanoma. Although all three types have UV rays as the main culprit, not all skin cancers are the same. BCC arises in skin basal cells. These cells are normally responsible for growing new skin cells to replace old ones. Undetected or detected but left untreated, BCC can inch deeper underneath the skin and spread to neighboring healthy cells. It is said that lighter-skinned folks with lighter eye color are at higher risk for BCC due to less melanin in skin and eyes and less UV protection. That said, proper protection can go a long way and do a lot of good. As for SCC, it is the second most common form of skin cancer in North America. Thanks to progress made, the majority of SCC cases today are treatable.

Melanoma is a different beast. Compared to other skin cancers, melanoma is much more serious and tougher to tackle with therapeutic interventions. It is classified into four stages depending on severity and metastatic properties. To date, the melanoma five-year survival rate is 100 percent for Stage-1, 80 percent for Stage-2, 70 percent for Stage-3, but only 30 percent for Stage-4. Melanoma is malignancy of melanocytes. Melanocytes reside in the skin (also hair follicles, inner ear, and iris of the eye) and secrete melanin. A pigment protein, melanin is a complex polymer derived from tyrosine (one of twenty amino acids that are the building blocks of proteins). Aside from determining color of skin and hair, melanin also shields the skin from the sun's powerful rays. Melanin levels increase in response to skin's sun exposure, resulting in a tan. Extended exposure to the sun or artificial UV rays drives high levels of melanin production as a skin protection and results in a tan, which is nice and cool, but sun tan is actually a form of skin damage which, depending on frequency, duration, and the time and day of exposure, can lead to skin cancer. As Dr. Joe Schwartz—an expert-chemist and an able director of the McGill University Office of Science and Society (OSS) weekly digest—writes to remind readers that no suntan is ever safe (https://www.mcgill.ca/oss/article/

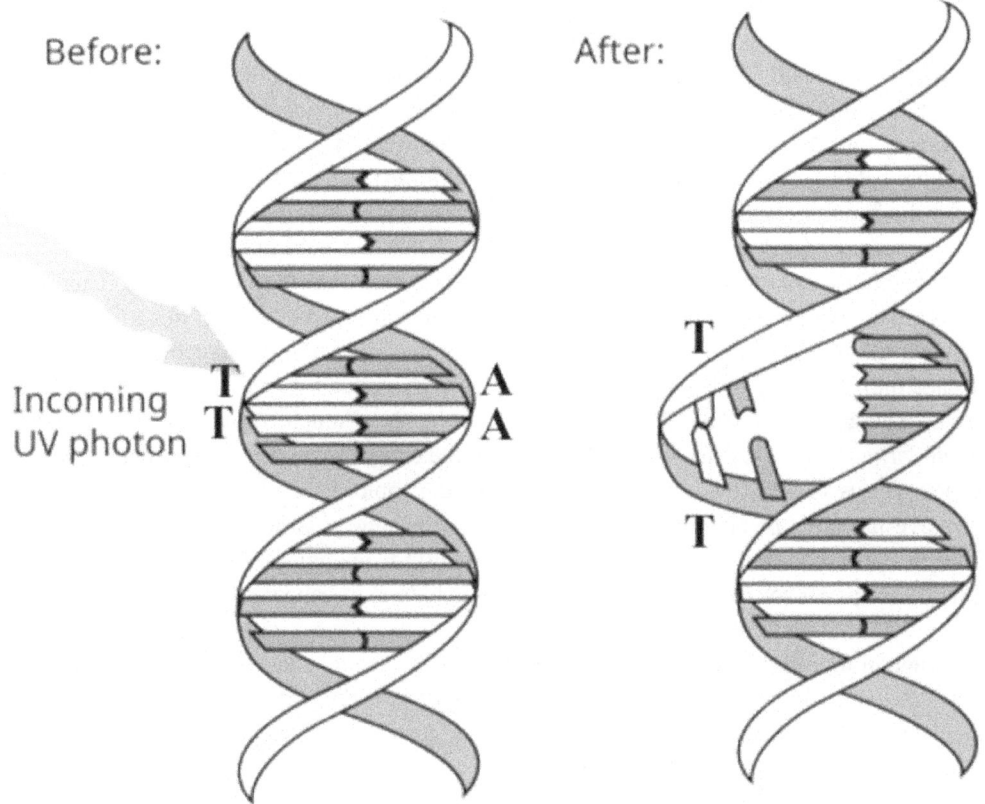

Image 73 UV disrupts DNA. Wikimedia Commons File: DNA UV mutation.svg.

medical-critical-thinking-environment/there-are-safe-sunscreens-no-safe-tans). How is UV skin damage linked to skin cancer?

UV and immune suppression. Being the largest organ and the frontline of immune defense, the skin possesses its own satellite immune system, in parallel to the central immune system. To be exact, the satellite system consists of the whole nine yards of immune barrier, innate arm, and adaptive arm of immunity shown in the following figure (for a detailed description, please refer to *AN ATLAS OF IMMUNE BIG PICTURE*, pages 5–6). The skin immune system covers both the *epidermis* (the outermost skin layer) and an immediate deeper layer termed the "*dermis*." There are also local nodes that channel lymph called "skin-draining lymph nodes." How does UV damage affect skin immunity? For one thing, harmful UV absorption stunts activation of T cells. T cells, especially KT cells, are the movers and shakers of fierce immune elimination of unwanted cells, including cancer cells. Absence or inadequate KT participation in immune battleground spells immune defense failure.

Tanning stations: A crazy idea! UV rays occur naturally, such as those from solar radiation. UV rays can also be generated artificially, for example, in tanning stations. It is said that ultraviolet A (UVA) rays emitted in tanning stations can be up to twelve times more than those from natural sunlight. The American Academy of Dermatology (AAD) states unequivocally the harmful effects of tanning stations on skin health, especially for young people. The ACS describes UV rays as a major cause of melanoma. Several professional healthcare agencies call for a ban of tanning stations. An uphill battle.

Embrace sunscreen! UVA has a longer wavelength that can penetrate the skin more deeply than UVB. For skin protection, resort to sunscreens. The *titanium dioxide* (TiO_2) and *zinc oxide* (ZnO) in the sunscreens collectively build a protective layer, indicated by the thick horizontal line shown in the figure below. This protective layer serves two purposes: as a physical shield and as a reflector to scatter the harmful UV rays.

No, tattooing does not cause cancer, but . . . Not a personal fan of tattooing. That said, live and let live. Quick googling tells a list of eight chemicals embedded in tattoo ink ranging from harmless (such as water and glycerin) to potentially harmful (such as cadmium, lead, and arsenic). You may ask: Why only "*potentially*" harmful for the latter chemicals described above? Thoughtful question. The answer resides in "how much" and "how often," hence the dictum "*The dose makes the poison*," coined by the Swiss physician and Father of Toxicology, Dr. Paracelsus (1493–1541). Okay, returning to the topic at hand here: despite the long and extensive mixtures of chemicals present in tattoo ink, there is no evidence of an association between tattooing and skin cancer, according to a leading skin cancer specialist from MSKCC (https://www.mskcc.org/news/can-tattoos-hide-skin-cancer-advice-msk-how-stay-safe).

Too much of anything is undesirable. Does it mean one should avoid the sun at all costs and at all times? *Na-dah*! Direct sunlight helps convert a type of skin cholesterol to vitamin D, an important molecule involved in hundreds of bodily activities, also indispensable for bone health and good moods. As always, the dose makes the difference.

Special note: The original version of this essay was published in the McGill University Office of Science and Society weekly digest.

Food for thought:

1. UVC is blocked off Earth's atmosphere by ozone.
   A. True
   B. False

2. Both UVA and UVB can damage DNA that leads to skin cancer.
   A. True
   B. False

RADIATION AND CANCER (3): INDELIBLE AUGUST OF 1945

A true saga: Of the three military infrastructure-heavy Japanese cities slated for attack by the atomic bombs to end the Second World War, Hiroshima was the primary target, and the detonation took place on August 6, 1945. Three days later, when the US B-29 bomber was heading toward the second target Japanese city of Kokura, the weather reconnaissance planes ahead of the bomber reported thick clouds mixed with heavy smoke blanketing the city sky with zero visibility. Kokura was spared. The second atomic bomb was dropped, instead, over the third target city of Nagasaki, 95 miles away from Kokura. The fate of an infant boy from Kokurahad was changed forever as a result of inclement weather. Later, he completed doctoral studies in theology in the United States and became an accomplished professor at a premier college on the East Coast.

Black rain. The death toll from the two cities amounted to close to 200,000, estimated a few months post the devastating detonation from the sheer force of direct hit and acute radiation sickness. The dense fiery ashes seeded the clouds in the atmosphere and produced a rainy condensation made up of thick black ashes mixed with deadly radioactive fallout materials that were collectively named the "black rain," bombarding a second hit to the poor survivors who were crawling over decimated soil, this time with radioactivity, silent but with a blaring long-term health impact of cancer in particular.

The rise of blood cancers. Both United States and Japanese agencies established research stations to conduct long-term follow-up studies of the survivors. Three types of cancer incidence excelled on the chart: leukemia, lymphoma, and multiple myeloma. All are blood cancers that arise from WBCs, which are designated cells for immune defense. Quick recap: There exists four major types of ionizing radiation powerful enough to break DNA—alpha particles, beta particles, X-rays, and gamma rays. The latter two are the most debated. The predominant form of high-energy radioactivity that befell on the survivors of Hiroshima and Nagasaki was reported to be gamma rays, capable of penetrating through the human body, leaving a trail of destruction of DNA, cells, tissues, and organs. Cumulative DNA damage that failed to be repaired timely and accurately drives normal cells to lose their cell growth restraints, turning them into wild cells recalcitrant to growth regulations. As a result, one mutated cell divides into two, two becoming four, and four turning into eight, and the expansion goes on. The exponential cell doubling leads to a tumor mass. When the tumor mass breaches the boundaries of the original primary site to invade other healthy cells, tissues, and organs, it has entered the territory of malignant tumors, also termed as metastatic tumors, or simply *cancer*. Back to blood cells: Why are they so vulnerable to harmful radiation? Even though similar concepts have been discussed elsewhere in this book, it's always a good idea to review.

Bone marrow is the most vulnerable. Distributed in the vertebrae, bones of the pelvis, sternum, and ribs, bone marrow is a cell- and blood-forming organ responsible for the supply of all cell types required for normal body functioning. It is widely acknowledged that cells that are less differentiated, well-nourished, and high in metabolic activity are the most sensitive to high-energy radiation damage. Bone marrow fits every criterion of the above benchmark. The concept of "undifferentiated" refers to cells in their original undefined stem state. Indeed, the bone marrow houses blood stem cells termed "hematopoietic stem cells" (HSC) capable of becoming specialized into all cells including blood cells. These blood stem cells are constantly working to fulfill their designated roles. A healthy adult person, for example, is estimated to generate 500 billion blood cells on a daily basis to maintain homeostasis and sustain normal physiological functions. A summary table of cells by degree of vulnerability to radiation damage is listed in the following figure:

The pattern is clear: the more constant and faster the cells divide, the more heightened the cells are in susceptibility to molecular havoc wreaked by high-energy radiation.

Radiation sickness, treatment, and remedies. Typical symptoms associated with radiation sickness range from mild to severe, including dizziness, headache, fever, nausea, diarrhea, low blood pressure, hair loss, infections, and internal bleeding. Radiation sickness treatment consists of external and internal contamination platforms. For external contamination, the first order of business is to reduce the extent of contamination by removing clothes and shoes, followed by washing off contaminated skin with soap and water. Internal radiation contamination treatment agents include (1) *potassium iodide* that saturates the thyroid gland absorption sites, leaving no room for radioactive iodine to bind; (2) *Prussian blue*, a chemical dye that binds to two forms of radioactive elements termed "cesium" and "palladium" and excreted as fecal matter; (3) *DTPA* (di-ethylene-tri-amine penta-acetate acid), a chemical that binds to radioactive particles of "plutonium," "americium," and "curium" for elimination through urine excretion.

Destruction of bone marrow severely compromises the production of the needed immune cells for health defense. As a result, radiation sickness victims are extremely prone to infections. To ameliorate the condition, a protein called "G-CSF" (granulocyte colony-stimulating factor) is prescribed to strengthen the patient's immune system by promoting WBC growth. So far, three types of G-CSF drugs have been approved by the FDA. These are *Neupogen* (by Amgen,

CELL TYPES	CELL RENEWAL FREQUENCY	RADIATION SENSITIVITY
Stem blood cells	Very high	Very high
Egg cells & sperm cells	High	High
Intestinal cells	High	High
Skin cells and hair follicles	High	High
Salivary gland & thyroid gland	Moderate	Modetate
Muscle cells & nerve cells	Slow	Low

Image 74 Human cell types and ionizing radiation sensitivity. Assembled by Dr. Nancy Liu-Sullivan.

Thousand Oaks, CA), *Zarxio* (by Sandoz, Princeton, NJ), and *Nivestym* (by Pfizer, Manhattan, NY). All three drugs are also used to help boost WBCs in cancer patients who have undergone chemotherapy treatment.

Rewinding back to 1945: Residents of the city of Kukora were unaware of just how close they were to being spared of the destructive A-bomb until much later. A new saying, *Kukora's Luck*, has since been added to the Japanese vernacular. The city of Kukora also declared itself a nuclear-free peace city. Hope *Kukora's Luck* is forever bestowed upon every corner of planet Earth.

Food for thought:

1. Blood cancers are the most frequent cancers that arise from high-level exposure to ionizing radiation.
   A. True
   B. False

2. Potassium iodine protects people from radioactive iodine destruction by occupying all binding pockets in the thyroid gland, leaving no room for radioactive iodine to be absorbed.
   A. True
   B. False

RADIATION AND CANCER (4): PANTHEON'S ETERNAL COUPLE

Modeled after the Roman Temple of All Gods, the Pantheon French National Cemetery located in the Latin Quarter of Paris houses starry French luminaries such as Rousseau, Voltaire, Zoila, and many more. Among the constellations is a special science couple: Marie Curie and Pierre Curie. Unique to Madam Curie's casket is the encasing of a thin layer of lead, a high-density metal that blocks ionizing radiation.

Madam Curie coined the term "radioactivity." A series of seminal discoveries in nuclear physics were unveiled around late nineteenth and early twentieth centuries, exemplified by the identification of X-rays by Wilhelm Conrad Röntgen in 1895, followed by the revelation of uranium-emitted uranic rays by Henri Becquerel in 1896. Two years later, in 1899, in-depth and studious scrutiny by the Curies led to the discovery of two brand new chemical elements, polonium and radium that emitted far more powerful radioactive rays than uranium. Madam Curie also coined the very term of "radioactivity." These pioneering physicists were awarded the Nobel Prize in Physics in 1901 to Wilhelm Conrad Röntgen and in 1903 jointly to Henri Becquerel and the Curies.

The glow had a catch. Uranium was first extracted from a mineral deposit called pitchblende. To the Curies' amazement, the mineral mixture emitted substantially elevated levels of radioactivity compared to uranium alone. They hypothesized that there must be additional elements in the pitchblende that were radioactive. Indeed, the Curies discovered not just one but a pair of such elements, which they named one "radium" and the other "polonium" (in memory of Madam Curie's ancestral country of Poland). Unaware of the dangers of radioactivity, Madam Curie routinely kept sample bottles of radium and polonium inside her desk drawer, in her pocket, and on the nightstand at home. As discussed in **RADIATION AND CANCER (3): INDELIBLE AUGUST OF 1945**, the most vulnerable human cells to radiation damage are the stem cells in the bone marrow due to their high rate of growth and metabolism. Years of exposure to an environment in the lab and at home replete with harmful rays led to Madam Curie being diagnosed with a blood cancer called "aplastic pernicious anemia." Her bone marrow essentially stopped producing blood cells, red or white. Madam Curie passed away on July 4, 1934, at the age of sixty-six.

In the old days before mankind became aware of radiation harms, no one was spared, from scientists and engineers to everyday folks. In addition to the X-ray shoe stores we have described, there was another major radioactive incident in the 1920s in the United State involving glow-in-the-dark hand watches. The dials and hands of the popular watch were hand-painted by women workers in factories in New Jersey, Connecticut, and Illinois. The paint contained a mixture of radium powder, water, phosphorus, and glue. To ensure meticulous painting, the workers were instructed to make the paintbrush pointed using their mouths and lips! Now, radium emits all three types of ionizing radiation: alpha particles, beta particles, and gamma rays. Alpha particles can be blocked by intact skin; however, when ingested, such as *"licking the brush to make the end pointed for fine painting of the dials,"* alpha particles were in direct contact with components of the oral cavity. Beta particles can readily penetrate intact skin for 0.8 centimeters. And of course, so powerful that only lead and thick concrete can block, gamma rays cut through the skin and through the body like a knife through butter. As the rays enter the human body, they commit molecular "slash and burn" to the DNA of any cells, particularly bone marrow blood stem cells, in their path. Not surprisingly, several dozen of the watch painters died of radiation poisoning; others suffered from gruesome damage to their teeth and bones. One worker had horrific damage to her jaw such that her entire jawbone had to be surgically removed to preserve her life. The beautiful green glow emitted at night from the watch had a terrible catch!

Half-life and radio decay. Madam Curie worked indefatigably on studying radium and polonium her entire life until shortly before her passing in 1934. Her body and her laboratory notebooks, the legacy of her scientific career and the treasure of mankind, however, all got contaminated with radioactive substances. Now, radioactive elements do undergo a decaying process calculated as a unit time associated with a 50 percent reduction of radioactivity termed as "half life" or "t1/2." Radium has a half-life of close to 1,600 years, meaning it takes 1,600 years for the radium to lose 50 percent of its radioactivity, another 1,600 years to lose half of the remaining 50 percent, and so on. An eternity for us mortal humans! To protect visitors of the Pantheon, Madam Curie's casket is covered with a radiation-blocking lead shield. Visitors are required to sign a liability waiver and to wear protective gear.

The sacrifice of Madam Curie and her contribution make it possible to turn radiation into a main pillar of cancer treatment. In fact, Madam Curie was the first to envision radiotherapy to destroy cancer cells. Indeed, radiation treatment has saved so many by delaying cancer progression and extending patients' lives. For that, the Curies have fundamentally changed the world. Allow me to dedicate a selective excerpt of an elegant poem, *The Life That I Have* (by Leo Marks), to the marvelous science couple. Mr. Marks, a British cryptographer during the Second World War, wrote the poem in memory of his sweetheart, who unexpectedly died in a plane crash. Each word, line, and stanza echoes the life, love, and the pursuit of science forever cherished by Maria Sklodowska-Curie (1867–1934) and Pierre Curie (1859–1906).

The life that I have
by Leopold Samuel Marks (1920–2001)
The life that I have
Is all that I have
And the life that I have
Is yours.
. . .
For the peace of my years
In the long green grass
Will be yours and yours and yours.
Notes: Unable to locate ownership of the above poem, I decided to quote here only the first and the last stanzas, in deference of poet Leo Marks' intellectual property rights. Hope that suffices.

RADIATION & CANCER (5): A DOUBLE-EDGED SWORD

Radiation beams obliterate cancer cells and shrink tumors. The same powerful rays can also damage healthy cells, giving rise to secondary cancers, that is, cancers caused by radiation treatment. The treatment gives rise to the same disease the treatment is targeting. Ironic, but bleakly true.

Traditional radiation therapy is imprecise. In spite of meticulous mapping and conforming to the tumor, traditional radiation therapy tends not to be very precise. Specifically, while zapping out cancer cells by destroying their DNA, the high-energy beams invariably leave a trail of "collateral damage" to healthy cells adjacent to the tumor and along the exit path on the other side of the patient's body. While it is true that healthy cells possess DNA repair capabilities much more robustly than those of cancer cells, the long-term impact of healthy cell damage by radiotherapy is nonetheless unavoidable, so much so that it induces secondary cancers. The sites of secondary cancers are closely associated with organs near the site of radiation. Hodgkin's lymphoma patients, for example, receive radiotherapy to the chest, and secondary cancers tend to arise in the breast or the lungs. In a similar vein, radiation treatment to the abdomen tends to give rise to cancers of the stomach, liver, and pancreas. The following side-by-side figures illustrate extensive damage to healthy tissues by the tumor as indicated by the cross signs; by contrast, the tumor treated by proton beam therapy has predominant radiation beams targeted on the tumor. More about proton beam therapy next.

Proton beam therapy comes to the rescue! Unlike traditional radiation that relies on high-energy *photon beams* produced by bombarding electrons against a tungsten plate, *proton* beams are generated by separating protons from hydrogen atoms and accelerating them in a synchrotron or a cyclotron (both are particle accelerators). The first attempt at proton beam therapy (PBT) took place at Lawrence Berkeley National Laboratory in 1954. Since then, proton beam centers have been on the rise (***LET THEM EAT CAKE: ON CANCER CARE DISPARITY,*** page 119)

Proton unmatched superiority. Two key features of PBT make this radiotherapy more superior to traditional radiation therapy: First, 80–95 percent of the energy is released at the end of the

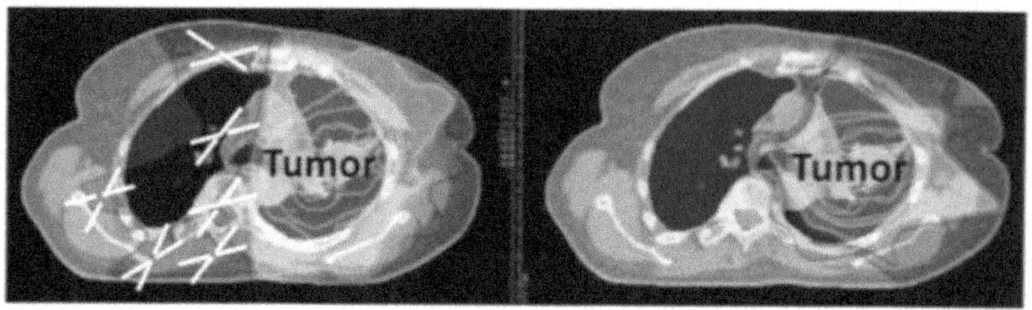

Image 75 Traditional radiotherapy vs. proton beam therapy. Adapted from http://www.cancer.gov/news-events/cancer-currents-blog/proton-therapy-safety-versus-traditional-radiation

beam's path. Second, proton beams do *NOT* pass through the body but instead all the high and formidable energy is deposited directly in the tumor. This means that more energy is focused on the tumor while maximally sparing healthy cells. On average, cancer patients who undergo proton beam treatment receive 60 percent less radiation, in stark contrast to traditional radiotherapy. Magnificent technology, but it also comes with an extremely dear price tag: $225 million per treatment center. The cyclotron particle accelerator itself occupies a space that size of a hockey field. There are forty-five proton beam centers in the United States, as shown in the map adopted from *Proton-Therapy.org*.

A wide range of cancers are treated by proton beam therapy, from cancers of the brain, breast, and prostate to cancers of the lung, head and neck, and cancers of soft tissues called sarcomas. Consistent with the high expense of building a proton beam center, treatment costs are also much higher than conventional radiotherapy. More about this topic is discussed in **HOUSTON, WE HAVE A PROBLEM** (page 99).

Food for thought:

1. The double edges of radiation therapy reside in the fact that the same radiation can destroy cancer cells to shrink tumors, but patients who have undergone high doses of radiation therapy can also develop secondary cancers defined as cancers that arise as a result of radiation treatment.
    A. True
    B. False

Proton Beam Centers Info: > than 100 in the world			
United States	46	Mexico	1
Japan	14 - 19	Thailand	1
China	5	South Africa	1
France	5	Argentina	1
Germany	5	Egypt	1
Singapore	3	Saudi Arabia	1
The Netherlands	3	Switzerland	1
UK	2	Spain	10 in planning for 2026
South Korea	2	Australia	WIP
Sweden	1	Canada	WIP

Image 76 Proton beam centers in the world. Assembled by Dr. Assembled by Dr. Nancy Liu-Sullivan.

2. Our understanding of radiation and its application to healthcare has come a long way. A more in-depth understanding can help improve the technology to maximize treatment efficacy while minimizing adversary effects.
   A. True
   B. False

RHAPSODY OF RAS (1): THE BIG BEGUILING MOLECULAR WOLF

Initially isolated from a rat RNA tumor virus, Ras genes have captivated the time, dedication, and intellect of several generations of cancer scientists, including my very own PhD mentor, Dr. Dafna Bar-Sagi. What has earned Ras an indisputable spot on the pedestal of cancer molecular biology? The reason is simple but at once complex: Ras is the most recognized *"big, bad, and beguiling molecular wolf"* that drives 95 percent pancreatic cancer, 50 percent colorectal cancer, and 30 percent lung cancer.

Three flavors. Owing to the association with "Rat sarcoma," the rat virus was so named "Ras." Small in size but coming from a big family with several dozen members, Ras is classified into three types: H-Ras, K-Ras, and N-Ras, respectively. An extensive list of cancer types harbor Ras mutations, including pancreatic cancer, colorectal cancer, lung cancer, thyroid cancer, and leukemias. Of these, the presence of Ras mutations in pancreatic cancer is the most outstanding, at a whopping 95 percent—*Ras on mutational "triple espresso."* Ras is found in normal cells as well, responsible for cell growth, differentiation, metabolism, and movement. In molecular genetics, the normal healthy copy of a gene is called "wild type" (the norm); the counterpart is "mutant" (anomaly). Mutant Ras genes produce mutant Ras proteins. Recall that amino acid chains are folded into three-dimensional species to be inducted as fully functional proteins. Ras mutant protein inflicts a serious defect: It holds the protein in a forever "Active" position, as if a car in permanent "Drive" mode. In molecular jargon, the "Active" position of Ras is called "*GTP-bound*," and the "Inactive" position is called "*GDP-bound*," as illustrated in the following figure:

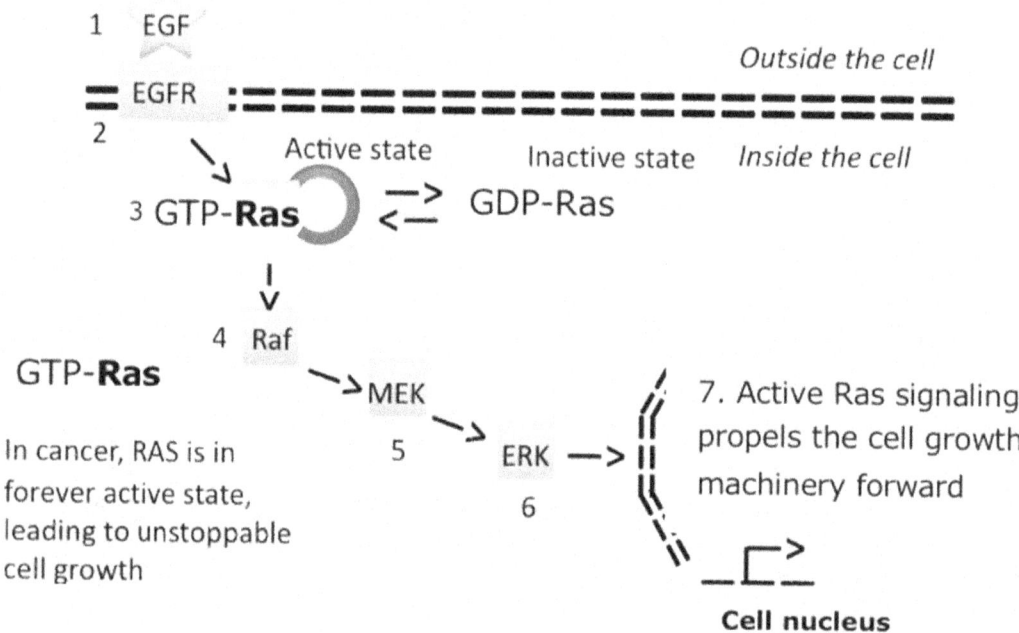

Image 77 Ras propels cell growth machinery. By Nancy Liu-Sullivan.

As shown above, the "Active" *GTP* mode drives the Ras signaling cascade and keep on going, driving the cell into a forward-going peddling mode of churning out more cells as well as proteins. By the way, GTP stands for guanosine triphosphate whereas GDP for guanosine diphosphate. Ras-GTP is the equivalent of a car in "Drive" gear, whereas Ras-GDP is in "Park" gear. Allow me to tell a grad school trivia: one of my doctoral thesis experiments involved purification of a Ras molecular "cousin" called Rho. Several months of hard work were finally beginning to see the long-awaited light at the other side of the tunnel. Then the 2003 Northeast blackout happened. I still remember vividly of that August midafternoon when the entire research building was ordered to evacuate. I was in the cold room working on the last step of the experiment. No way was I going to give up months of work. I calmly stayed, completed what was needed to be done by flash light, then walked out of the building, feeling so accomplished.

The Ras signaling cascade. As shown in the figure above, Ras is situated in the inner space of the cell membrane, acting like a relay station to pass signaling from the cell-surface receptor protein downstream all the way to the cell nucleus. That is what happens in healthy cells. In cancer, the hyperactive GTP state locks Ras in forever active mode and the "Grow-Grow-Grow" signal keeps on propelling downstream through Raf, MEK, and ERK to drive the cell cycle machine forward. No surprise that all major components along the Ras pathway are cancer-promoting proteins or oncoproteins. The extensive involvement of additional proteins adds momentum to Ras but also creates opportunities for therapeutic interventions. After all, suppressing any protein along the Ras cascade shuts down the entire chain of actions. Small molecule inhibitors against Raf have recently received approval by the FDA for the treatment of melanoma.

Epiphany over the Longfellow Bridge. February 5, 1978, a nor'easter blanketed the greater Boston region. The entire city was shut down. Treading along the Longfellow Bridge that leads to the Massachusetts Institute of Technology (MIT) was a determined young fellow, one step after another, through the historic blizzard, heading for his cancer research laboratory located on the other side of the Charles River, while pondering the ongoing project of how to identify *THE DNA* segment from bladder cancer cells shown to be capable of transforming prim-and-proper normal cells into unsettling and aggressive tumor cells. As the pristine snowflakes were coming down, one by one, each unique, each with a character... Suddenly, *AHA*! How about screening the DNA segment one at a time, just like the snowflakes falling one after the next? Dr. Robert Weinberg murmured. A din started as a hum and grew into a grand symphony. The revelation worked! One year later, a milestone discovery stunned the cancer research community: the discovery of the very first human oncogene, H-Ras! Subsequently, K-Ras and N-Ras cancer-causing genes were also discovered in human cancer cells. Instrumental to the discovery processes, alongside the Weinberg Lab at MIT, are the Wigler Lab at Cold Spring Harbor Laboratory (CSHL), the Weiss Lab at the Institute of Cancer Research in London pioneered by Chris Marshall and Alan Hall, the Cooper Lab at Harvard University, and team Barbacid and Aaronson at the National Institutes of Health (NIH).

***Src*, the first brick of cancer molecular scaffolding.** Paving the road to human oncogenic Ras discoveries is the paradigm-shifting discovery of the *Src* gene from a viral origin that regulates normal cellular processes but also capable of going awry to wreak molecular havoc that drive the initiation of cancer! The two scientists who made the seminal discovery and won the 1989 Nobel Prize in Physiology or Medicine are Dr. Michael Bishop and Dr. Harold Varmus. I am taking the liberty to dedicate the following note to Dr. Varmus: Aside from helming MSKCC as President and CEO (2000–10), Dr. Varmus served two terms as director of the National Cancer Institute (NCI) from 2010–15. An extraordinary mind, Dr. Varmus is talented in natural sciences, also gifted in the humanities. He devoted his undergraduate studies to English literature and poetry. Legend has it that working on a joint grant proposal with Dr. Varmus is akin to going to school on science and English, for in addition to suggestions on more rational experimental design and sounder methodology, the lucky co-author would receive returned pages peppered with red ink corrections on syntax, semantics, diction, even spelling!

The next two essays describe an instrumental role played by oncogenic Ras in the tumor microenvironment (TME) and the hunt for a potent anti-Ras drug plus work-in-progress on a Ras vaccine. Stay tuned!

Food for thought:

1. Ras mutations are found in nearly 100% of all forms of pancreatic cancer.
    A. True
    B. False

2. Ras consists of three isoforms designated as H-Ras, K-Ras, and N-Ras.
    A. True
    B. False

RHAPSODY OF RAS (2): IN THE EYE OF CANCER STORM

If cancer were to wail a sob story, the two top topics are sugar shortage and oxygen deprivation. When the two defects mingle, however, a monstrous gene becomes full-blown. You've guessed it: the gene is oncogenic Ras and the consequences exclusively favor cancer. Let's catch a closer glimpse.

Mutant Ras boosts cancer fuel supply. Cancer cells are in constant need of glucose to make cellular fuel to sustain constant growth and expansion. When demand exceeds supply, a crisis is in the making. What are cancer cells to do about the dearth of glucose? An intriguing observation was made where cancer cells that harbor mutant Ras show high levels of a protein responsible for shuffling glucose Morley core into cancer cells. This glucose receptor molecule is termed "glucose transporter 1" (GLUT-1). More GLUT-1 leads to more glucose to feed cancer cells, which confers a survival advantage for them. Worth mentioning is that GLUT-1 and its glucose transporter "cousin" called GLUT-4 have had their respective crystal structures solved by Dr. Nieing Yan, paving the way for in-depth analysis of the physical properties that can shed light on rational drug design against overactive cancer glucose gates. Interesting to point out that Dr. Yan was mentored by Dr. Yigong Shi, who was the protégé of Dr. Joan Massagué, who directs the Sloan Kettering Institute (SKI) of MSKCC). Speaking of passing on the torch!

Mutant Ras rescues cancer cells from an oxygen crisis. We described above that since cancer growth outpaces new blood vessel formation, cancer cells are in a constant state of oxygen deprivation, also termed *"hypoxia."* **Quick Word Anatomy:** *Hypo* = under, *Oxia* = oxygen; together *Hypoxia* = oxygen deficiency (to tissues). Unable to confront the oxygen crisis head-on, cancer adapts, and mutant Ras plays a key role. In specific, mutant Ras promotes the expression of VEGF which translates to *vascular endothelial growth factor*—a molecule instrumental for forming blood vessels.

How does⟩ ⟩ mutant Ras initiate this molecular feat? Think about what is done to release water out of a dam for field irrigation: Just release the gate and channel the water through a network of canals that reach the fields. Metaphorically, mutant Ras engages in something very similar by pressing the *ON* button of a key vessel-forming molecule HIF1a (*hypoxia inducing factor 1 alpha*). By the way, the biomedical jargon for vessel formation is *angiogenesis*. **Quick Word Anatomy:** *Angio* = vessel, *Genesis* = creation; together *Angiogenesis* = blood vessel formation. What is the biological consequence of activating *HIF1a?* The aim is crystal clear: To augment VGEF which in turn boosts *angiogenesis*. Now, we have completed sketching the **Cancer ↔ mutant Ras** feedback loop as summarized in the following interconnected tiles in the molecular game of dominoes:

Cancer growth outpacing blood supply as the initiating event:

- *Leads to* Poor oxygen (hypoxia) in tumor core, *which*
- *Leads to* Action by mutant Ras, *which*
- *Leads to* Activation of HIF1a gene, *which*
- *Leads to* Augmentation *of* VGEF gene, *which*
- *Leads to* CANCER ANGIOGENESIS

Not surprisingly, the big bad beguiling cancer-causing gene of Ras is situated in the eye of the cancer storm, as illustrated below in a highly simplified fashion. Of course, for cancers where Ras mutation is not center stage, other mechanisms may evolve as part of the overall selective pressure within the tumor microenvironment (TME) which confers cancer survival advantage.

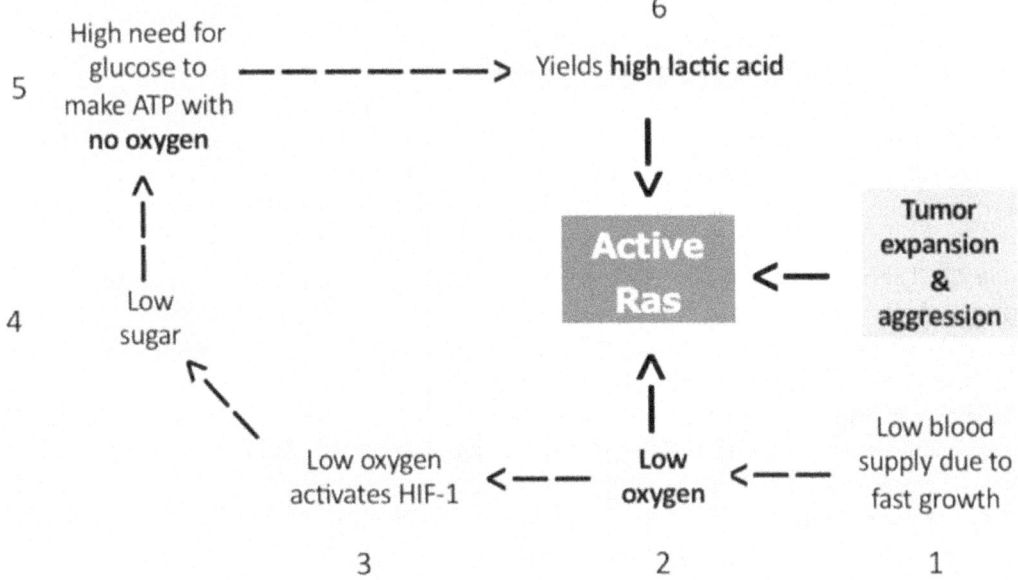

Image. 78 Ras at center stage of tumor village. Assembled by Dr. Nancy Liu-Sullivan.

At this point you must be asking: Given the long "molecular wrap sheet" of Ras mutations, are there anti-Ras cancer drugs available? The answer is YES AND FINALLY! Indeed, it has taken several decades and several generations of Ras pioneers to brainstorm and tinker with assorted ideas in developing a drug that jams cancer-causing Ras. The hard work has finally yielded the long, long-awaited fruition: not one but two Ras inhibitor drugs have received FDA approval, while in parallel, a Ras vaccine is also on the horizon. Good things happen in threes! More discussion next

Food for thought:

1. Mutant Ras facilitates cancer cells in making new blood vessels to sustain cancer's unstoppable growth and expansion.
   A. True
   B. False

2. The reliance on surviving in a low oxygen environment drives cancer to pursue making cellular fuel ATP in the absence of oxygen.
   A. True
   B. False

RHAPSODY OF RAS (3): HOOKED, FINALLY!

The hunt for an anti-Ras drug potent enough to disable the entire Ras signaling cascade and to gut cancer at its very root has been a long battle and the dream mission for several decades. Why has it taken so long?

No holds on the climbing wall. Imagine an indoor climber climbing a wall, grabbing onto the holds with hands and feet, one after another, moving upward toward the destination. Now imagine a climber stuck at the foot of the wall with NO HOLDS to grab onto! This is exactly the conundrum Ras scientists confronted: NO molecular HOLDS for the prospective drug to sink into to jam Ras. There was a promising breakthrough in 2013, but it was not until 2021 when the perfect-on-paper design was eventually turned into a real-life product and also received FDA approval for emergency use for the treatment of lung cancer. Let's look more closely at what made the turning point in this hard-to-come-by drug.

Codon 12: The mutation hotspot. RNA is a single strand made up of codons, with each codon consisting three of the four four bases of A (adenine), U (uracil), G (guanine), and C (cytosine), such as "AUG" or "UGG." Each codon represents an amino acid and all twenty amino acids have designated codons, shown in the following diagram:

As shown above, on the "wheel of RNA codons," there is a first-tier central ring of A-U-G-C surrounded by a second-tier ring of G-A-C-U, divided into four quarters followed by a third-tier ring of G-A-C-U consisting of a cluster of six that corresponds to each of the four quarters of the second-tier ring. To translate each RNA codon into an amino acid, one simply follows a very procedural process: First, select a base from the first-tier ring, then select a base from the second-tier ring, followed by selecting a base from the third-tier ring. Let us have a practice run for the amino acid *methionine*, which corresponds to the START codon. Here we go:

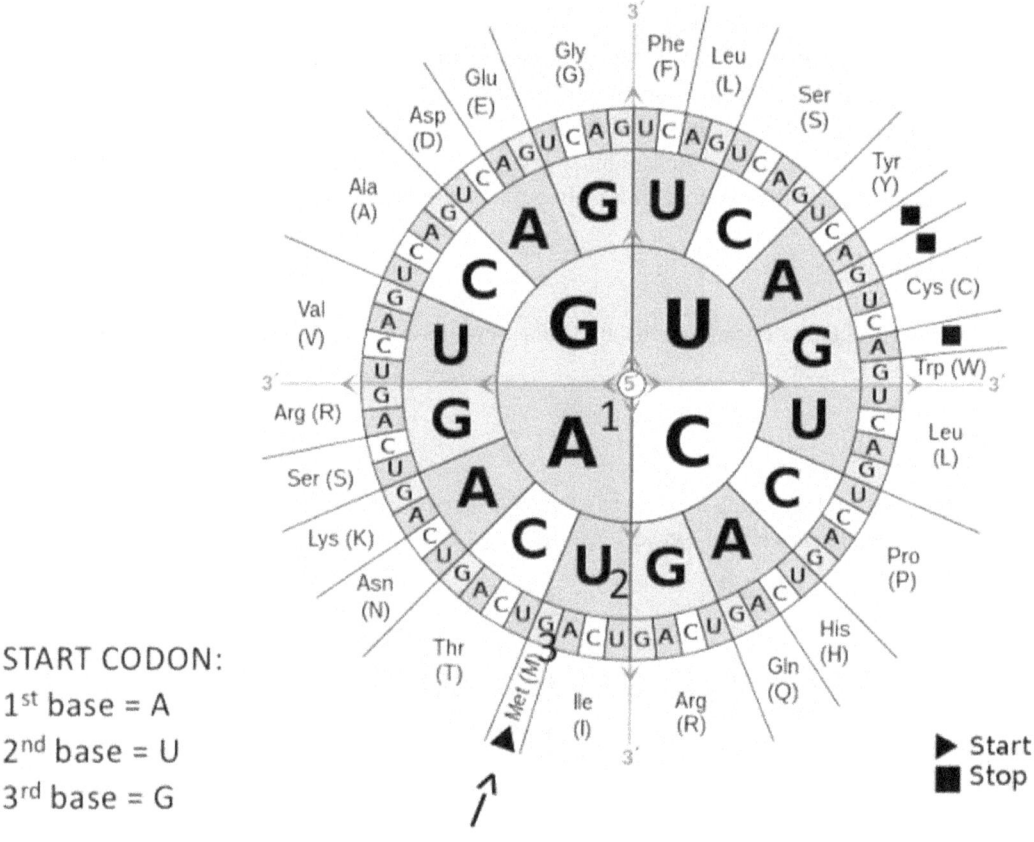

START CODON:
1st base = A
2nd base = U
3rd base = G

Image.E 79 The RNA code. Wikimedia Commons File: Amino acids table.svg.

Step 1: Select A from the central ring;
Step 2: Select U from the second-tier ring;
Step 3: Select G from the third-tier ring

There it is, we now have **AUG,** the RNA codon that codes for the amino acid methionine! A cakewalk. If one really wishes to pin down why AUG is designated for the leader position of the amino acid chain, here is a fun game of free association that I applied to help make an unforgettable mental note as I was hitting the books for my molecular genetics class final years ago: *Augustus was the first Roman emperor*! AUG, alpha in Roman history, is also an alpha RNA codon.

Here is a more germane question: How many RNA codons are there from the four bases of A-U-G-C with three bases per codon? Well, a simple plug-in is $4\wedge 3 = 64$, read as "4 to the power of 3 yields 64" possible codons. Why the need for sixty-four codons while there are only twenty amino acids? The answer is molecular spare tire. Certain amino acids have more than one RNA codon to their name. The answer is written in the wheel of RNA codons. Try it out and have fun!

Mysterious mutant Ras Codon 12. Having walked through interesting aspects of RNA codons, let's take a look at the mysterious Ras mutant RNA codon 12. Which Ras form? K-Ras. What type of mutation? A *substitution mutation* as Kras-G12C, where the original amino acid at the twelfth position is supposed to be G for glycine, but is substituted by another amino acid C which represents "aspartic acid." This hot spot mutation is particularly dominant in pancreatic cancer, lung cancer, and colon cancer.

Skating ahead of the KRas-G12C puck! A popular motto among biologists goes like this: Search and search again, leaving no stone unturned. Recall that Ras works like a "binary" system of *ON* (for GTP) and *OFF* (for GDP), akin to "1" and "0." One way of preventing Ras from latching onto GTP is to lock Ras in its inactive state of GDP. Easier said than done! Even if locking Ras in GDP could be achieved, how to prevent Ras from bouncing back from GDP to the active state of GTP? Scientists did find a way that allows them to skate ahead of the mutant Ras puck next landing spot that allowed scientists to pour molecular concrete into it such that when Ras is ready to slide into the GTP molecular pocket, the pocket is no longer there because it has been filled up with no more room for Ras. BRILLIANT! The indefatigable team of scientists who deserve every credit for the wondrous work is from Amgen, a leading biotech company located in the San Francisco Bay Area. Specifically, they designed a chemical drug that acts like a molecular concrete that occupies the GTP binding pocket, hence preventing mutant Kras from getting into the GTP *ON* position, which permanently locks mutant KRas in its GDP *OFF* position. Well done! The name of the drug is "AMG 510." The mechanism of action is illustrated below:

Ras meets its match, finally! How good is the AMG 510? The proof is in the clinical pudding. A Phase I clinical trial participated in by lung cancer patients reported 31 percent response rate; that is. One-third of the patients responded to the treatment. Phase II reproduced the result of 32 percent. A few lung cancer patients achieved CR and are cancer-free! Since receiving emergency status approval from the FDA in May 2021, AMG 510 has also been granted permission by the European Union (EU).

Now after forty years of perspiration and inspiration, mutant Ras, the big bad beguiling "molecular wolf" is finally confronting a tough "house" not made by mushy straws, not by flimsy sticks, but by rock-solid bricks. Just as the fabled "wolf" was no longer invincible, so is oncogenic mutant Ras! Since AMG 510 (also called "*Sotorasib*"), there has been another new drug ("*Adagrasib*") that also targets KRAS-G12C from another biotech company. Finally, a potent molecular arsenal that targets cancers that harbor Kras mutations is available. Bravo!

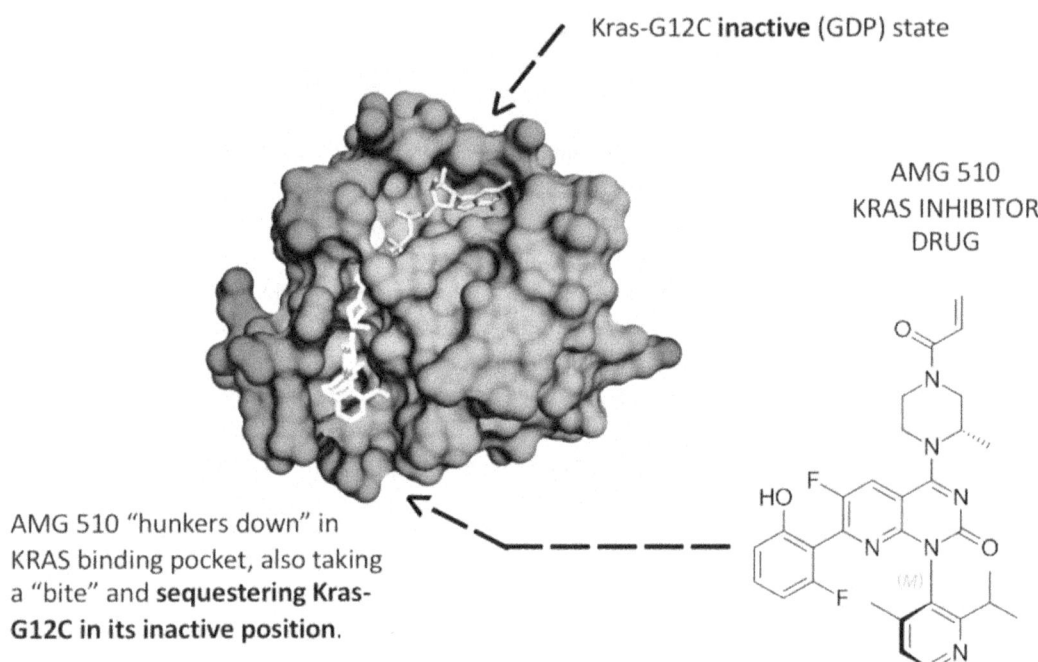

Image. 80 The Ras blocker. Wikimedia Commons File: KRAS protein G12C mutant with GDP and sotorasib 6OIM.png and Wikimedia Commons File: Sotorasib structure.svg.

Equally exciting, an experimental anti-Ras vaccine against lung cancer and CRC is in the making with surprisingly encouraging Phase I clinical trial outcomes, yielding more than 80 percent favorable patient responses. Carry on!

Food for thought:

1. The newly approved mutant Ras inhibitor drugs are for the treatment of lung cancer and colorectal cancer.
   A. True
   B. False

2. A Ras mutant therapeutic vaccine has entered Phase I clinical trial stages.
   A. True
   B. False

RISK REDUCTION OF CANCER PENTALOGY (1): SUCCESS IS THE GRAND SUM OF SMALL STEADY STEPS

Ad nauseam but timelessly true: *An ounce of prevention is worth a pound of cure*. While not yet an etched-in-stone mantra of "If you do ABC, you can *confidently prevent cancer*" owing to cancer's extremely complex facets, there are ways to reduce cancer risks. Let's zero in on a few examples.

Minimize toxin exposure. Cancer risk enhancers can occur naturally, with examples ranging from radon gas, benzene from car exhaust, UV damage from excess and unprotected sun exposure, to man-made factors that include PFAS and tanning station UV rays. As a "side effect" of modern industrialized lifestyle, it is next to impossible to completely stay away from certain toxins: the simple act of soaking a bag of tea leaves in a saucer of hot water leaves a silent trail of food toxins from PFAS-infused tea bags. The presence of water-resistant PFAS in the tea bag prevents the bag from crumbling down in the hot water. How convenient. But here, convenience has an inconvenient catch! A detailed description of PFAS is in my upcoming book. Many environmental toxins are DNA breakers, leading to mutations and weakening immune defense—the combination is a lethal force that drives cancer.

Kick bad habits. The first link between tobacco smoking and most lung cancers was reported by Richard Doll and Tony Bradford from the UK in a 1950 seminal paper. Decades of research and concerted public education efforts have finally made it widely accepted that tobacco smoking (first- or second-hand) is an unquestionably causative factor of smoking-related lung cancer. How many chemicals are generated in tobacco smoke? The answer, buckle up, is more than 7,000 assorted chemicals from the uncool rings of puffs. Out of those chemical, seventy are known or potential carcinogens—cancer-causing toxins. A major one contained in cigarette smoke is polonium-210, a high-energy element that emits radioactive alpha particles which, when inhaled, can wreak havoc in DNA. More about alpha particles is discussed in ***RISK REDUCTION OF CANCER PENTALOGY (3): WINTER, ALASKA, AND RADON GAS*** (page 170). Another carcinogen from cigarette smoke is *benzo[a]pyrene* (BP), also a DNA destroyer, as detailed in ***RISK REDUCTION OF CANCER PENTALOGY (2): COAL TAR, CANCER, AND THE MYSTERIOUS LINK*** (page 168).

Eat smart. There is more than one way to eat smart. A warmly welcomed way is the Mediterranean style of olive oil whipped in balsamic to dip plain whole wheat pita in, or hummus decorated on a plate of garden-fresh greens surrounding a thick slice of lightly grilled salmon. Yum and healthy! Among the different versions and variations of *Eat Smart* recipes out there, a common denominator is a *Balanced Diet* that typically consists of whole grains, fresh greens, and good protein, devoid of trans fat, saturated fat, sodium in moderation, and sugar in conservative quantities (because excess sugar is converted to fat that gets stored in fat cells in our bodies).

Worry not and be happy! Topics under healthy lifestyle extend to emotional health distilled as *Don't worry; Be happy*—more than a pet phrase for comfort but with science-backed proof of support for immune balance and immune defense. The details are described in ***REDUCTION OF CANCER PENTALOGY (5): MILLION DOLLAR SMILE*** (page 175).

Get thy lymph going! All the smart choices and good practices described above aim at one important goal: to boost immune defense capacity to preempt cancer in the bud. As for how to boost the immune system, two simple words: *Get Moving,* because movement propels lymph to move faster, and a fast-moving lymph system is more effective at moving immune cells to the immune battleground where they are needed. A detailed discussion is in ***NODES THAT CHANNEL LYMPH: STRONGHOLDS OF TRUSTED IMMUNE RADARS*** (page 127). The next few essays of this series are devoted to specific topics on cancer risk reduction. Read on.

Food for thought:

1. There are too many toxins in our living environment and in our diet that it is next to impossible to build a strong immune system.
   A. True
   B. False

2. A fast-moving lymphatic system sets the stage for a robust immune system.
   A. True
   B. False

RISK REDUCTION OF CANCER PENTALOGY (2): COAL TAR, CANCER, AND THE MYSTERIOUS LINK

In 1775, English surgeon Dr. Percival Pott observed unusually high incidence of cancer cases in chimney sweepers. Soot was the suspected culprit, but there was no direct evidence. The proof of the existence of cancer-causing carcinogens was not available until 1915, when two physician-scientists in Japan made their findings.

The historic bunny experiment. Dr. Katsusaburo Yamagiwa, a Japanese pathologist at Imperial Tokyo University, and his research assistant, Dr. Koichi Ichikawa, carried out an experiment in which they *repeatedly* painted the inner side of 101 rabbit ears with coal tar for 150 days. Coal tar, the liquid byproduct generated during coal gasification (also called coking), is the precursor to soot, which is a byproduct generated from incompletely burned coal. Instead of painting rabbit ears with the liquid dark coal tar just once, the two scientists carefully designed the experimental steps so that they would peel off the previous dried layer of coal tar from the rabbit ears before applying a fresh layer. The painting-peeling off-painting process lasted for 100 and 50 days, and meticulous notes were taken. On day 35, some rabbits began to show initial signs of cancer; 12 days after that, some rabbits developed full-blown cancer, and by day 150, cancer was evident in all experimental rabbits. The cancer turned out to be squamous cell carcinoma, the same cancer that arises in sun-exposed areas of the human body.

Coal tar is a carcinogen. Data on initial skin irritation followed by benign tumor which deteriorated to full-blown skin cancer demonstrated unequivocally that coal tar is a cancer-causing agent. What is the leading chemical in coal tar that gives rise to cancer? The full name is benzo[a]pyrene with the acorn of BP. What links BP to skin cancer? The answer is DNA, or more precisely DNA damage. It has been revealed that BP has a particular molecular penchant of latching onto DNA to form extensions called *DNA adducts*. The associated DNA extensions alter the original structure—any alteration to DNA is, by definition, a mutation. Ordinarily, p53 would spot DNA errors and call for DNA repair crew to fix the errors. But the 101 rabbits whose ears were repeatedly painted with toxic coal tar did not have the blessings of their p53. Even if p53 may have been activated initially to try to correct the wrong, the constant exposure to coal tar from *repeatedly* painting fresh layer after peeling off the dried layers added an unimaginably high potency of coal tar. This is also part of the reason (the other reason being rabbit skin is uniquely sensitive and ready to absorb coal tar) why it took only 150 days for all 101 experimental rabbits to develop squamous cell skin cancer, as carcinogenic exposure at lower levels and with less frequency would typically take a much longer period of time to develop from DNA damage to permanent mutations that ultimately lead to cancer.

A quick recap of the types of DNA damage that can be caused by carcinogens such as BP (from coal tar but also petroleum products such as crude oil and diesel exhaust) or free radicals (produced by harmful ionizing radiation).

Type 1: Breakage of DNA backbone made up by sugar and phosphate chemical groups,*Type 2*: Breakage between G—C *Type 3*: Breakage between A—T.**Coal tar in shampoo, seriously!** Knowing how potent coal tar can be, many are unpleasantly surprised when they learn about a medical shampoo that harbors the very chemical compound in the ingredient list. Well, coal tar is pretty effective at regulating the growth rate of skin cells; hence, its presence in shampoo helps ameliorate skin conditions such as dandruff and psoriasis. Per the FDA, coal tar of 0.5–1 percent is safe to use. It is, however, generally recommended not to wash hair using coal-tar shampoo for more than once a week. Whole coal tar-based shampoo is readily allowed in the United States, United Kingdom, and Canada; however, it is strictly banned in the EU out of concern about the presence of a known carcinogen, albeit in low amount. Oh well, to each their own. There are shampoos that use coal tar substitutes such as apple cider vinegar, coconut oil, and tea tree oil. All sound ideas. A quick survey reveals that coal tar is present in our everyday products beyond shampoo. Sealant contains three asterisks because it has been strictly banned in states like New York, the District of Columbia, Minnesota, and Maine; it is also restricted in Massachusetts, Pennsylvania, Maryland, Illinois, Michigan, Texas, Kansas, Wisconsin, North Carolina, and South Carolina. Here is a summary table:

Coal tar found in everyday products	
Food	Certain food dyes
	Certain butter
	Certain candy
	Certain artificial sweeteners
Supplements & OTC meds	Synthetic vitamin B1
	Certain psoriasis ointment
Bodily products	Certain shampoos
	Certain perfumes
Construction materials	Certain paints
	Certain sealants***

Image. 81 Coal tar-containing products. By Nancy Liu-Sullivan.

Food for thought:

1. The coal tar rabbit experiment demonstrated for the first time that chemical toxins can act like carcinogens to drive cancer formation.
   A. True
   B. False

2. Benzo[a]pyrene (BP) found in coal tar and certain petroleum products damages DNA by forming adducts defined as DNA extensions.
   A. True
   B. False

RISK REDUCTION OF CANCER PENTALOGY (3): WINTER, ALASKA, AND RADON GAS

The link between cigarette smoking and lung cancer is indisputable. Yet, not everyone who smokes gets lung cancer, and not everyone who gets lung cancer is a smoker. In fact, one type of lung cancer is non-smokers' lung cancer. How does this happen? The answer, my readers, is blowing in the wind that harbors a harmful gas.

Radon comes from uranium. The world is all too familiar with uranium. *"Fat Man"* and *"Little Boy"* were the two atomic bombs dropped over Japan in August 1945 to end the Second World War. The immeasurable radioactive power came from uranium, a naturally occurring element. Uranium was first discovered by German chemist Martin Heinrich Klaproth in 1789, but its radioactive property was not appreciated until 1896 by French physicist Henri Becquerel. The revered Polish-French physicist/chemist Madam Curie discovered two sibling radioactive elements, *radium* and *polonium*. Madam Curie also coined the term "radioactivity" that best captures the core property of the powerful energy.

Elements undergo radioactive decay due to inherent elemental instability. During the decaying process, some ephemeral, others lasting an eternity. Eventually, the ancestry element settles to its stable state but has transcended to an entirely different element. Uranium 238 (U-238), for example, decays into *lead* (Pb-206) after (fasten your seatbelt) 4.5 billion years! Lead is a stable element with very high density and an ideal material to shield off harmful radiation including rays from U-238. A case of what comes around, goes around.

Granite, shale, and limestone. Along the very extensive journey of uranium decay is radon gas, one of many intermediary products. Where there is uranium, radon is bound to be present. Invisible and odorless, radon gas readily seeps into our living space. Excess inhalation is known to increase risks for the so-called non-smokers' lung cancer. The three "champions" of natural radon gas emitters are granite, shale, and, as a surprise to many, limestone, as illustrated in the following figure.

Radon damages DNA. Radon gas is radioactive and emits alpha radiation. A quick brush-up: high-energy radiation can be manifested as alpha particles, beta particles, gamma rays, and X-rays. The respective penetrating power and associated shielding materials are presented in the following figure:

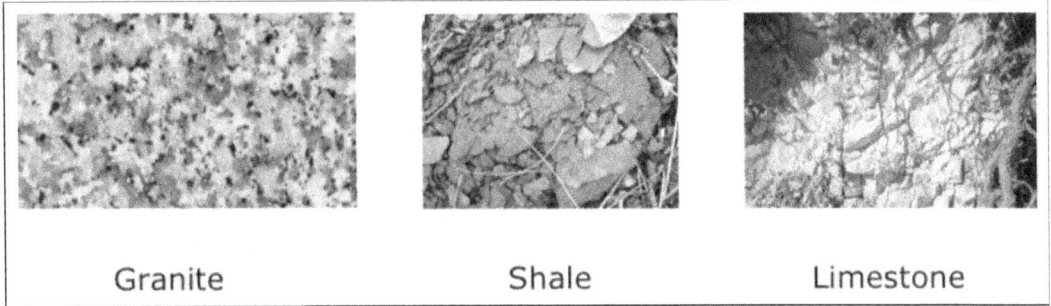

Image. 82 Radon gas from nature. File: Bianco Sardo Granit mit polierter Oberfläche.jpg. File:Shale 8040.jpg. File: Limestone Eocene deposit at Sinj Stari grad—Dalmatia—Croatia IMG 20210820 083857.jpg.

Radiation Shielding Materials and Cautions		
Alpha particle	Outer skin layer, thin shield of paper, aluminum foil, plastic, or clothing	CAUTION: Despite low penetrating power, inhalation of alpha particles leads to tissue damage.
Beta particle	Can pass through paper but can be shielded by aluminum sheet, plastics, or acrylic glass	CAUTION: Do not shield beta particles with lead as it can produce harmful X ray (bremsstrahlung)
X ray, Gamma ray	For medical lead apron (0.5 mm), also lead gloves/thyroid wear/eye wear; for nuclear facilities, lead (3.2 mm)	CAUTION: Be ware of lead dust; never fold lead garments to avoid cracking; carry out routine checks for lead wear integrity.

Image. 83 Ionizing radiation shield table. Assembled by Dr. Nancy Liu-Sullivan.

As shown above, the upper left-hand corner sign is the international symbol of ionizing radiation (IR). Alpha particles can be blocked by a piece of paper; the printed form of the *New York Times* (*NYT*) will suffice. Intact skin can also block alpha particles. Beta particles can readily go through the *NYT* paper and into intact skin for a tiny bit of distance but can be blocked by an aluminum sheet. Gamma electromagnetic waves, together with X-rays (not shown), are exceptionally powerful, capable of cutting through paper and aluminum like knife through butter. Both gamma and X-rays are shielded by lead, although not 100 percent. Back to alpha particles emitted from radon gas: While it is true that they are too bulky to penetrate intact human skin, they can enter the human body through inhalation.

Radon wreaks havoc on the lungs. Once breathed in, radon gas becomes unhinged in causing DNA damage by breaking molecular bridges that hold atoms together in DNA. DNA stretches are segmented to code genes; hence damaged DNA, if not repaired properly and timely, can trigger a mutation. Cumulation of mutations in five critical genes sets the perfect molecular storm for cancer formation. It is estimated that radon gas-associated lung cancer accounts for 12 percent of all lung cancer diagnoses in the United States annually. How does radon gas sneak into the house? Check the basement!

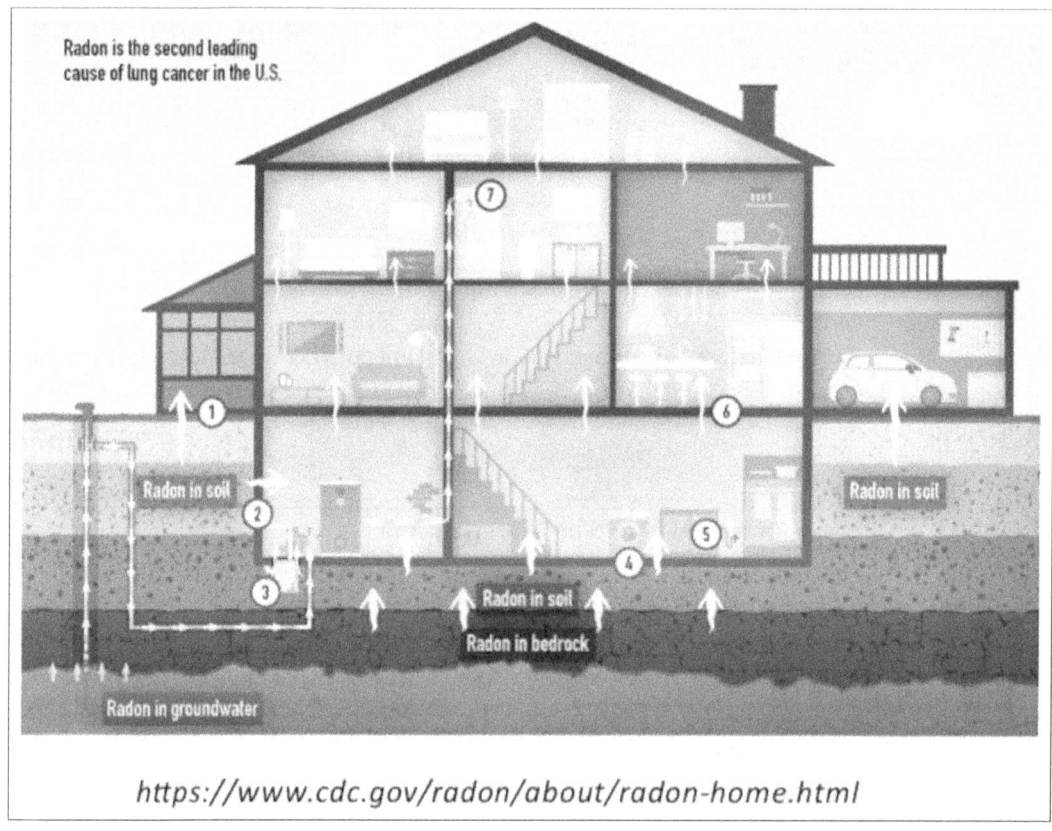

Image. 84 Radon gas entry into houses. https://www.cdc.gov/radon/about/radon-home.html

As shown above, radon gas can be emitted from the rocks of your house's foundation, leaked into air, and inhaled by people. Once in lung tissues, alpha particles emitted from radon gas begin their destructive trail to break DNA, generate mutations, and drive lung cancer.

Winter, Alaska, and high radon. Radioactivity is measured in picocuries per liter of air (pCi/L). On average, in North America, outdoor levels are around 0.4 pCi/L, whereas indoor levels are higher, at roughly 1.3 pCi/L. Which state has the highest radon level in the United S? The answer is Alaska. This is related to the extensive deposits of uranium-rich granites. Uranium decay leads to radon gas emission. This explains why radon level in outdoor Alaska is more than twenty times higher than the national average: 10.7 pCi/L. Of course, here, we are talking about the average radon gas level in Alaska, whether in winter or other seasons. Slightly shy of #1 Alaska are #2 South Dakota, #3 Pennsylvania, #4 Ohio, and #5 Washington State.

Back to Alaska. From October through April, the long, chilly cold with below freezing temperature of 5–30°F (degrees Fahrenheit), Alaskan winter increase indoor pressure that results in more air being sucked in from the ground. Winter houses are also better insulated to keep warm air in, which at the same time prevents radon gas from getting dissipated. It is recommended that protective measures be taken *IF* indoor radon levels are above 4 pCi/L, pronounced as pico curies per liter. The US Environmental Protection Agency (EPA) and the Center for Disease Control (CDC) offer instructions on proper protocols to follow and suitable measures to be carried out. For details, please check out their website (www.epa.org and www.cdc.org).

One more note about radon gas-linked lung cancer: In parallel to radon gas exposure, there are also additional factors at play: genetics, lifestyle choices, and immune strength. Cancer is not built in a day, nor by a single factor.

What about that beautifully polished granite countertop in your kitchen? No worries, as traces of radon gas emitted are negligible, relative to ambient air amount, especially in properly ventilated homes. *Bon Appétit*!

Food for thought:

1. Generated as an intermediary product during uranium decay, radon gas emits harmful radioactive rays which, when inhaled at a level higher than 0.4 pCi/L, act as a contributing factor for non-smokers' lung cancer.
   A. True
   B. False

2. Discard all granite products in your house to avoid radon gas poisoning in order to prevent lung cancer.
   A. True
   B. False

RISK REDUCTION OF CANCER PENTALOGY (4): RED MEAT AND HIGH FLAMES DO NOT MIX

Midsummer afternoon, the sky is blue, the air crisp, and the backyard barbecue is in full swing. The flames are high, the short ribs marinated in spicy sweet sauce are sizzling, a mug of Heineken in hand, and everyone is cheerfully munching and imbibing. You feel so tempted to join in the feast, but then the din in your head begins to get louder: I heard red meat is linked to cancer. Truth or myth?

Why is grilled steak so yummy? To many folks, the aroma of a steak cooked to perfection is so captivating that the best thing to do is to simply succumb to the temptation. Why is cooked red meat so palatable? What's the secret "red meat chemistry"? The answer has everything to do with French. French chemist, Dr. Maillard, was curious about the same question of what gives cooked food the intense flavor. It turned out that the aroma comes from a "quartet" of amino acids, sugar, fat, and high flames.

The tangible proof of the aroma is written in the telltale brown hue: slightly burnt steak, golden french fries, and pale brown glazed donuts rolling out of the conveyor; the list goes on. The chemical reaction is named after Dr. Maillard as "the Maillard Reaction," or the browning process.

Steak in hot flames sets off carcinogen alarm. Well, there is an unexpected catch that spoils the aroma: Two types of carcinogens are produced in the heat of the flames. Each has a long and complicated name; here, we'll resort to the acronyms of "HCA" and "PAH." For those curious about the full names, HCA stands for "heterocyclic amines" and PAH for "polycyclic aromatic hydrocarbons." Both chemicals are classified by the World Health Organization (WHO) as "probable carcinogens," meaning there is evidence to point to a definitive "cause" between HCA or PAH and cancer. This short essay focuses primarily on HCA.

Steak is *bona fide* muscle meat. Muscles are rich in proteins; hence, rich in amino acids, since amino acids are the building blocks of protein. Muscles are also endowed with a special molecule called "creatinine" that serves as the energy source to pump our muscles. What "catalyzes" the reaction to produce the final and unwanted carcinogen HCA? "Fire," or to be exact, high flames. Here is an easy-to-follow formula:

Amino acids + creatinine + fire → HCA

A common HCA produced from high-flame red meat is 2-amino-1-methyl-6-phenylimidazo[4,5-b] pyridine (PhIP), which is a carcinogen capable of disrupting DNA stability and causing damage, as illustrated in the following figure.

Some may argue that HCA breakage of DNA shouldn't be an astounding alarm because broken DNA can be fixed anew. Indeed, our body is equipped with powerful DNA repair machinery that constantly scans for DNA errors. The moment an error is spotted, a repair crew is dispatched for a quick fix, much like our local electrical power supply company that offers all-weather repair service 24–7, 365. Our DNA repair crew works just as hard. Besides, from DNA damage to the eventual biogenesis of cancer, it does not happen overnight, nor in a fortnight, but takes years. Still, one should avoid or minimize carcinogen intake where possible. What about the yummy steak? Can we have our steak with the annoying HCA? The answer is a cheerful yes, as discussed below.

Remedies to rescue yummy steak. How you cook the steak matters. Since HCA is only produced in steak over high flames, it occurs within a range of flame temperatures from high 200s to the low 300s in degrees Celsius. Knowing this narrow range of HCA production, all we need to do is avoid high temperatures. The National Cancer Institute (NCI) recommends cooking temperatures below 300 degrees Celsius. So retire the barbecue stand, put away the high flame-resistant wok, and turn to your oven or the slow cooker. As long as there are no blazing high flames, HCA from the steak can be under control. Since beef is not the only "red meat of interest" when it comes to "muscle meat," other animal protein sources such as pork, lamb, bison, chicken, and even fish, are also capable of producing HCA if prepared over high flames. Know the science; eat smart.

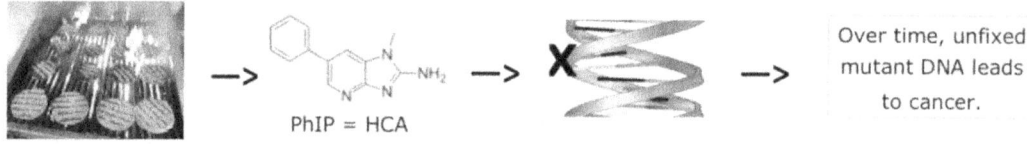

Step 1: Yummy barbecue & HCA carcinogen molecules ingested.

Step 2: HCA becomes highly reactive and breaks DNA.

Step 3: Un-repaired DNA becomes a mutation.

Step 4: Cumulative mutations cause cancer over time.

Image 85 Red meat on high flames—not a yummy idea. Wikimedia Commons File: Charbroiler-operations-cooking 1.JPG and Wikimedia Commons File: PhIP.svg assembled by Dr. Nancy Liu-Sullivan.

Food for thought:

1. HCA is produced in animal meat cooked over high flames.
   A. True
   B. False

2. Animal meat, especially red meat, should be avoided at all costs in our diet.
   A. True
   B. False

RISK REDUCTION OF CANCER PENTALOGY (5): MILLION DOLLAR SMILE

Many moons ago in our golf phase, my spouse and I spent a few weekends on the links. One midsummer Sunday, we were paired with a Japanese couple as a foursome. Japanese people are known for their formality and polite bows. On the first shot, the Japanese husband drove the ball into the ground. While my husband and I were trying to offer a consoling word, the Japanese wife burst out with hearty laughter. "Take a mulligan," my husband suggested. The Japanese husband tried again and this time, he sliced the ball 30 yards into the woods. His wife laughed again. The laughter must be contagious, as the couple began laughing together. An adorable duffer couple having an awesome time. Why not?! After all, golf is only a only game for us amateurs.

A *DOSE* of feel-good molecules. Laughing is an unfiltered expression of happiness and relaxation. Laughter comes in assorted shades, shapes, and styles. Some laugh heartily with their mouths open, others laugh somewhat subdued without showing their teeth. To each their own. Styles aside, laughing actually produces several feel-good hormones in our bodies, according to *Harvard Health*. The four hormones, after linking the first letter of each word, become *DOSE*, which stands for dopamine, oxytocin, serotonin, and endorphins.

Dopamine is a hormone released by our brain when we are happy and relaxed. It is also a neurotransmitter that connects feel-good activities with pleasurable rewards and motivation. To experience the sense of reward again, we are drawn to repeat the same activity that enables us to feel good again. A good example of this scenario could be a student who has received kudos for being in good academic standing and is motivated to maintain the good record with the expectation of additional positive reinforcement. Laughing makes it much simpler. No sweat, no burning the midnight oil, all you need to do is laugh a little.

Oxytocin is typically a hormone released in large quantities in pregnant mothers to facilitate giving birth. Yet, pregnancy is not the only stimulus for oxytocin production. Music can also do the trick. One study showed that listening to slow music increases the level of oxytocin in the saliva in addition to reducing heart rate. Somber with a hint of melancholy and sporadic crescendos, Beethoven's *Moonlight Sonata First Movement* hums gracefully in oxytocin positivity.

Serotonin is a neurotransmitter that enhances communication among brain cells and regulates a myriad of bodily and brain activities including mood, attention, and memory. Insufficient serotonin levels are a widely acknowledged culprit for depression or lack of cheerfulness. Laughter can modulate serotonin levels in the brain, elevate our moods, and give us a shot of positive energy.

Endorphins are the most exquisite of all four happiness hormones produced by laughter. *Quick Word Anatomy: Enco = endogenous or internal, Orphin P = morphine, together Endorphin =* Morphines from within (produced by our brain). Morphine from nature was first isolated from opium poppy by a German chemist. Endorphins enhance a sense of pleasure and well-being. As an opioid medication, morphine is used for pain management, including alleviating excruciating pain in late-stage cancer patients.

By the way, aside from laughter, there are other means for endorphin enhancement. Exercise, whether intense, moderate, or light forms of exercise all achieves the same effect. Perhaps "laughing yoga" was created to combine laughter with exercise to double the effect on endorphin production? Your guess is as good as mine.

Laughter triggers the release of four precious hormones—dopamine, oxytocin, serotonin, and endorphins. These happy hormones, in turn, help de-stress our body and mind by taming stress hormones such as cortisol. And stress reduction boosts the immune system. A strong immune system lays the

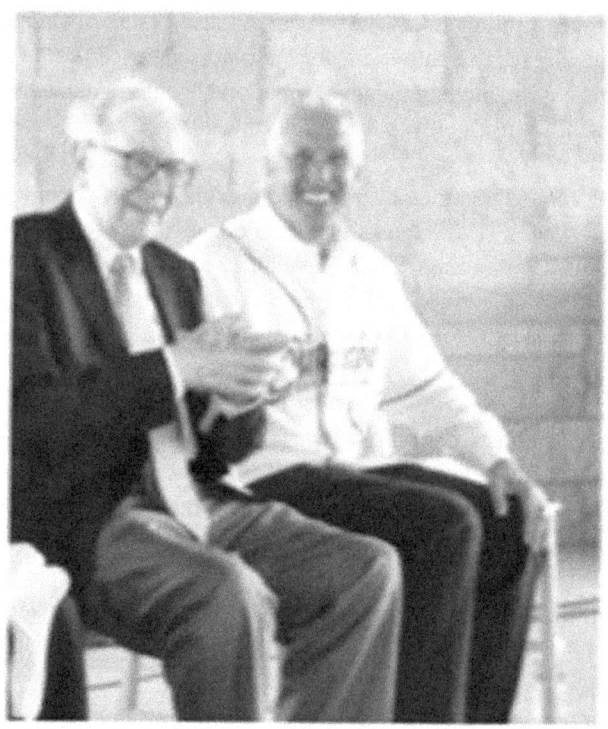

Mr. Warren Buffet with Mr. Gary Green at a news conferences, both smiling and sassy.

Image 86 Warren's smile. Wikimedia Commons File: Storm Chasers press conference.jpg.

foundation for good health. We don't necessarily have to laugh all the way to the bank, like Mr. Buffet and Mr. Green—*Laughing all the way to the bank* or just laugh, LOL, for laughter is the best medicine!

Food for thought:

1. Laughter produces happy hormones. It also reduces stress and strengthens immune systems.
   A. True
   B. False

2. Stress, by contrast, triggers the release of cortisol which weakens overall immune strength.
   A. True
   B. False

RENOWNED NOBEL WITH A SUGAR TWIST

The 2022 Nobel Prize in Chemistry has been announced, with a sugar twist.

Honorable to the sweet success are three chemists, Dr. Carolyn R. Bertozzi, Dr. Morten Meldal, and Dr. Barry Sharpless. Interestingly, Dr. Bertozzi's pioneering innovation was built upon a path paved by Dr. Sharpless. Joining Dr. Sharpless in this endeavor was Dr. Meldal. Heroes think alike! Great thinking, here, leads to sugar. Let's dig some more.

Sugars are ubiquitous in our diet, in both simple and complex forms. All complex sugars are eventually broken down in our body to the simplest form called glucose. Glucose is indispensable for cellular activities.

Sugars are versatile in their functions, also excellent at multitasking. Aside from serving as cellular fuels, sugars are also "decorators." Before delving into how and why sugars possess such a function, a quick recap of how proteins are made by our cells. It all starts with DNA housed in the cell nucleus. Genes that encode proteins are first transcribed from DNA to messenger RNA (mRNA), followed by mRNA exiting the nucleus to the cytoplasm (the space between the nucleus and cell's outer membrane) where mRNA gets translated to the "precursor" proteins constructed by twenty-two types of amino acids. These precursor proteins are two-dimensional linear structures and are useless in their current form. To function biologically, they must be folded into three-dimensional species. Indispensable to protein three-dimensional folding is a modification process by attaching "sugars" or "glycans" to the precursor protein surface.

Wait, sugar modifiers? Are they glucose molecules? The answer is no, they are not glucose, but related to glucose. Simply put: glucose is the simplest sugar (also called monosaccharide). Glycans is a generic term for complex sugars (or polysaccharides). A more jargon-friendly term is carbohydrates. A distinction between glycans and carbohydrates is that all glycans are carbohydrates, but not all carbohydrates are glycans. Examples of complex sugars include starch (found in potatoes) and cellulose (the tough parts of plants and vegetables indigestible by humans but, for our pet rabbit, a walk in the park, owing to specially powerful digestive enzymes unique to rabbits but not to humans).

Back to protein sugar modification: adding glycans to precursor proteins is no easy feat. A process called glycosylation, it involves eleven different types of monosaccharides that get attached to eight different types of amino acids catalyzed by multiple enzymes! In my graduate school days several moons ago, I devoted many hours trying to figure out how a glycosylated protein contributes to the clustering of acetylcholine receptors essential for robust neurotransmitter acetylcholine activities at the neuromuscular junction (where nerve endings interface with skeletal muscles).

When a glycan sugar group is added to a protein, the protein becomes a glycoprotein. Every organism under the sun has a sugar coating, and more than 50 percent of proteins in us humans are decorated with complex sugars. Okay, we know the form; what function does the sugar coating serve?

First and foremost, without proper sugar addition, the precursor proteins freshly made in our cells would not function. How? Because a functional protein needs a prerequisite: it must be assembled into a three-dimensional structure via a process called protein folding. Without sugar decoration, protein folding would not be successful in two scenarios: the precursor protein either becomes folded wrongly (or misfolded) or correctly folded but unstable. Neither scenario leads to a functional protein.

Glycans, the complex sugars, are also intimately associated with our RBCs. On the surface of RBCs reside different types of proteins decorated with different types of complex sugars. Such sugar coating provides a protective layer to RBCs, also serving as a cellular "barcode" that determines and distinguishes our blood type, whether Type O, Type A, Type B, or Type AB. Blood type compatibility is of utmost importance when it comes to blood transfusion. A mismatch is a matter of life or death.

Glycans also play a role in cancer by controlling how fast cancer cells grow, how extensively cancer cells metastasize to adjacent healthy cells, and how effectively cancer cells build new blood vessels to travel to tissues and organs far away from the primary tumor site. The significant contribution of Dr. Carolyn R. Bertozzi's work on protein sugars that won her the 2022 Nobel Prize in Chemistry has paved the way to study sugars on cancer cells. A picture is worth a thousand words. To characterize sugar activities, scientists need to develop a method to visualize sugars in action. Here is how it is carried out: a chemical group is inserted into the complex sugars on the cell surface. A fluorescent dye is tagged to the chemical group. Under the microscope, where it glows indicates where sugars are localized.

There is a fancy name tag for this innovative technology: Bio-orthogonal Chemistry. Orthogonal is typically defined as two perpendicular lines that form right angles. Orthogonality in the cellular context refers to two functional groups that would interact with each other without involving other molecules that may trigger secondary (unwanted) biological activities. This very discreet aspect of bio-orthogonality ensures the reliability of observations confined to sugar activity with high specificity. This remarkable tool has led to successful imaging and tracing of how sugar groups behave in several cancer types, including breast cancer and prostate cancer. Not surprisingly, new cancer drugs that target sugars are a rapidly developing field of study. Of course "Click Chemistry," independently innovated by Dr. Sharpless and Dr. Medal, played an instrumental role in the success of "bio-orthogonality" by Dr. Bertozzi. Click Chemistry allows discreet interaction of two molecules in the absence of unplanned secondary effects. Warm congrats to the three scientists and to mankind for another achievement in broadening our understanding of nature. Looking forward to sweet success in combating the sugar conundrum of cancer!

Special Note: This essay appeared in McGill University Office of Science and Society (OSS).

"RUBY RED DEVIL" RUINS CANCER DNA

Once upon a time in the thirteenth century in southeast Italy stood a magnificent castle with a crown connection. Some 700 years later, an Italian pharmaceutical research team discovered a special chemical compound from a strain of soil bacteria near the castle. Remarkably, a French research team identified the same chemical compound around the same time, although from another site. The two teams joined hands and named the newly found compound "Doxo-rubicin." "Doxo" represents a tribe that settled near the castle while "rubicin" was French for "red." Red is becoming in this context: the compound itself projects a red hue and turns patients' palms and soles gory red, earning the nickname of "ruby red devil."

"RUBY RED DEVIL" RUINS CANCER DNA

Survival of the best endowed. In the bacterial world, survival is an everyday matter due to limited resources. To kill your rivals that competes for food off your plate, you'd better possess potent weapons in the form of "antibiotics." Coined by a scientist by the name of Salman Waksman in 1941, "antibiotics" are chemical compounds that counteract microorganisms. As a *bona fide* antibiotic, doxorubicin was also found to be capable of vanquishing cancer cells.

Two lethal arrows against cancer in doxorubicin's quiver bag. Doxorubicin is abbreviated as Dox. The first arrow aims at cancer cell DNA. Specifically, Dox molecules latch onto DNA strands like a wedge, making DNA stuck in space and unable to make chromosome copies to replicate more cells. Death soon ensues in these cancer cells. The DNA "wedge" metaphor along with the consequence is illustrated in the following figure:

In addition to bringing direct destruction to cancer DNA as a wedge, Dox is also capable of causing indirect damage to cancer DNA by producing free radicals, particularly reactive oxygen species (ROS). ROS attacks cancer cell DNA, causing damage, even breakage, followed by the death of the cancer cell. This Dox 1–2 punch does an effective job of curbing cancer cell growth.

As one could imagine, a potent antibiotic such as doxorubicin against cancer cells can also exert side effects on normal cells. A major area of concern is toxicity to the heart. Nonetheless, Dox is a standard line of chemotherapy approved by the FDA to treat several cancers ranging from certain types of leukemia, lymphoma, breast cancer, bladder cancer, and soft tissue sarcomas. The strategy of combination therapy is likely favorable in reducing Dox toxicity since the synergy of Dox plus one or more other cancer drugs can lead to a reduced level of Dox, thereby decreasing toxic side effects. It would be interesting to find out to what extent AI can optimize algorithms to best predict synergistic effects against cancer.

Food for thought:

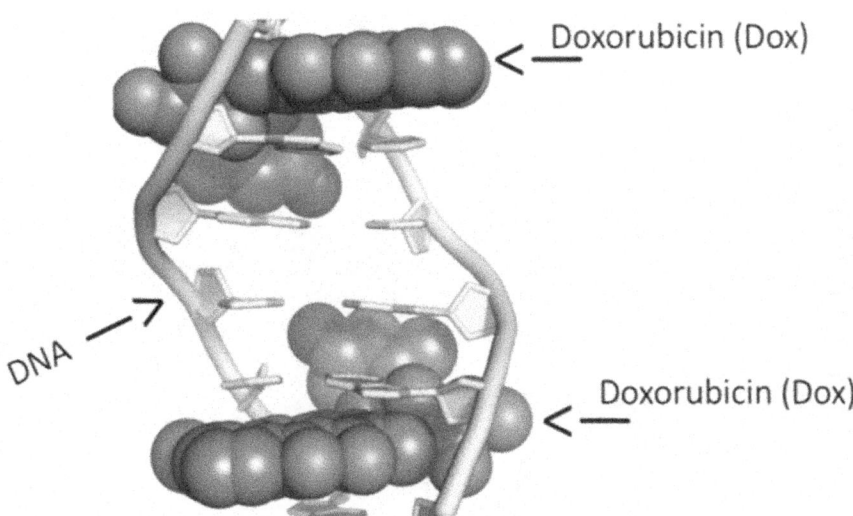

Dox acts as a wedge to jam up DNA, leading to breakage and cell death.

Image 87 Dox jams up DNA. Wikimedia Commons File: Doxorubicin–DNA complex 1D12.png.

1. Doxorubicin, a potent antibiotic, was originally isolated from soil near an Italian castle
   A. True
   B. False

2. Dox is capable of halting cancer growth by interfering with cancer cell chromosomes in addition to dispatching free radicals termed "ROS" to bring about more cancer damage.
   A. True
   B. False

S

SELF OR NON-SELF: A TOUGH IMMUNE QUESTION!

At the core of rampant cancer cell growth machinery are immune cells that live shoulder to shoulder with cancer cells. These immune cells that have breached into cancer quarters are termed as tumor infiltrating lymphocytes (ITLs) center stage to TILs are CD8-Killer T (KT) cells. What makes KT cells so tame in front of cancer?

Immune cells' "excuses." Consider the following *soliloquy* by immune Killer T (KT) cells:

We single out "non-self" cells by their "calling cards" that look "alien." We are on high alert because alien antigen means "danger." We put up a good fight, and we often win. Cancer cells are more deceptive: coming from normal cells a long time ago, they probably look nothing like normal cells anymore, but we immune cells are programmed not to gauge the entire target cell but only telltale red flags that signal suspect cells as "alien." Cunning cancer cells are clever at hiding their alien ID cards to keep us in the dark. So, what's us immune cells to do?!

Fair point. Indeed, wildly deformed in shape, in size, and in possession of more than one cell nucleus of exponentially enhanced replication power, cancer cells look nothing like normal cells. The conundrum confronted by immune cells is that they can only catch cancer cells by checking on "alien" ID displayed on cancer surface antigens. Cancer cells do carry molecular ID badges except most of these badges bear a remarkable resemblance to those from normal cells, since, once upon a time, cancer cells were normal cells before they went awry and manically. These shared ID antigens are called tumor-associated antigens (TAA), an example of which is CD 19 molecules found in all B cells, tumor as well as normal. There are, however, cancer ID antigens that are *uniquely cancer*—the so-termed tumor-specific antigens (TSA)—but they are hard to catch! Commonly found TSAs and TAAs in several cancer types are summarized in the following figure:

CAR-T leads the way. To lend a guiding hand to wandering Killer T (KT) cells that are present but inactive, CAR-T cell therapy has been developed by taking T cells (a mixture of CD8-T and CD4-T cells) from the patient, inserting relevant genetic markers that confer high potency and superb stability, and infusing the "engineered" T cells back into the patient. Several CAR-T therapies have been approved by the FDA for the treatment of blood cancers. By precisely spotting cancer cells with the engineered molecular keys, T cells find cancer cells with precision and annihilate cancer cells without hesitation. A detailed description of *CAR-T THERAPY* can be found in the CAR-T series of essays (page 48–67).

The hunt for additional tumor-specific antigens (TSA) is challenging but not mission impossible. The success of ongoing pancreatic cancer mRNA vaccine clinical trials is largely built upon patient-tailored pancreatic cancer antigens of twenty in total from resected cancer tissues. In light of how each cancer patient has their own cancer "universe" in terms of gene mutation patterns and individual immune background, cancer immunotherapy guided by personalized cancer antigen biomarkers is the direction and the future, with all certainty. For details about the MSKCC-BioNTech pancreatic mRNA vaccine, please visit *CANCER VACCINES (6): IMMUNE WRITING STENTORIAN FROM THE MESSENGER* (page 46).

Tumor markers	Full name	Cancer
Bence-Jones protein		Multiple myeloma
B2M	Beta 2 microglobulin	Severity test for multiple myeloma, Chronic lymphocytic leukemia, certain lymphomas
BRCA1/2	Breast cancer antigen1/2	Breast cancer
CA-125	Cancer antigen 125	Ovarian cancer
CA 15-3	Cancer antigen 15-3	Colon cancer, endometrial cancer, lung cancer, ovarian cancer, pancreatic cancer
CA 19-9	Cancer antigen 19-9	Bile duct cancer, colon cancer, stomach cancer
CA 27-29	Cancer antigen 27-29	Advanced breast cancer
CEA	Carcinoembryonic antigen	Breast cancer, ovarian cancer, cervical cancer, lung cancer, thyroid cancer
CFP*	Complement factor properdin	Gastric cancer, lung cancer
hCG	Human chorionic godadotrophin	Breast cancer, ovarian cancer, cervical cancer, lung cancer,
Her2	Human epidermal growth factor receptor 2	Her2 breast cancer
HPV E6/E7	Human papilloma virus E6/E7	High-grade cervical cancer
M-Protein	Myeloma protein	Multiple myeloma
PSA	Prostate-specific antigen	Prostate cancer
Thyroglobulin		Thyroid cancer

Image 88 Tumor ID: a growing list. Assembled by Dr. Nancy Liu-Sullivan.

Food for thought:

1. Tumor-associated antigens (TAA) are found both on cancer cells and normal cells.
   A. True
   B. False

2. Tumor-specific antigens (TSA) are uniquely expressed on cancer cells.
   A. True
   B. False

SPONTANEOUS TUMOR REMISSION: A FEVERISH CONNECTION

A true story: A lymphoma patient was sent home after all treatment options had been tried but failed. That was early March 2020. The patient subsequently contracted Covid-19. By the time the patient had recovered, his viral infection was gone, so was his metastatic lymphoma! Below are the patient's CT/PET scan images side by side of before and after the viral infection. Truly remarkable. It turned out that it wasn't an isolated event.

The earliest account of tumor spontaneous remission was said to be in the sixteenth century. Two centuries later, Dr. William Coley of Sloan Kettering Hospital, New York, made a similar observation of a sarcoma patient with a large inoperable tumor on his neck. The poor man then came down with a deadly bacterial skin infection called "erysipelas" or "red skin" in Ancient Greek. In addition to nasty skin rashes, the patient also had very high fevers. Like the lymphoma patient who spontaneously recovered from lymphoma described above, the sarcoma patient also experienced "infection gone, tumor gone."

High fever as a key link. Both tumor spontaneous recovery cases involved high fever associated with a deadly infectious disease. High fevers are known to stimulate the release of immune signaling molecules called "cytokines," particularly of interleukin-1 (IL-1), interleukin-6 (IL-6), interferon

Tumor Spontaneous Remission Cases Reported	
Blood cancers	Certain leukemias
	Certain lymphomas
	Certain multiple myeloma
Solid malignant tumors	Certain sarcomas
	Certain lung cancers
	Certain melanomas
	Certain colon cancers
	Certain kidney cancers

Image 89 Spontaneous tumor remission reported in multiple cancer types. *Assembled by Nancy Liu-Sullivan.*

gamma (IFNg), and tumor necrosis factor alpha (TNFa). All are potent pro-inflammatory cytokines known to promote the activation of innate immune cells (including neutrophils, dendritic cells, macrophages) which are pivotal in activating elite immune T and B cells. High fever serves as a highly plausible immune weapon that led to the complete disappearance of a deadly malignant tumor, as sketched in the following figure:

Three black boxes. As shown above, viral (or bacterial) infection induces high fever, which stimulates cytokines that promote inflammation, leading to activation of a cascade of immune cells that swept through both battlefields of infection and tumor with victory. The molecular water is very deep, replete with missing links—the three "black boxes" pertaining to (1) do inflammatory cytokines work independently or in coordination? The latter would likely yield synergistic effects in sounding "danger alarms" all over the town of immune cell communities. (2) Infections typically produce infectious bug-specific immune reactions. How then are immune cells supposedly to have been activated in response to viruses or bacteria attack end up destroying cancer cells? Was it intended or merely an accident? (3) In cases of viral infection-associated tumor spontaneous disappearance post-infection, did the viral particles provoke an anti-tumor campaign that drove cancer to self-implosion? What is unmistakably clear is the power of the immune system against cancer. The amazing immune power has been translated into clinical fruition by Team Rosenberg at the National Cancer Institute (NCI), as described in *LES TROIS PIONEERS OF MODERN CANCER IMMUNOTHERAPY (3): STEVEN A. ROSENBERG* (page 117).

Food for thought:

1. There are quite a number of documented accounts of cancer patients whose malignant tumors remitted after they had survived a deadly infection.
   A. True
   B. False

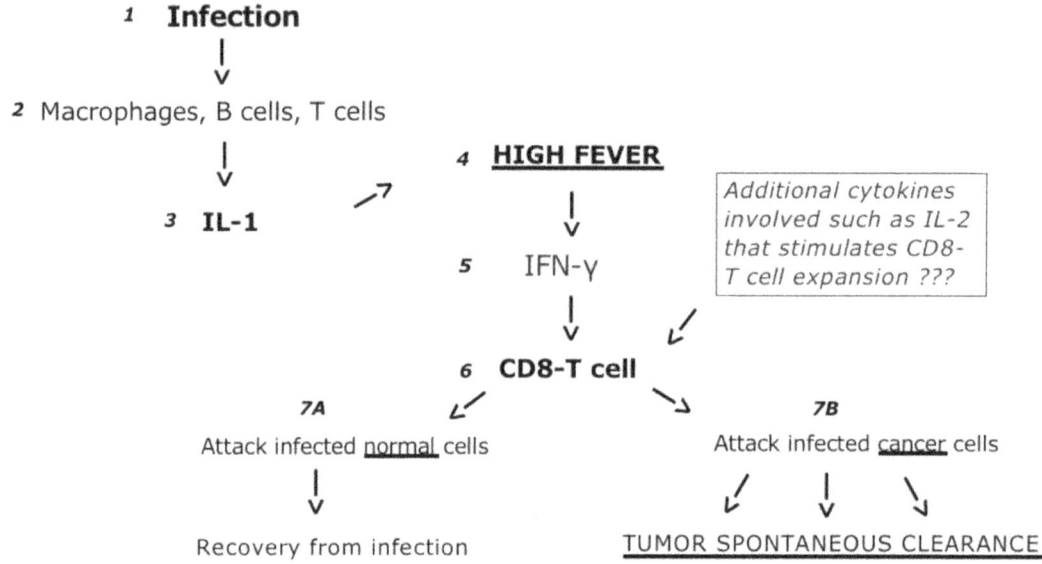

Image 90 The link between infection and tumor disappearance. By Nancy Liu-Sullivan.

2. Among inflammation-promoting cytokines, interleukin 1 (IL-1) induced fever.
    A. True
    B. False

SUGAR SONATA AND TUMOR TAG

Sugar! The sweet, versatile ingredient that we can't do without but can't afford to have too much of, either.

Sugar is gasoline to cells. Glucose gets broken down to make cellular ATP in a three-step process, with each glucose molecule yielding thirty-two molecules of ATP. Normal healthy cells utilize all three ATP-making steps, with the first step carried out in a hypoxic (no oxygen) environment and the second and third steps relying on oxygen. As discussed in *CANCER TRICKS AND TRAPS* series (page 25–36), cancer cells prefer exclusively the first step of making ATP without oxygen. This is not because cancer abhors oxygen; rather, cancer is oxygen-poor as a result of constant growth and expansion so voracious that it simply is unable to build new blood vessel highways to ship the needed nutrients to cancer cells. You might be asking: What's hypoxia and oxygen-poor got to do with sugar? Everything! Cancer's reliance on making ATP using Step-1 only requires cancer to have large quantities of glucose supply. Cancer's sugar craving is driven by its predilection for making ATP without oxygen. Since this way of producing ATP is terribly inefficient, cancer cells must have excess amounts of glucose to compensate for the low efficiency. The more sugar cancer cells imbibe, the less sweet cancer's living quarters become as a result of the sour byproduct of lactic acid. In fact, the cancer "village" (tumor microenvironment, TME) is often inundated with a flash flood of acids. Cunning cancer cells adapt to survive the harsh living environment while at the same time subjecting cancer-fighting immune cells to the unlivable acidic state. This is a chief mechanism by which cancer cells manage to keep immune fighter cells at bay.

High-sugar diet, obesity, and the link to cancer. While sugar gives us joy, excess sugar intake can render us joyless. For starters, our body can only digest a certain amount of sugar; the daily allowed sugar recommended by the FDA is 33 milligrams (mg) for men and 30 mg for women. Any excess sugar not needed to sustain bodily functions is put in "safe deposit boxes" in our body called "fat cells," with a formal name "adipose cells," which make up the fat tissues in our body. Excess sugar is stored in fat cells, not as sugar, but as "fat." The greater the amount of excess sugar, the bigger the fat cell becomes, leading to weight gain and, over time, to obesity. In addition to adding pressure to the cardiovascular system, obesity is also an inducer of inflammation. Chronic inflammation, as we now know, has a direct link to cancer. It turns out that fat cells also possess a pool of estrogen, the female hormone primarily produced by the ovaries. Well, estrogen can also be secreted by fat cells, perhaps as backup stock. The more spacious the fat cell, the more estrogen it contains. It is now an established fact that excess estrogen increases breast cancer risks. According to the Cleveland Clinic, Cleveland, Ohio, for every ten breast cancer diagnoses, eight patients test positive for excess estrogen receptor proteins (https://my.clevelandclinic.org/health/diseases/10312-estrogen-dependent-cancers). This is also the reason why the current recommendations do not encourage the use of estrogen replacement therapy to alleviate menopausal symptoms. That said, not all women who take estrogen supplements develop breast cancer, just like not all smokers develop lung cancer. Genetics, especially DNA damage repair capacity, environmental toxin exposure, dietary choices, metabolic proficiency, and immune state all vary from individual to individual.

Sugars also serve as tumor ID badges. There is actually a less known but indispensable sugar feature in the context of cancer. Sugars decorate the superficial layer of proteins that reside on the outermost layer of cells. Under both healthy and cancerous conditions, these sugars act as essential messengers that connect cells to their neighbors.

The logical question you may ask: If sugars are found on both healthy and cancer cells, how do they function as tumor ID? Great question. Indeed, if the same marker is found on both healthy cells and cancer cells, our immune fighter cells can get confused and end up letting cancer cells go to avoid killing healthy cells by mistake. So, for immune cells to identify only cancer cells, the marker protein must be *unique* to cancer but not found on healthy cells. Since cancer cells are basically healthy cells gone awry, they continue to share lots of sugar-coated biomarkers with their healthy cell counterparts. A detailed discussion is described in ***SELF OR NON-SELF: A TOUGH IMMUNE QUESTION!*** (page 181).

Not always a villain. The moment we take a bite of chocolate fudge fresh out of the oven, we get melted in the soft, moist, slightly chewy sweetness; our duress dwindles, anxiety clears, and stress subsides. The world is a wonderful place again, all because sugar bestows an indescribable sense of glee through the production of good-mood enhancers—dopamine, oxytocin, serotonin, and endorphins, the four foundations of happiness. More about good moods in ***REDUCTION OF CANCER PENTALOGY (5): MILLION DOLLAR SMILE*** (page 175).

Food for thought:

1. Excess sugar from diet gets converted to fat and is stored in adipocytes.
   A. True
   B. False

2. Sugar chemical groups that serve as surface IDs are only found on cancer cells.
   A. True
   B. False

T

T CELL PENTALOGY (1): AUDITION BITE TEST

Unsparingly brutal, auditions put performers to no-nonsense tests for "talents" and "suitability." Our disease-fighting immune T cells are also subjected to "auditions." The goal is to select and retain the most qualified T cells to be honed to "shoulder" assorted immune tasks down the road, each unique and working collectively to form and sustain a major pillar of immune defense. This process is coined as "T cell selection."

The bite test. T cells, including Killer T (KT) cells, were born in the bone marrow and were dispatched to the thymus for an audition that defines the fate of "to live or to die" in a molecular "bite" test. Markers from self body cells designated as "antigens" are presented to each T cell to kick off the bite test. There are three scenarios of T cell "fate":

   Scenario 1: If a T cell bites too tightly to a self antigen, that T cell receives a score of "negative selection," meaning an F for bad performance, and is marked for elimination. Why? Because biting to a self antigen too tightly indicates that the T cell would end up mistaking healthy self body cells for dangerous entities and marking them for destruction. Interestingly, 95 percent of T cells undergoing the bite test audition end up being selected out. A tough test!
   Scenario 2: If a T cell takes a soft bite without "tooth marks" at the self antigen, that T cell receives a score of "positive selection," becomes a winner of the audition, and is retained as a "keeper" to carry out future immune tasks. The gentle bite indicates that the T cell will steer clear of self body antigens and live in peaceful co-existence with healthy self body cells. Only less than 1 percent of T cells pass muster for positive selection with flying colors. Another tough test!
   Scenario 3: "Middle-of-the-roaders" exist in almost every situation; T cells are no exception. These T cells would bite into a self body-cell antigen not too tightly but not comfortably smooth either. Surprisingly, this cohort of T cells also scores a "positive selection" but under one condition: They will be sent for special training to learn how to tame overactive immune situations to help maintain immune homeostasis, that is, immune balance. How is this task achieved? A special gene in these T cells is turned on, leading to a molecular transformation of becoming "regulatory T cells," abbreviated as "Tregs." Thanks to these Tregs, our immune system is able to return to baseline when an immune battle has been completed with success. Guess what? Many cancer cells take advantage of this exquisite Treg mechanism by recruiting Tregs to the tumor site and having Tregs do the nefarious work of keeping anti-cancer host Killer T (KT) cells at bay. The details are described in CANCER TRICKS AND TRAPS: THRIVING IN LOW OXYGEN (page 28). The three T cell audition outcomes are illustrated in the following figure:

As shown above, T cells that have passed the bite test undergo another selection process to eventually become CD4+ T cells and CD8+ T cells; that is, they display CD4 or CD8 receptor proteins respectively as their "calling cards." CD4 T cells are also called helper T (T-h), and indeed their role is to facilitate

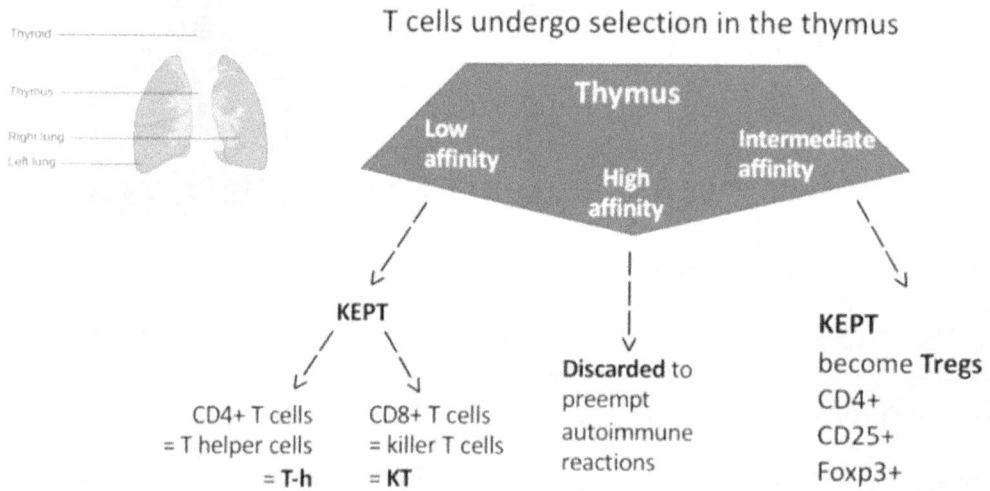

Image 91 T cell bite test. Wikimedia Commons File: Diagram showing the position of the thymus gland CRUK 362.svg modified by Nancy Liu-Sullivan.

CD8 T cells to progress to become Killer T (KT) cells when activated in response to invading dangers from infectious bugs. Tregs, on the other hand, express on their surface a triplet of three receptor proteins: CD4, CD25, and Foxp3. As for the category of T cells that are excessively "smitten" with antigens of self body cells, they are unhesitatingly discarded to obviate chances of wreaking havoc in the host body down the road. The road, however, is not always smooth and even, as described next.

Food for thought:

1. T cell selection takes place in the bone marrow.
    A. True
    B. False

2. The rubrics of T cell selection are based on biting strength: T cells that bite self antigen too rightly are eliminated, T cells that bite mildly are retained to develop into CD4 T and CD8 T respectively, and T cells whose biting strength is in the middle are also retained to become Tregs.
    A. True
    B. False

T CELL PENTALOGY (2): A TALE OF TWO TANGOS

Like new college grads who have completed all required coursework, proudly obtained the coveted baccalaureate diploma, but still need guidance in taking the next step of their professional career path, immune T cells, too, need molecular guidance to prepare them to be immune "combat" fit. Why? Because these are still "naive" T cells that have not yet "seen" the world of stormy and tempestuous immune jungles of infectious bugs or incipient cancer cells. What's a T cell to do? The operative word is "wait"—waiting for an invitation for an immune tango.

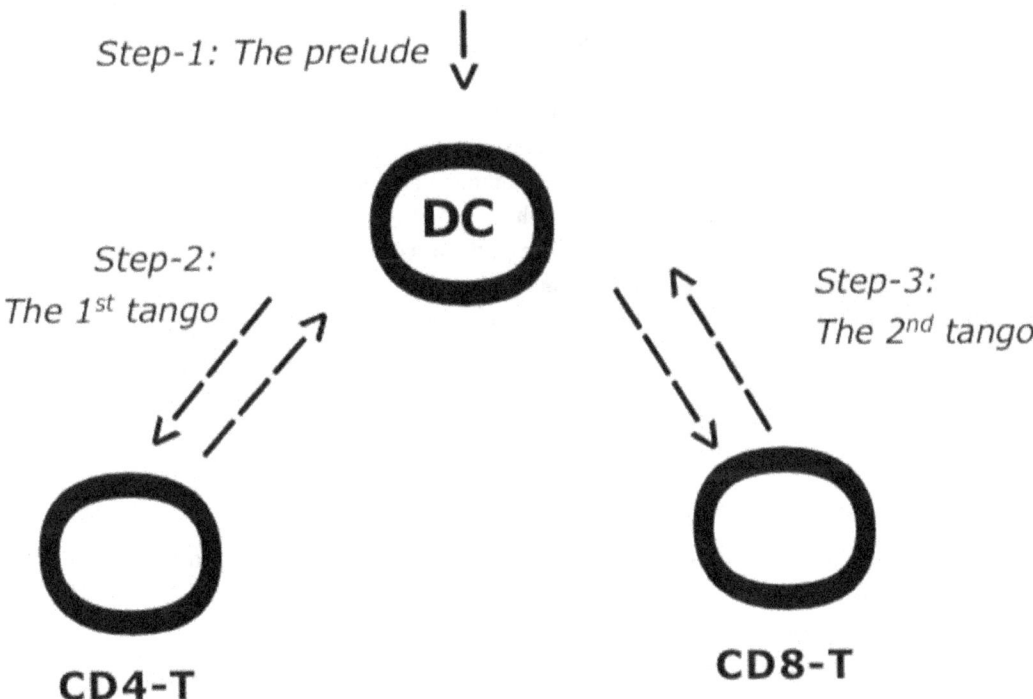

Image 92 TWO tangos to ignite CD8-T. By Nancy Liu-Sullivan.

Two unique immune tangos. As described above, T cells come in two flavors: CD4 T cells and CD8 T cells. It turns out each type of T cell needs to "dance" a separate immune tango to propel the collective immune response forward. The first tango occurs between dendritic cells (DC) and CD4 T cells, and the second dance occurs between DC and CD8 T cells. The first tango promotes the second tango for quicker and more dexterous steps. Both tangos involve immune "enemy" intel exchange, as shown in the following figure:

As shown:

Step 1: A disease-causing bug shows up unannounced but quickly spotted by DC cell.

Step 2: DC literally chews up the bug and spits out a tiny bit to display on a molecular silver platter called "MHC II." Quick note: MHC, by the way, stands for "major histocompatibility complex" first discovered in mouse models. The human equivalence of MHC is termed as "human leukocyte antigen" (or HLA). MHC and HLA are touted as the "gate to immune battlegrounds," for, all "immune intel" (the bug slice) presented to T cells or B cells must be presented on MHC or HLA, which I have taken the liberty of "coining" it as the "immune silver platter." MHC consists of two classes as "MHC-I" and "MHC-II" with the former paired with CD8+ T cells and the latter with CD4+ T cells. One trick I share with my students in how to unmistakably remember the correct pairing is "MHC class I × 8" and "MHC class II × 4" since both yield a sum of "8." Balance is key to the beauty of symmetry, without being too much off on a tangent.

Step 3A: The cargo of "MHC-II + bug slice" is recognized by CD4+ T cell antenna called "TCR" (T cell receptor). This is the first tango! The goal is clear: To activate CD4+ T cell.

Step 3B: Activated CD4+ T begins to secret a motivational molecule to give a boost to CD8+ T cell.

Step 3C: The cargo of "MHC-I + bug slice" is prepared and recognized by CD8 T cell antenna, also called "TCR" (T cell receptor). This is the second tango! The goal is lucid and steadfast: To activate CD8+ T cell (or Killer T, KT cell).

Step 4: Now, CD8+ T cell is activated and ready to hit the ground running toward the bug-infected self-body cell or an incipient cancer cell although the latter is a more complex story.

Step 5: CD8+ T cell is now face to face with the infected cell (or cancer cell) and unleashes the "1-2 punch" with one enzyme poking holes on the infected cell to allow the other enzyme to enter and ignite the cell-death engine in enemy cells.

Step 6: Infected cell is defunct and defeated. Immune defense mission accomplished!

Amazingly coordinated events that procedurally carry out immune defense in two elegant two sets of molecular tangos! *"Play it again, Sam!"*

Food for thought:

1. Dendritic cell (DC) relays enemy antigen *Intel* (on a molecular silver platter termed as HLA) to CD4 helper T cells, followed by DC direct interaction with CD8 Killer T cells that leads to CD8 T cell activation.
    A. True
    B. False

2. Cancer cells hide their HLA to make it impossible for DC or CD8-T cells to spot cancer antigen *Intel* that results in cancer cells hiding in plain sight in front of host immune troops.
    A. True
    B. False

T CELL PENTALOGY (3): SEE HOW THEY ROLL!

We have learned that CD8-T cells receive enemy antigen *Intel* from DC in lymph nodes. This exchange prepares CD8-T cells to be ready to confront infected cells such as those infected by the Covid-19 SARS-CoV-2 virus or early-stage cancer cells. These unwanted cells can be located anywhere in the host body. How do combat-ready CD8-T cells travel to immune frontlines? They roll!!

See how they roll! From lymph nodes, a CD8-T must cross two "waterways"—the white lymphatic brook and the crimson bloodstream—which is too much for a CD8-T to handle alone; hence, it takes a village! First, a series of molecules form "molecular bridge piers" to help CD8-T cells glide and roll along the blood flow toward their destination. The chief molecular piers are made up of two families of proteins called "selectins" and "integrins." To facilitate CD8-T cells squeezing through blood vessels with less strenuous effort, a type of signaling molecules collectively termed "cytokines" comes to the rescue by increasing the permeability of blood vessels, that is, to make the vessels porous to allow CD8-T cells to meander out of blood vessels to land on the immune battlefield, be it the site of infection or tumor, as shown below:

A cold welcome. Having traversed through two waterways to finally arrive at the tumor homestead, that is, the tumor microenvironment, CD8-T cells confront a cold reality: although it is effortless to spot and kill infected cells, spotting cancer cells is not at all a walk in the park! The detailed descriptions of cancer tricks and traps to hide away from CD8-T can be found in the ***CANCER TRICKS AND TRAPS*** series of essays (pages 25–36). Innovative scientists outwit cancer cells by engineering a molecular GPS to guide CD8-T cells to the front door of the cancer cell house with high precision, termed CAR-T cancer immunotherapy. For intriguing details, please refer to ***CAR-T THERAPY*** (1–10) series (page 48–68).

Food for thought:

1. CD8-T cells travel to sites of infection or cancer by rolling with the help of structural molecules and cytokines.
   A. True
   B. False

2. CD8-T cells are versatile and able to eliminate both infected cells and cancer cells with the same ease.
   A. True
   B. False

T CELL PENTALOGY (4): THE DEATH PUNCH

How exactly do CD8 Killer T cells annihilate unwanted cells that pose imminent danger to the host body? The short answer is the death punch aided by two potent enzymes. Let's find out how.

Enzymatic dynamic duo and the 1–2 punch. An enzyme is a type of chemical made by living cells that functions to "catalyze" (or boost) chemical reactions. Familiar enzymes that aid digestion include *Amylase* found in saliva that helps turn starch (such as baked potato) into simple sugars that our body can absorb easily, or *Trypsin* from the small intestine that dissembles complex proteins down to their component parts of "amino acids," or *Lipases* in the gut that breaks down fat. When it comes to tackling cancer, two outstanding enzymes are *Perforin* and *Granzyme B*. **Quick Word Anatomy**: To *perforate* = to poke holes, *Grand* = big, of course. Granzyme B is too bulky to enter cells, so it needs perforin to poke holes in the cell surface to pave the way for Granzyme B entry. Thanks to this exquisite 1–2 punch, CD8-T cells are ready to take the next step.

Switch on the death button. What happens next after Granzyme B marches to the interior of unwanted cells? This enzyme is a cool customer: It slays with no mercy but without blood, pushing a molecular death button that triggers the so-called "programmed cell death," also termed as "apoptosis." Why would cells possess an intrinsic machine for self-dismantling and clearance? Likely an evolutionary vestige as a way of removing cells that are too far gone to be resurrected. The cellular death pathway is very elaborate, consisting of a cascade of molecules, each relaying the death decree to the next post until it reaches the "executioner" molecule termed "Caspase 3" (or Casp3). In an instant, the entire cell shrivels up and turns into a thousand apoptotic bodies from an implosion. Mission accomplished! The detailed steps are illustrated below:

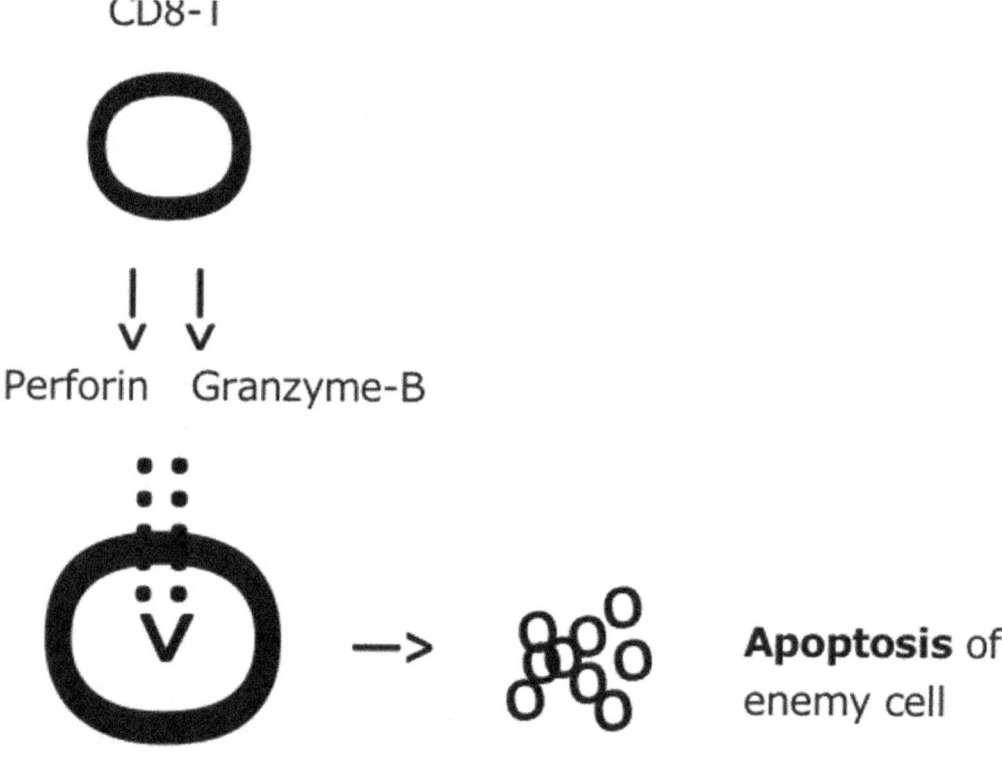

Image 93 Programmed cell death by mighty T lymphocytes. By Nancy Liu-Sullivan.

Food for thought:

1. CD8-T cells destroy unwanted cells via apoptosis.
   A. True
   B. False

2. The way to apoptosis is paved by an enzymatic 1–2 punch carried out by *Perforin* and *Granzyme B*.
   A. True
   B. False

T CELL PENTALOGY (5): A BUG TO REMEMBER

T cell memory versus memory T cells. Not a deliberate tongue twister but a reflection of an immune unvarnished truth: T cell memory lasts a lifetime, yet individual memory T cell lifespan is up to merely five months. Sounds paradoxical but there is a logical explanation.

It turns out that when it comes to immune memory, what matters is the "memory" as opposed to the actual physical presence of individual T cells that harbor the memory. How is this realized? The answer resides in the dynamic nature of T cell memory. While it is true that individual memory

T cells quickly reach the pinnacle of their lifespan in a matter of days, they are replenished with replica memory T cells that carry the same memory. This reminds us of wave movement where, from a distance, individual waves appear to be in a moving "forward" motion, whereas closer scrutiny reveals that individual waves simply serve to propel the collective wave motion forward. Like the motion of eternal waves, T cell memory is also everlasting despite high turnover of individual T memory cells. Of course, T cell memory enables the host immune system to mount a more swift immune retaliation should the same infectious bug dare to show up again.

Memory B cells are superior. The discussion on memory T cells and T cell memory naturally leads to similar functions by T cell immune cousins—B cells. In contrast to memory T cells, which have a life span of a few months, memory B cells can last for years, even decades. A favorable dwelling for memory B cell gathering is a niche area in our gut called *Peyer's Patches* (named after the Swiss physician who discovered it). Why are patches a strategic immune location for memory B cells? Because the patches continuously confront assorted gut antigens. How durable are our memory B cells? For folks who were immunized against infectious smallpox when they were young, memory B cells specific for smallpox are detected in those folks half a century later. Very impressive memory!

The same persistence also applies to memory B cells generated from natural infections such as influenza. This leads to our next question: If memory B cells against the flu are so long-lasting, why is there a need to have annual flu shots? The answer resides in the nature of the flu virus being RNA viruses, which are highly unstable and prone to constant alterations such that new strains keep being evolved seasonally. Back at MSKCC, all scientists and staff are required to get annual flu shots, and for who opt not to must wear a face mask upon entering the hospital cafeteria to protect patients. Cancer patients are particularly susceptible to infections, including the flu, as a result of their immune system being weakened by cancer, in addition to the immune system being subjected to a second toll from chemotherapy and radiotherapy. Delighted that MSKCC, in parallel to providing unparalleled cancer care, also offers a wide range of patient welfare care through complementary services such as acupuncture and music therapy.

Food for thought:

1. Memory T cells last a short time but can divide and pass on immune memory that is long-lasting.
    A. True
    B. False

2. Memory B cells from vaccination and natural infections are capable of a lifetime.
    A. True
    B. False

TEARS: LET THEM STREAM DOWN THY CHEEKS

Under Woody Allen's at times angsty but always elegant pen, the audience is directed to a rhetorical question, *"Tears of sorrow, tears of joy, aren't they the same tears?"* (*Malinda, Malinda*). Actually, from a physiological perspective, these may very well be different tears.

Tears come in three flavors. Slicing an onion on the cutting board, suddenly you feel a sting in your eyes and immediately tear up. These are "reflex tears." My husband and I both teared up at the scene in *A Million Miles* when astronaut Jose Hernandez's inspiring elementary school teacher paid a surprise visit before the launch of the spaceship Discovery. These are "emotional tears." There is a third kind of tear called "basal tears" that lubricate our eyes, during the day, at nights, and when our eyes confront germs.

The eye is endowed with immune privilege. Here is the excerpt of a formal letter by the FDA to the CEO of a major healthcare product company that was required to withdraw a product due to health concerns, dated *9/11/2023*. Sensitive company information is masked by XXX.

> *Your "XXX Health Pink Eye Relief Drops" product is especially concerning from a public health perspective. Ophthalmic drug products, which are intended for administration into the eyes, in general pose a greater risk of harm to users <u>because the route of administration for these products bypasses some of the body's natural defenses</u>.*

In stating the risks of harm from substandard eye drops due to contamination, the FDA letter alluded to the immune vulnerability of the eyes. This vulnerability stems from "immune privilege." The eyes are endowed with the privilege of not being subjected to fierce attacks by our own immune system. A cut on the foot leads to local inflammation so much so that the foot would be temporarily dysfunctional. The person would resort to a walking cane or crutches. If the same disability were to occur in our eyes from a debilitating inflammatory response launched by our immune system, our eyes would become temporarily out of commission, and we cannot afford that, not even for a nanosecond. The following figure illustrates a sophisticated field map of the human eye. Images that we see start with (1) light being converted to electrical impulses and relayed to the brain, and (2) the brain then converts electrical signals into images of the world that we see. The same logic explains why we are unable to see in darkness devoid of light.

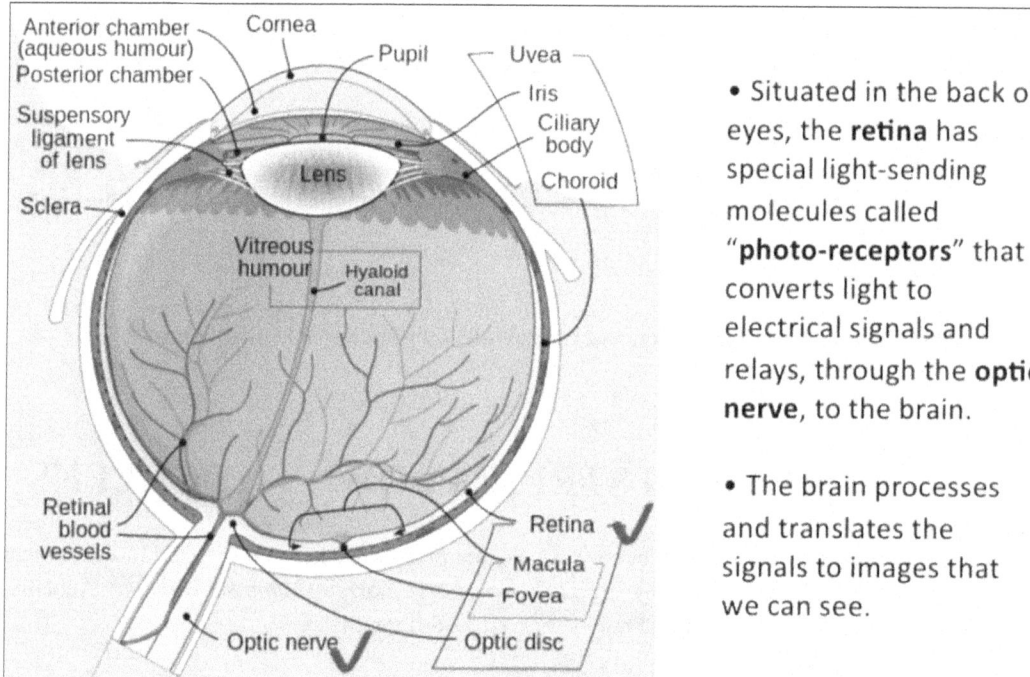

Image 94 A brief overview of eye anatomy. Wikimedia Commons File: Schematic diagram of the human eye en.svg.

Two core tactics to ensure eye immune privilege. Fortunately, we creatures of evolutionary adaptation have advanced to demarcate our eyes as a site of "immune privilege" to be shielded from immune storms. To make sure that our eyes steer clear of strong immune attacks, several arrangements are organized. These include (1) the absence of "lymphatic drains" so no immune cells come near to invading germs, and (2) Absence (or non-detectable presence of) "immune whistle blower" protein termed "human leukocyte antigen" (HLA), which normally signals CD8-T cells "Danger! Come and fight!" By clearing the above two robust immune energizers, our eyes are now safely nestled in peace and quiet to perform their designated function: to give us vision.

Tears come to the rescue. You might ask: If no immunity is associated with our eyes, how do we fend off germs that invade our eyes? Good question. The answer lies in our tears. Our everyday basal tear harbors ~1,500 different types of molecules for assorted forms of eye protection. Three particular active ingredients stand out. (1) *Lysozymes* are enzymes that kill germs such as bacteria. Dr. Alexander Fleming, who discovered the first antibiotic, showed in a paper published in 1922 that lysozymes isolated from tears readily dissolved some bacteria. (2) Antibodies called "*IgA*" in tears also help rid germs from our eyes. Quick notes on nomenclature: "Ig" stands for "immunoglobulin" which is another name for antibody. "Globulin" refers to the globular shape of the antibody. IgA molecules exist as an entity of "joint identical twins," and the jargon term is "dimer." Think of a pair of chopsticks that makes it handy to pick up food off a dinner plate, IgA dimer molecules also make it easy to take care of germs on our ocular surface, which brings in the third active ingredient of precious basal tears: (3) *Neutrophils*. You might ask: Neutrophils are immune cells from our innate immunity. Is the existence of neutrophils conflicting with the eye's immune privilege? The answer is no because the eye is part and parcel shielded from any major immune networks capable of triggering havoc-wreaking "cytokine immune storms"; besides, neutrophils exist in specially designated areas of the eye and work in conjunction with IgA dimers for eye pathogen elimination.

A special note on emotional tears. Produced in response to sorrow, joy, fear, anger, or pain, emotional tears come in different shades and properties. Scientists have proposed that "emotional tears" harbor hormones that are absent in "basal tears" or "reflex tears." For example, rich in emotional tears is a stress hormone called "*leu-enkephalin*" and it is speculated that the release of such a stress hormone helps us tone down heightened emotional stress levels to the baseline. It would be interesting to sort out the unique properties associated with "tears of sorrow" versus "tears of joy" by Woody Allen's barbed quill. More crying research will tell.

Food for thought:

1. Tear consists of three categories as basal, emotional, and stress.
    A. True
    B. False

2. Our eye is a designated immune privileged site to best preserve eye function.
    A. True
    B. False

THE "OLD" MAN AND THE VACCINE

For many, a single seminal discovery suffices to cement a claim of fame on a hallowed science pedestal, deservedly so. For Dr. Lloyd Old (1933–2011) who made so many original discoveries (as reflected in 700+ publications) that have reshaped the field of "tumor immunity"—a term coined by Dr. Old—the question is: Which discovery is the most groundbreaking? Here, let's focus on his visionary experimentation to repurpose existing infection-combating vaccines that paved the way to the very first approved therapeutic cancer vaccine.

Reigniting the torch of cancer immunotherapy. Back in the 1880s, Dr. William Coley, a bone surgeon at Memorial Hospital (the historic name of MSKCC, started experimenting with a potentially deadly infectious bacterial agent to treat inoperable cancers of the soft tissues called "sarcoma." It was met with remarkable initial success, but the situation became complicated with other physicians jumping onto the bandwagon by imitating the same method mixed with their own renditions. In the absence of regulatory procedures, the results were inconsistent: some patients saw their tumors disappear, others experienced no effect, and a few unfortunate patients succumbed to severe infection from the very bacterial toxin used to treat their tumors. With a strong belief in the power of revitalizing patients' own immune systems to fight cancer, Dr. Old picked up the baton and carried on. Among a host of accomplishments,

- *1959:* Discovered that Bacillus Calmette-Guerin (BCG) vaccine against TB killed cancer cells in laboratory mice with high potency, laying the groundwork for BCG being repurposed as a treatment for early-stage bladder cancer approved by the FDA.
- *1968*: Identified a surface protein on Killer T (KT) cells instrumental in orchestrating KT into immune action against dangerous cells, including cancer cells. The protein has gone through several naming steps and was finalized as the famous "CD8," as CD8-T cells.
- *1976–1979*: Discovered antibody proteins that combat cancer cells in the blood of cancer patients, laying the groundwork that immune cells are capable of spotting and slaying cancer cells.
- *1979*: Co-discovered p53, a small molecule that serves a big role in DNA damage repair and in suppressing insidious tumor cells. The discovery was independently carried out, aside from Dr. Old's group at MSKCC, by three other United Kingdom and United States research laboratories including team Dr. David Philip Lane and Dr. Lionel Crawford, team Dr. Daniel Linzer, and team Dr. Arnold Levine. Also worthy of mention are scientists instrumental in the characterization of p53 and core components of the p53 signaling pathway: Dr. Bert Vogelstein, Dr. Carol Prives, and Dr. Scott Lowe.
- *1980s*: Discovered an important cytokine called "tumor necrosis factor" (TNF) that could turn cancer cells into dying debris.
- *1997*: Identified a family of unique surface marker proteins found only in normal and cancerous testis cells but not in other cell types. The existence of testis-only protein markers makes it a feasible reality to design drugs that preferentially target testicular cancer cells without causing collateral damage to healthy cells in other parts of the patients' bodies.

These discoveries are fundamental in carving new paths and exciting vistas in basic immunology and tumor immunology. Unfortunately, cancer cut Dr. Lloyd Old's life short in 2011 at the age of 78. The impressive list of important discoveries to Dr. Old's name is several lives' worth. Hats off to the "Old" Man who was instrumental in the repurposed cancer-killing vaccine!

THERANOS: THE FIRST BLOOD THAT NEVER WAS

Theranos, the once starry start-up lab test company in Silicon Valley established in 2003, after more than two decades of fanfare, finally fell off the pedestal in 2018 with the founder's sentencing in December 2022 as a sad afterthought.

Air castle. Elizabeth Holmes, a Stanford bioengineering student, grew a fanciful idea of screening a few drops of blood on an attaché-sized machine to analyze over 200 substances and biomarkers to signify assorted arrays of diseased conditions ranging from infections to cancer. Her unparalleled charismatic power of persuasion convinced angel investors and celebrities to pour funds and support. Before long, she became the rising star helming a company with $9 billion in assets. Frequently appearing on high-tech platforms in a signature black turtleneck, Elizabeth was touted as the female version of Steve Jobs.

Appearance is easy to imitate; substance an entirely different matter. The company Theranos soon confronted problems—serious problems. Relying on a tiny volume of finger-prick blood, test results were inconsistent and unreliable. Instead of going back to the drawing board to revisit the science, *Theranos's* top management chose to cover up the scandalous tech blunders. Out of desperation, *Theranos* purchased leading instruments on the market to obtain results that claimed to be from *Theranos's* mini-analyzer named *Edison*. Mendacity *par excellence*!

Small is not necessarily savvy. A few drops of blood are adequate to run basic lab work tests such as blood sugar and cholesterol but unsuitable for detecting an extensive range of disease biomarkers. To start with, the tiny sample volume may not suffice to reflect a complex collection of disease or cancer molecular IDs. Second, a finger-pricked blood sample of a tiny volume may harbor injured cells that contaminate the blood sample and can easily obscure testing results from a tiny blood sample. Indeed, *Theranos* claimed that its proprietary analyzer, capable of detecting over 200 diseases under the sun turned out to be filled with inaccuracies. The company's downfall was inevitable from day one.

Lessons learned! On the part of investors: (1) Get to know the basics of science, or hire a qualified scientific review panel to scrutinize and ensure the soundness of the science behind any claims, no matter how outstanding. (2) Visit the company's physical site (not website!) and request a live demo from A to Z to check validity, reliability, sensitivity, and specificity—the whole 9 yards of clinical lab testing standard operating procedures. (3) Last but not least, "fast and easy" at the expense of "accuracy" and "reliability" is taboo in general practice, but especially when it comes to clinical and medical laboratory sciences where errors could be a matter of life and death for patients.

In the meantime, good science continues to advance. Recent news from the cancer screening front describes a new high-throughput cancer screening test that boasts detecting fifty different cancer types. The story so far is a mixed bag, although the positives outweigh the negatives. The jury is still out.

U

URANIUM ROCKED STATEN ISLAND

South of Manhattan, east of New Jersey, connected to Brooklyn on the northeast edge via the magnificent *Verazzano-Narrows* Bridge, Staten Island, holds a special chapter in the book of American independence. The Staten Island Battle took place in 1777, led by Major General John Sullivan of the Continental Army. Despite a crushing failure, the fighting spirit and the patriotic legacy are remembered on every July 4th.

Staten Island chapters are not always sanguine. One such chapter concerns *Fresh Kills Landfill* that haunted Staten Island's soil, water, and air for more than half a century. Residents, local officials, congressional representatives, and state officials alike joined together with a singular voice, the voice loud and clear: Shut down the toxic waste land, ASAP! My respected colleague recalls how, in order not to miss any demonstration events, she put her infant girl in a baby carriage and the mother-and-daughter team joined the demonstrations, rain or shine. Intense outcry finally resonated and led to the permanent shutdown of the toxic site in 2001.

Who could imagine that the finishing touches of one ugly chapter only led to the opening of another and even uglier chapter imposed upon Staten Island? This time, in contrast to the open toxin-replete landfill, the site and the associated saga were deeply hidden from three generations of Staten Islanders for more than half a century!

The "Manhattan Project." A stupendous undertaking from 1942–1946, the historic *Manhattan Project* was embarked upon under the remarkable helmsmanship of General Leslie Groves fused with the able mind of physicist Robert Oppenheimer. The mission was secretive but steadfast: to develop atomic bombs. The source material of superbly enriched uranium must start from uranium ore, the rocks that harbor uranium.

Incognito cargo. In 1938, a shipment of 1,200 tons of high-grade uranium ores out of the Belgian-Congo uranium mining company left for the East Coast of the United States. In 1939, the cargo was transferred to a secret warehouse on Staten Island near the magnificent Bayonne Bridge and stayed there until 1942. The project was so secretive that even the Staten Island borough president had no inkling at the time. In September 1942, the entire stockpile of 1,200 tons of uranium ore was shipped out of Staten Island, destined for Los Alamos, the research hub for the Manhattan Project. Thank goodness for the stockpile; it helped the Manhattan Project secure the majority of top-quality uranium-235 (U-235) needed for purification on short notice. To the local folks on Staten Island, especially those who reside in the vicinity of the warehouse, the rocks have left a jarring radioactive trail.

Kept in the dark. According to the Preliminary Assessment report conducted by the US Army Corps of Engineers in 2011, the warehouse covers 1.2 acres, and within 1 mile of the site houses "*9 schools, 5 hospitals, and 32 daycare centers*" with a total of close to 30,000 people in the vicinity. Back in 1980, one on-site study was conducted by the US Department of Energy (DOE) and detected a radioactive contaminated area of 20 × 40 square meters within the warehouse site, based on testing results from six soil samples. The specific type of hazardous substances identified is summarized in the table below.

Radioactive substances	U-238	Ra-226
Level	1,187 pCi/g	1,102 pCi/g
Half life	4.5 billion years	1600 years
Decay type	Alpha	Alpha
Annual exposure limits	10 microCi for ingestion; 0.4 microCi for inhalation	5 pCi/L

Image 95 Uranium and radium half-life. Assembled by Dr. Nancy Liu-Sullivan.

As the table summary indicates, uranium-238 (U-238) and radium-226 (Ra-226) levels detected in the contaminated slot of the warehouse are close to 200 times higher than the annual exposure limits designated by the US Environmental Protection Agency (EPA).

Dark secret unburied. Most alarming is that neither the "warehouse history" nor the "contaminated slot" was made known to the Staten Island residents. It took a serendipitous event to uncover the dark secret. The local heroine is Beryl Thurman, President of the Port Richmond Civic Association on Staten Island. In 1999, while hosting a local community event, Ms. Thurman learned about a deserted local warehouse. Leaving no stone unturned, she embarked on a crusade for truth. Thanks to Ms. Thurman's tireless effort and steadfast determination, this "surprise page" of the Staten Island chapter finally got a fighting chance to be heard by government agencies. The circuitous journey took more than two decades. The encouraging news finally came in 2020 that an executive plan for toxic clean-up was finally in the making. The table below summarizes key events concerning the Staten Island contaminated site in terms of requests, recommendations, and actions or lack of actions (indicated by the blank boxes in the table):

Alarmingly high cancer incidence on Staten Island. According to the New York State Cancer Incidence Report for the Staten Island Study Area conducted in August 2019, as part of the *Governor's Cancer Research Initiative*, the borough of Staten Island has an unusually high cancer incidence, compared to the other four boroughs of New York City—Manhattan, Bronx, Queens, and Brooklyn—and to New York State (excluding the four boroughs), in all cancers but particularly in thyroid cancer, as shown in the following figure:

Which straw broke the camel's back? Thus far worldwide, more than two hundred types, each associated with cancer subtypes, have been identified. It is commonly acknowledged that human cancer results from irreversible mutations of at least five critical genes. As for what drives genetic mutations, there is a growing list of risk factors ranging from exposure to environmental toxins, high-energy radiation (naturally occurring or man-made), industrial pollutants, first- or second-hand tobacco smoking, alcohol, poor diet, and aging. It is unlikely that any single risk factor makes a dominant difference in driving genetic mutations unrelated to inherited mutations. That being said, a

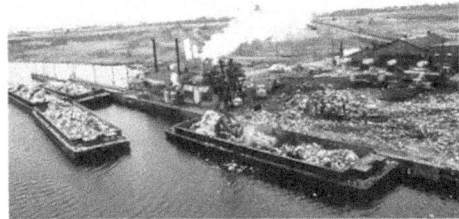
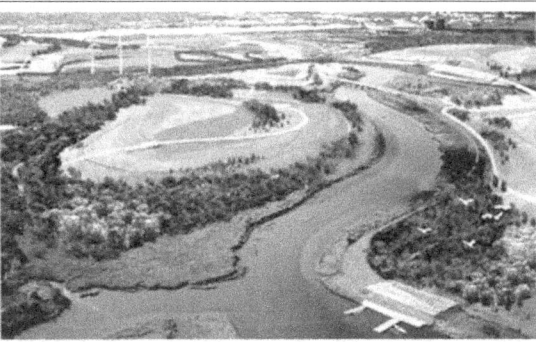

Staten Island Fresh Kills: Yesterday's Landfill transformed into today's bucolic eco-park.

Image 96 Staten island fresh kills: Yesterday's Landfill Transformed into Today's Bucolic Eco-Park). Wikimedia Commons File: Fresh Kills Park.jpg. Wikimedia Commons File: Garbage scows bring solid waste, for use as landfill, to fresh kills on Staten Island, just east of Carteret, NJ-NARA-548315.jpg.

	Staten Island cancer rates (2008–2019)	
	All cancers	Thyroid cancer
Compared to the 4 boroughs of NYC (Manhattan, Bronx, Queens, Brooklyn)	16% higher than NYC	76% higher than NYC
Compared to NYS (excluding NYC 4 boroughs)	3% higher than NYS	**63% higher than NYS**

Image 97 The Staten Island case: Thyroid cancer alarmingly high. Assembled by Dr. Nancy Liu-Sullivan.

risk factor presented as high in frequency, chronic in exposure, and elevated in amount could well serve as a leading risk factor that triggers a cancer flashpoint—the equivalent of the camel back-breaking straw. Adding another dimension to the cancer landscape is the immune system. It is indisputable that a compromised immune system is open season for vulnerability to cancer development.

As for what might account for Staten Island's unusually high overall cancer and thyroid cancer rates, none of the investigational reports identified leading factor or factors. Patterns of Staten Islanders' tobacco smoking, alcohol consumption, dietary choices, and aging processes are not particularly different compared to data sets collected from residents of other NYC boroughs or counties in New York State. The only two factors that do stand out for Staten Island are the long-term exposure to toxic air from Fresh Kills Landfill—an open garbage mountain of not only regular residential trash but also industrial waste including medical waste—and from radiation contamination from the vestige of the Second World War uranium warehouse. As for what roles these two outstanding factors have played in contributing to Staten Island's high cancer incidence, the jury is still out there.

It was reported that the last shipment to Staten Island Fresh Kills Landfill was in March 2001. Then came 911 that shocked the world. Without hesitation, Staten Islanders agreed to have more than one million tons of debris from the fallen twin towers transported to the Landfill—a selfless step instrumental for the recovery operations. Hats off to selfless Staten Islanders!! Today, the landfill has been transformed into a borough park that welcomes the return of golden finches, hawks, and snapping turtles, as my esteemed ecology colleagues have reported.

As for the uranium ore warehouse from Second World War, the Army Corps of Engineers was dispatched for cleanup in November 2023. Two months and $1.8 million later, all radioactive soil was removed. Finally!

The two chapters are officially closed but remain special in the history of Staten Island—buried but not forgotten.

Food for thought:

1. Although highly radioactive uranium ore was transported out of the Staten Island warehouse, harmful radioactivity was detected fifty times higher than average background levels.
    A. True
    B. False

2. Thanks goodness the once infamous Fresh Kills Landfill has been sealed up and transformed into a park and a wildlife sanctuary.

    A. True
    B. False

V

VICTORY LAP PROUD YET HUMBLE

Born to a surgeon's family in 1942, Tasuku Honjo completed medical school training at Kyoto University. Instead of practicing medicine, Dr. Honjo took a research career path as a molecular biologist, spent decades between research labs in Japan and the United States, and finally settled down at his *Alma Mater* Kyoto University, as professor and leader of molecular biology. In 2018, Dr. Honjo became the co-recipient of the Nobel Prize for Physiology or Medicine for his contribution to PD-1, an immune checkpoint protein that has been translated into life-saving cancer medications. In his Nobel Biographical, Dr. Honjo shares his inspirations on science and life distilled into six characters as curiosity, challenge, courage, concentration, continuation, and confidence. I am taking the liberty to feature it as Dr. Honjo's *6-C Motto*.

1. **CURIOSITY.** As Dr. Honjo advised his students, curiosity should be the primary force that drives those who choose to devote their intellect to science—the curiosity to find new paths that lead to the unknown world. Dr. Honjo describes his own mission of satisfying intellectual curiosity in a vivid metaphor as wading deep into big mountains in search of the source of water. Indeed, driven by that curiosity, Dr. Honjo discovered a previously unknown gene termed *"programmed cell death 1"* (PD-1). Residing on the surface of immune T cells, PD-1 maintains the checks and balances of immune response and deters T cells from over-exuberant activities.
2. **CHALLENGE.** Dr. Honjo also encourages his students to "embrace challenge," however daunting. He leads by example. To determine the function of PD-1 protein, Dr. Honjo and a team of scientists under his leadership journeyed using a "knock out" experimental method termed *loss-of-function* (LOF) studies. The scientists observed that laboratory mice with PD-1 gene erased developed inflammatory conditions of joints (arthritis) and kidneys (nephritis). Both medical conditions arise from the individual's own immune cells attacking one's own joints and kidney tissues—collectively defined as "autoimmune conditions." Absence of PD-1 driving autoimmune conditions is prima facie evidence that PD-1 is a negative regulator of immune T cells. In other words, when PD-1 functions normally, autoimmune conditions are prevented because PD-1 effectively restrains T cells from causing self-harm. It turned out that confirming PD-1 as a negative immune regulator only revealed one side of the molecular coin. What's on the other side?
3. **COURAGE.** It took several decades for PD-1 from the initial discovery to being turned into a high-efficacy anti-cancer antibody drug. The courage to carry on and follow through in spite of setbacks has made it possible, as shared by Dr. Honjo. The same courage was instrumental in the identification of PD-1's "other side."
4. **CONCENTRATION.** With laser-like focus, Dr. Honjo led his team to pursue the other side of the coin regarding the functional role of PD-1. Diligence was awarded with fruition: When PD-1 was deleted in laboratory mice that bore malignant tumors, tumor size considerably shrank or completely disappeared! To show that blocking PD-1 could reduce tumors in humans, Dr. Honjo set the next goal.

5. ***CONTINUATION.*** The search for the source of the waterway buried deep in endless mountain ranges is invariably a pinnacle mixed with lots of treacherous troughs along the journey. Setbacks come in different flavors. Deviating onto the wrong path or getting stuck in a *cul-de-sac* is one kind; being bogged down with politics is quite another. Remaining clear-headed to see through the fog and focus on science propels the scientist and the science forward. Lamenting is useless—like riding a rocking chair, it keeps one busy but goes nowhere!
6. ***CONFIDENCE.*** *Good better best, never let it rest; till good is better, and better best*! The timeless saying applies perfectly to Dr. Honjo's journey of PD-1. To block a protein situated on the cell surface, the best strategy is to develop purified antibodies that bind and impede the activities of the target protein. In collaboration with another group, anti-PD-1 antibodies were successfully developed, tested on cancer patients, and obtained surprisingly encouraging clinical outcomes. Following the approval of the first PD-1-targeting antibody drug in Japan in 2014, the PD-1 antibody drug received subsequent approval in the United States, European Union, and China. Former president Jimmy Carter was successfully treated with the drug and achieved CR of his late-stage melanoma that had metastasized to the brain. Science saves!

Decades of perseverance in the tireless pursuit of science have led to the victory lap. Instead of self-glowing, Dr. Honjo shares with all pupils the detours and setbacks encountered along the paths of discovery. Humility is a virtue. For a detailed description of the 6-C motto and Dr. Honjo's journey of scientific discovery, please visit NobelPrize.org.https://www.nobelprize.org/prizes/medicine/2018/honjo/biographical/

W

WATER: BLISSFUL JOY; *ELEGANTLY DESTROY*

Water . . .
It wets my foot, but prettily,
It chills my life, but wittily,
. . .
In perfect time and measure
With a face of golden pleasure
Elegantly destroy.

Pithy lines on the dual nature of water by American thinker, preacher, and poet Ralph Waldo Emerson (1803–1882).

Indeed, water that covers 71 percent of Earth's surface and 60 percent of the human body is a vitally nourishing part of our lives. Water also has a tempestuous side to it and can even act as an enabler to promote mutations. Let's zoom it.

Water is bent. Composed of one oxygen atom in the center bonded to two hydrogen atoms (hence, H_2O, as shown in the lower right-hand corner of the following figure), water is not linear but bent and polar with partial negative charge on the oxygen and partial positive charge on the two hydrogens. Water exists in one of the three phases: *liquid* (in which water molecules move freely), *solid* (as ice, in which movement is restricted), or *gas* (such as steam, in which water molecules are chock-full of energy in motion or kinetic energy, as exemplified by Watt's steam engine). The interchangeable states of water phases are also best exemplified by Watt's steam engine, where water is turned into steam (gaseous state) by heating to drive the piston, followed by condensing the steam back to liquid (liquid state) such that a partial vacuum is created to be filled with steam, thus keeps on driving the piston.

Water is interactive. Water's polar structure also renders it a near universal solvent, meaning water is capable of dissolving many molecules that are polar. Examples of water-soluble substances at our dinner table include simple sugars (glucose or fructose), table salt, vitamins B (1, 2, 3, 6, 9, 12), vitamin C, and delightful of all, soluble fiber, notably oats.

Water turns radical. Water can be strong enough to form form giant waves, raging storms, and perilous flash floods. At the same time, water can also be vulnerable and fall apart, especially when it comes to harmful radiation. Ionizing radiation (IR) such as gamma ray and X-rays can dismantle water molecules to form hydrogen peroxide (H_2O_2) and hydroxyl radicals (-OH). Now, -OH possesses unpaired electrons and is therefore unstable and has the penchant to snatch electrons out of DNA molecules—the outcome of which is *bona fide* DNA damage. You might ask: How does hydrogen peroxide cause damage to DNA since it is not a free radical? Excellent question. Indeed, H_2O_2, with fully happily paired electrons, has no need to steal electrons from its neighbors and therefore is not defined as a free radical. However, H_2O_2 can readily interact with certain metals (such as copper and

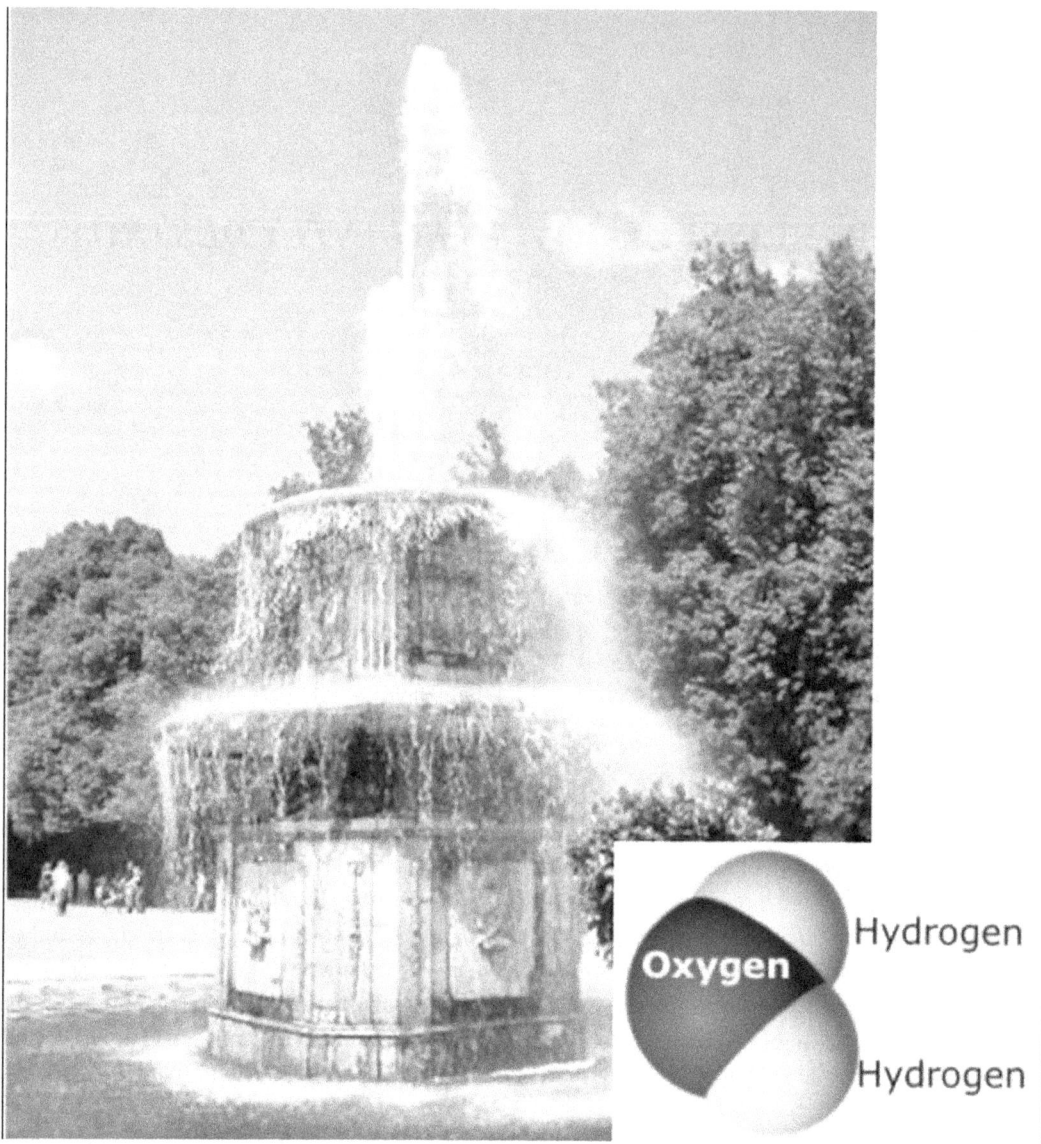

Image 98 Water fountain. Wikimedia Commons File: Rimsky Fountains Peterhof.jpg Wikimedia Commons File: Water molecule 3D.svg.

iron) to generate -OH or hydroxyl radicals. In short, both products of water destruction by ionizing radiation can harm DNA.

Antioxidants come to the rescue. Free radicals, harmful as they are, can be rectified with antioxidants, which altruistically donate an electron to free radicals to pair up the lone electron in the valence (outermost electron orbit) shell to tame free radicals from wreaking havoc on molecules. Blissfully, antioxidants naturally exist in many food items, and compounds with antioxidant properties include beta carotene (richly endowed in carrots), vitamin C (in citrus fruits, apples, and many berries), and vitamin E (abundant in almonds, peanuts, and avocados).

Water can heal. Water can also kill. Respect its charm but also be vigilant about its harm, as hymned by Emerson:

Well used, it decketh joy,
Adorneth, doubleth joy:
Ill used, it will destroy

Food for thought:

1. Water can be ionized by high-energy radiation to form free radicals that can damage DNA by snatching electrons out of DNA.
   A. True
   B. False

2. Antioxidants can readily make free radicals less reactive by donating electrons to them.
   A. True
   B. False

WONDERFUL LAND OF MILK, HONEY AND BEYOND

The King James Version of the Bible, Exodus 3, describes "land of milk and honey" as "promised land of Judaism." Our close family friend, a devout believer and an accomplished scholar (who claims to have never stepped into a Synagogue—another story, another time, perhaps), shared with us how conventional Judaic practice against "milk" had nothing related to religion but had everything to do with how eons ago, before Louis Pasteur's pasteurization method was available, milk spoiled very readily in the cracks and crevices of wooden bowls and turned bad very easily. Of course, since the advent of pasteurization, milk has been bestowed with a much longer shelf life. Thanks to science!

The milk scare. Rich in vitamin D and other vitamins and minerals, milk nourishes. In the early to mid-1950s, however, there was a "milk scare" in heartland states including Missouri, Utah, Idaho, and Montana. The worst of all scares was "milk and its link to cancer." It turned out that milk itself is not at all a carcinogen, none whatsoever. What tainted the reputation of local milk was the route of production. In the aforementioned states, nuclear bomb testing was carried out more often than necessary. After each test, as mushroom clouds were dissipating, the dust filled with radioactive substances also seeped into the grasses. Cows munched on the tainted grass, and humans consumed the milk from those cows. Before long, the radioactive materials got into people's blood as the blood traveled up and down the human body to deliver the needed nutrients. It was especially warned that young children should stay clear of milk sourced from those heartland states. Thank goodness nuclear testing eventually came to a halt, cows could freely roam again, and people were able to pour milk into their cereal bowls without being freaked out.

Honey quicksand for bad bugs. Don't mean to be sensational. This warning is meant for bacteria, not humans. It turns out that honey is a natural antibacterial agent. In the old days before refrigerators, freezers, and modern freezing agents such as liquid nitrogen and dry ice, our ancestors had to resort to nature for food preservation. Top on that list is honey. How does honey perform its trick on bacteria? It so happens that raw unprocessed honey has very high osmotic pressure, which literally sucks water molecules out of bacteria, disabling them from growing and eventually leading to their demise.

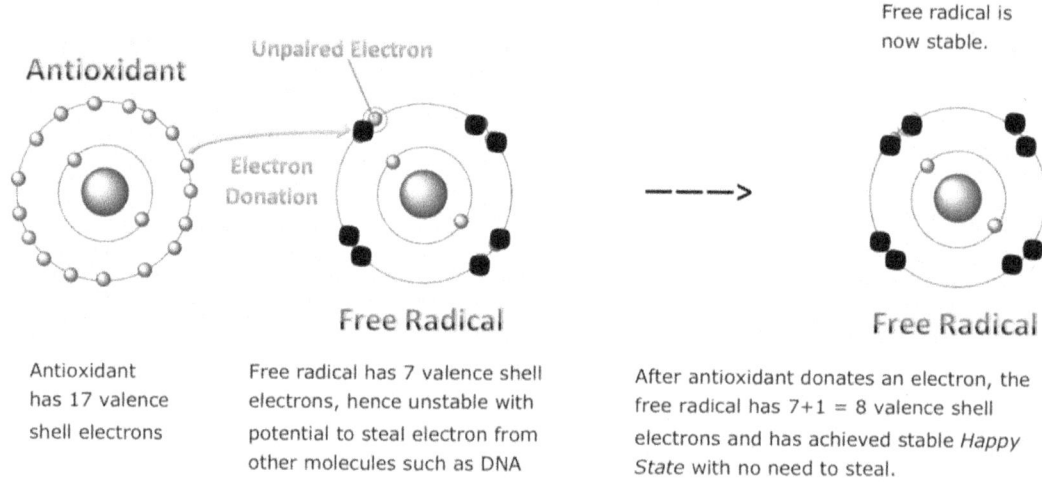

Image 99 Antidote for free radicals. Wikimedia Commons File: Antioxidants Free radicals Lobo et al.. Png modified by Nancy Liu-Sullivan.

Honey's healing power. Of course, honey possesses more power beyond pinning down bacterial bugs via high osmotic pressure. Honey is also a robust antidote against "free radicals," the harmful chemical compounds to human health. As is infamously known, free radicals can wreak havoc in DNA by breaking up the spiral strands. Why? Because free radicals are *a priori* molecularly "handicapped" in that they do not possess paired electrons in the outermost orbit (the valence shell) of an atom. Like a four-legged picnic table with one leg missing, free radicals, too, "suffer" from imbalance. To achieve balance, free radicals literally steal electrons wherever and whenever possible, and DNA becomes a vulnerable molecular victim. Fortunately, we have honey on our side. Richly endowed with healing chemicals, most notably flavonoids, honey is a powerful anti-free radical agent, which in chemical terms is also deemed as *antioxidants*. How does honey unleash its magic power? By shuffling an electron to an unstable free radical to restore balance in the free radical. Balance tames free radicals, and our precious DNA is protected.

You might ask: Missing electron? Imbalance? Shifting an electron to restore balance? Sounds Greek! With you. Here is an everyday example of how atomic balance is stored: table salt. A picture is worth a thousand words, so here it is, an example of how two "free radicals" combine to form a stable dinner table staple:

As shown above, as a stand-alone element, sodium (Na) and chlorine (Cl) are "free radicals" due to unbalanced number of electrons floating in the valence shell of an atom. After an exchange in which sodium donates its lone electron to chlorine and chlorine accepts an electron from sodium, table salt is created—a molecular win-win that brings out the flavor out of food and provides strength to us. As an added note, salt is not always a dietary villain. For one thing, sodium is one of four indispensable "electrolytes" (the other three being potassium, magnesium, and calcium) that work hard to maintain our metabolic balance. Besides, have you ever tried a dish with zero salt? It is tasteless! Of course, overindulgence in salt is also undesirable, especially for folks with cardiovascular risks.

So honey, go for it! Honey-glazed carrots, honey-flavored sweet and sour chicken, a hint of honey to tame bitter coffee, a personal favorite delicacy of peeled whole garlic marinated in balsamic and honey, . . . the yummy list goes on. A paper by a research team from the University of Toronto reports that two teaspoons of honey per day added to a good diet have broad effects against inflammatory conditions. Well, the catch here is a diet that is already healthy. Honey alone cannot do all the tricks. Also, since honey is a form of sugar, calories should also be kept in mind. Once again, the time-tested golden rule of balance reigns: Eat well, exercise regularly, stay happy and healthy. Cheers!

Food for thought:

1. Honey is an antidote against harmful free radicals.
    A. True
    B. False

2. Honey is also antimicrobial by literally sucking water out of bacteria that leads to bacterial death.
    A. True
    B. False

WONDROUS POISON AGAINST LEUKEMIA

Rumor has it that Napoleon Bonaparte died of arsenic poisoning as an unusually high arsenic level was detected in his hair sample. Arsenic's lethality is manifested in dismantling cells' energy machinery and disrupting oxygen-carrying RBCs—two vital lines of life. A common arsenic compound is arsenic trioxide (ATO, As2O3). Surprisingly, in September 2000, the FDA approved ATO for the treatment of "acute pro-myelocytic leukemia" (APL). Poison prescribed for patients? What's going on?

It's all in the dose! Worry not. According to the CDC, the potentially fatal dose of ATO is 1—2.5 mg/kg. By contrast, ATO standard dosing for treating APL is only 150 μg/kg/day, five days per week with a sixty-day limit; that is, the regimen continues until cancer remission is achieved, and in cases where, by day sixty, cancer remission does not occur, the treatment is halted.

Overall, arsenic trioxide is very effective in treating APL leukemia. According to a report published in the *Journal of American Medical Association* (JAMA) in 2021, ATO in pediatric acute promyelocytic leukemia (APL) shows a 97 percent disease-free rate for standard risk patients over two years and 83 percent disease-free rate for high-risk patients also over two years. The disease relapse rate was determined to be only 4 percent. Extremely encouraging news! Overall, ATO is safe to use, and common side effects include fever, fatigue, swelling of hands, legs, and feet, among others. The benefits of ATO clearly outweigh the side effects.

Arsenic arsenals against leukemia cells. The culprit of two mutations, one located on Chromosome 15 and the other on Chromosome 17, APL affects 1 in 250,000 people in the United States. Immature cancerous WBCs from the innate arm of immunity grow uncontrollably in the bone marrow that leaves no room for RBCs, lymphocytes (B, T, NK cells), or platelets. ATO helps immature WBCs to undergo differentiation (to become specialty immune cells), which pressures cancerous WBCs to return to their state of normalcy. Another remarkable achievement of ATO is triggering cancerous leukemia cells to die by a process called apoptosis, also called programmed cell death. An additional ATO trick against APL involves the generation of potent free radicals termed "reactive oxygen species" (ROS) that break leukemia DNA with no molecular qualms.

Instrumental in establishing ATO as a standard leukemia treatment are two Chinese physician-scientists, Dr. ZHANG Tingdong and Dr. WANG Zhenyi.

Back to Napoleon: A new theory has surfaced as death by stomach cancer. The mystery continues to unfold.

Food for thought:

1. Arsenic trioxide promotes APL leukemia cells to achieve maturation or differentiation, which helps revert APL cancer cells back to normal WBCs.
   A. True
   B. False

2. Arsenic trioxide can also activate apoptosis cascades in APL cells that lead to death of leukemia cells.
   A. True
   B. False

X

X: ENTERING DOMAINS OF CANCER UNKNOWNS

Residing in the English alphabet table at position #24, X represents the unknown quantity in algebra, symbolizes the horizontal axis in Cartesian coordinates, denotes the mysterious ray in nuclear physics, while being the equivalent of ten in the Roman numerical system. Coincidentally, ten also portrays the masterfully distilled Weinberg-Hanahan core hallmarks of cancer (***CRAB: THE NAME TELLS A VIVID TALE***, page 72). Here, let's venture into cancer unknowns—known unknowns, even unknown unknowns.

Toxin synergistic effects still unknown. Certain toxic chemical compounds are capable of driving genetic mutations that eventually convert normal cells into cancerous cells. Collectively, these toxins are classified as *carcinogens*, defined as "substances that cause cancer." The most comprehensive list of carcinogens is the one established by the *International Agency for Research on Cancer* (IARC) under the World Health Organization (WHO). As shown in the table below, IARC classifies cancer-linked carcinogens into different groups: Group 1, Group 2A, Group 2B, and Group 3. More detailed information can be obtained from the IARC WHO website (https://monographs.iarc.who.int/agents-classified-by-the-iarc/).

Great work! Extremely informative. What's missing, however, are potential synergistic effects of mixtures from Group 1, 2A, and 2B depicted in the above table. Take Group 2B as an example; exposure to heavy metal lead or jet fuel alone only serves as possible cancer risk factors according to the WHO. But what happens when individuals are suddenly subjected to frequent exposure to a combination of lead and diesel fuel (and possibly additional toxic metals and chemicals)? Do toxin mixtures confer synergistic effects that accelerate time taken to transform normal cells into cancer?! The answer in theory is that *we do not know*. In practice, American veterans exposed to frequent and high-intensity burn-pit toxins during the Iraq War came down with cancers (especially of the brain, lung, and thyroid) at more elevated rates when compared to everyday folks. Aside from benzene from jet fuel (used to ignite burn pits), the gigantic toxin piles also contained medical waste, assorted metals, rubber, plastics, paints, and solvents. Do combos of toxins and fumes serve to drive cancer flashpoints? A worthy known unknown for unraveling. The 2022 Promise to Address Comprehensive Toxics (PACT) Act is a good start.

Interplay between vaccine and cancer killing unknown. We discussed how the TB vaccine BCG was unexpectedly found to be highly effective at killing early-stage bladder cells. Good job by MSKCC scientists who gained the groundbreaking insight over vaccines repurposed against cancer (***THE OLD MAN AND VACCINE***, page 196) in addition to paving the road for deciphering mysterious codes that are embedded in BCG, capable of mobilizing potent cytokines against cancer cells (*Ibid*). What remains puzzling, however, is among a long list of cancer types tested, why BCG is preferentially effective against early-stage bladder cancer, but not early-stage lung cancer or colon cancer? Another known unknown worthy of unraveling.

	International Agency for Research on Cancer (IARC) Classification, WORLD HEALTH ORGANIZATION (WHO)	
Group 1	Asbestos / Ionizing Radiation / Ultraviolet (UV) / Benzene / Hepatitis B,C / HIV /HPV /Alcohol / Tobaco	KNOWN human carcinogens
Group 2A	Malaria / Red Meat / Talc / Very hot beverages > than 65-degree-Fahrenheit	PROBABLE human carcinogens
Group 2B	Diesel fuel / Gasoline / Bleomycin / Cobalt / Lead / Titanium dioxide	POSSIBLE human carcinogens
Group 3	Coal dust / Cholesterol / Caffeine / Vitamin K	Carcinogens UNRELATED to humans

Image 100 World Health Organization (WHO) carcinogens classified, assembled by Dr. Nancy Liu-Sullivan.

Precise link between high fevers and tumor spontaneous remission unknown. As for spontaneous tumor remission that occurs after cancer patient has recovered from a serious bacterial or viral infection that involved high fevers, what was the battleground like when the patient's immune cells were simultaneously battling against infectious bugs and cancer cells? Was the strategy of "speed and surprise" deployed to swiftly bombard the pair of "enemy" lines of infection and cancer from land, air, and sea? Another worthy known unknown waiting to be elucidated.

As for areas pertaining to *cancer unknown unknowns*, let's set them as a series of "X1, X2, X3, ... Xn" for now. The advent of AI will, with high confidence, offer unique executive assistance to scientists in quantum computing and multi-dimensional algorithms to aid vector meta-analyses of tons of temporal and spatial data sets involving genetics, epigenetics, genomics, metabolics, immunologics juxtaposed with environmental and lifestyle factors—the complex befuddling anarchical molecular chaos of *anything and everything all at once* of cancer. No easy task, especially considering how a one-centimeter cubed (1cc) tumor harbors one billion cancer cells! What's more, no tumor is formed by a single type of cancer cells, but consists of varied sub-populations termed "tumor heterogeneity." What's even more, a cancerous tumor is a moving train that constantly evolves in reaction to retaliations by immune cells or anti-cancer therapeutics or both. Despite cancer's enormous complexity in temporal and spatial dimensions, with talents and the helping hand of AI, turning all cancer stones is not a mission impossible. We shall make it to the finish line—a known known!

Food for thought:

1. A key challenging aspect of cancer complexity resides in the interplay of cancer cells with their environment.
    A. True
    B. False

2. AI is the only hope of solving the cancer mystery.
    A. True
    B. False

Y

YALOW: PRIDE OF THE CITY UNIVERSITY OF NEW YORK!

Her parents, first and second-generation immigrants to New York City, had a career plan for her: to become a school teacher. Inspired by her own school teachers, she first became keen on math, then chemistry, and then grew to be enamored with nuclear physics. In 1945, as the world was celebrating the end of the Second World War, Rosalyn Yalow became Dr. Rosalyn Yalow and wrote the history of the first-ever female graduate with a PhD degree in nuclear physics from the University of Illinois, Champaign-Urbana. Greater history was made in subsequent years by Dr. Yalow.

Following the footsteps of the Curies. Written by Irene Joliot-Curie, the biography about Madam Curie's life and science cemented young Rosalyn's penchant for nuclear physics. Most interestingly, in 1977, seventy-four years since Madam Curie won the Nobel Prize in Physics in 1903, Dr. Yalow was also inducted into the hallowed Nobel Hall. How did Dr. Yalow, a nuclear physicist, win the Nobel Prize in Physiology or Medicine? It all started with insulin.

Blood sugar and insulin. After a meal, blood sugar spikes. The raised blood sugar signals the pancreas to release insulin—a hormone that dispatches sugar out of the blood to cells. The sugar that enables cells to make fuel is the simplest form of sugar called *glucose*. Cells make fuel called "adenosine triphosphate" (ATP) by breaking down glucose. Each glucose molecule yields thirty-two molecules of ATP. For folks with type 1 diabetes (T1D), when blood sugar spikes, their body is unable to secrete insulin that helps shuffle sugar to tissues. Even though type 2 diabetes (T2D) folks are able to make their own insulin, they confront a similar insulin conundrum: Their body is insulin "insensitive," that is, the insulin cannot be used to transport blood sugar into cells. In both medical instances, absence or inadequate insulin activity poses a big problem for hungry cells: No glucose to make ATP. No ATP, no fuel, and the cellular "car" goes nowhere! The starving cells resort to another means of energy source: fat which can be metabolized to manufacture the sorely needed cellular energy. Burning fat for fuel may seem a convenient energy-gathering shortcut; however, it leads to an accumulation of ketone bodies in blood, a condition called *diabetic ketoacidosis* (DKA) that requires immediate medical attention. To avoid DKA, insulin must be injected into T1D patients and, depending on condition severity, also to some T2D patients. While today insulin shots and insulin pumps are standard care, the life-saving meds were not available until 1922, thanks to a Canadian surgeon and researcher as well as to mankind's best canine friend.

Canine, bovine, porcine, and human. In 1921, University of Toronto, a bone surgeon by the name of Dr. Frederick Banting set up shop for the very first insulin research laboratory in the world. Assisting Dr. Banting was Charles Best. Team Banting and Best also came up with an ingenious experimental design for the pursuit of insulin by tying up the pancreatic duct of an experimental dog (a procedure called *ligation* that cuts off blood supply to the ligated target of interest) and subsequently isolating canine insulin which was used to treat dog diabetes, with marked improvement observed. The team then switched to isolating insulin from cows. The bovine insulin was used to treat a dying fourteen-year-old diabetic patient by the name of Leonard Thompson, who was saved and lived to the age of twenty-six. Another patient of Dr. Banting's lived to celebrate her seventy-third birthday, having been injected with life-saving insulin since age fifteen for a total of 42,000 shots! Many more lives were also saved and extended. What happens to insulin after it is injected into the human body? That was the research question posed by Dr. Yalow and her scientific partner, Dr. Berson.

Insulin: amount tiny but role big. To learn about the physiological events of insulin injected into the human body, one must have a way of measuring insulin concentration in blood. This was no easy feat due to the minuscule level of insulin in blood. How minuscule? Pico-gram minuscule! Well, 1 pico gram = 1 trillionth of a gram, with the scientific notation as 1×10^{-12} grams. Ingeniously, Dr. Rosalyn Yalow and Dr. Solomon Berson, the scientific dynamic duo made up of a nuclear physicist and a biochemist at the Bronx Veterans Administration Hospital (VA Hospital) north of New York City, brainstormed and developed a precision method called *Radio-Immuno-Assay* (RIA), for which Dr. Yalow was awarded the Nobel Prize in 1977 (Dr. Berson had unfortunately passed away five years earlier). How exactly does RIA work?

Molecular musical chairs. July 4th weekend backyard party, a happy bunch of family friends gather to play a game of musical chairs. The participants walk around a circle of chairs as the music plays. As soon as the music stops, each is to grab the nearest chair and sit down. Those who fail to occupy a chair are invited out. Now, imagine two groups of participants, one dressed in an outfit with the "lightning" symbol, the other group dressed in a different outfit with a large symbol of a "triangle." Let the two groups run around eleven chairs formed in a circle. If you allow all "lightning" participants to play the game, when the music comes to a halt, all the chairs will be occupied by participants in "lightning" outfits. If, however, you mix eleven "lightning" players with twenty "triangle" players and let them compete, when the music ceases, more chairs will be occupied by "triangle" players. Why? Because of the sheer greater number of players dressed in "triangle" outfits. The RIA insulin measurement method developed by Dr. Yalow and Dr. Berson, believe it or not, is kind of related to the musical chairs game, as follows:

Let the "musical chairs" be insulin antibodies fixed in a well on a plate. Imagine the "lightning" players as insulin molecules, each carrying a radioactive isotope tag that emits "hot" radiation that can be detected by a gadget. Imagine the "triangle" players as plain, un-decorated insulin molecules not carrying any radioactive tags, and hence "cold" insulin. The raison d'être of insulin, hot or cold, is to snug onto insulin antibodies, just like each musical chair player is determined to occupy a chair. Now, if you mix eleven "hot" insulin molecules with twenty "cold" insulin molecules, then release them *en masse* to a pool of insulin antibodies, and let the game of "molecular musical chairs" begin! When the dust settles, more insulin antibodies will be occupied by "cold" insulin due to the sheer larger numbers (twenty) than "hot" insulin (eleven). Like the musical chairs game where players who fail to occupy a chair get eliminated, in the assay designed by Dr. Yalow and Dr. Berson, insulin, hot or cold, that fails to latch onto an insulin antibody protein, gets washed away. The above is illustrated in the following diagram:

Antigen keys latching into antibody "lock." As described in the series of *ANTIBODY PLAYBOOK* (pages 7–12), antigen binds to antibody very much like a key fitting into a lock. Insulin is an antigen that binds to insulin antibody but to the insulin antibody only, not the adrenaline antibody, not the dopamine antibody. Shaped like a tree, each antibody consists of a stem and two outward-pointing branches. The tip of each branch harbors the binding pocket, and each antibody possesses two binding

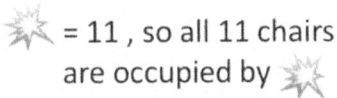
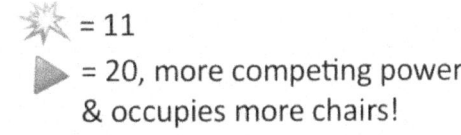
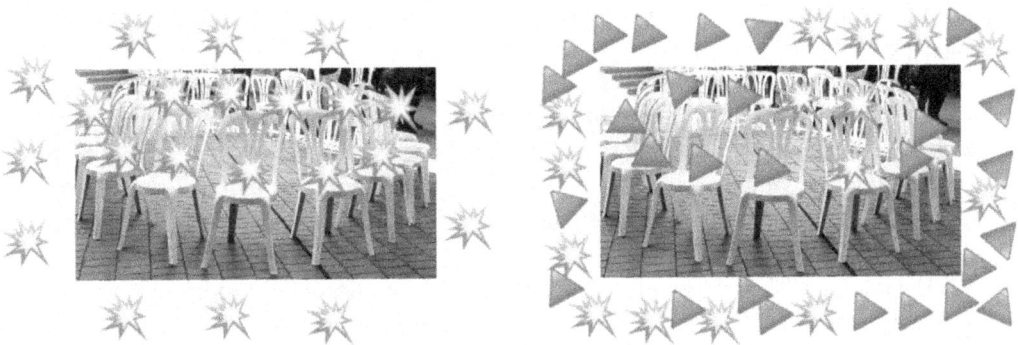

Musical Chairs Game

Image 101 A game of musical chairs. By Nancy Liu-Sullivan.

pockets. In a similar vein, each insulin antibody can accommodate two insulin antigens, as shown in the following figure:

RadioImmunoAssay (RIA) principle = Competitive binding

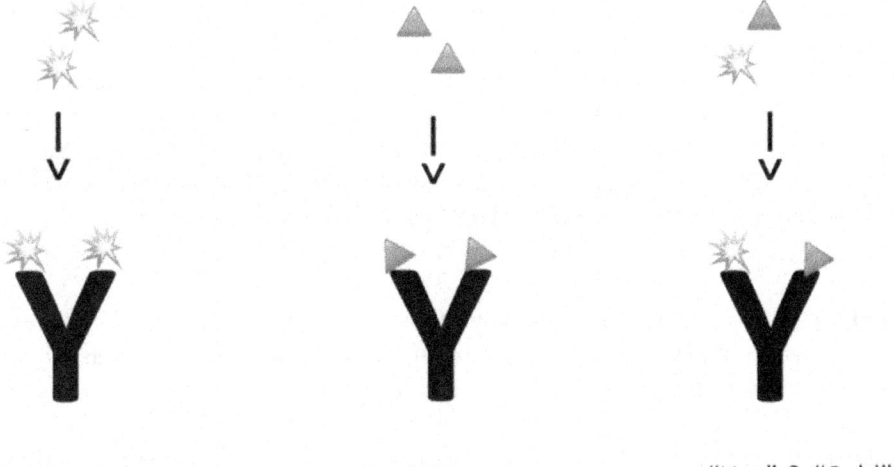

"Hot" insulin binds to insulin antibody

"Cold" insulin binds to insulin antibody

"Hot" & "Cold" insulins COMPETE to bind to insulin antibody

Image 102 Ria. By Nancy Liu-Sullivan.

Competition between "hot" and "cold" insulin. To prepare hot insulin molecules, Dr. Yalow labelled a pool of insulin molecules with radioactive *iodine 125* (I-125), which emits high-energy gamma rays that can be captured and measured by a gamma counter. The cold insulin molecules did not receive any radioactive molecular decorations. When these two pools of insulin are mixed together and poured into a plate of insulin antibodies, competition embarks!

Taking advantage of the *competitive binding* feature, team Yalow and Berson designed the following experiment by:

Step 1: Establishing the positive "control" by adding a saturating level of "hot" insulin to insulin antibodies such that every binding site on the antibodies is saturated by "hot" insulin as measured by 100 percent radioactivity—This is the baseline or benchmark of radioactivity with all antibody binding pockets being occupied. Of course, all floating unbound "hot" insulin molecules are washed off.

Step 2: Having established the baseline, the two scientists extended the experiment by including additional experimental groups where the same level of insulin antibodies and same level of "hot insulin" that produced 100 percent radioactivity were kept as exact replicas from the experiment described in Step 1.

Step 3: Once the additional replicas groups were set with each group showing 100 percent hot insulin bound to insulin antibodies, what happened next is absolutely ingenious: To the replica groups labelled as Group-1, 2, 3, . . . 7, in sequential steps each group was added with increasing amount of "cold" insulin to compete with "hot" insulin in binding to insulin antibodies in each group. The idea was that the presence of an overwhelming number of "cold" insulin would crowd in and kick off "hot" insulin already bound to insulin antibodies in each group. You might be asking: What?! "Hot" insulin molecules have already snugged in insulin antibodies, why are they so easily lifted up and replaced by "cold" insulin??? Fair question. The answer is affinity. Specifically, the affinity (or attraction) between "cold" natural form of insulin to insulin antibody is significantly higher than affinity between "hot" radio-labelled insulin and insulin antibodies, just like a child having higher affinity for mother over aunt. Nothing against aunts. :) The displaced "hot" insulin from each group leads to reduced radioactivity and by comparing to the known baseline radioactivity of 100%, team Yalow and Berson successfully measured the EXACT amount of insulin in the testing sample. The step-by-step displacement of "hot" insulin by "cold" insulin is illustrated below:

The standard curve! It is clear from the illustration above that there is an inverse relationship between amount of "hot" insulin displaced and the reduction of radioactivity. This relationship can also be represented as the standard curve in an X-Y coordinate system where Y is a function of X, as follows:

Blood insulin measured with precision. The standard curve serves as a reference table; each coordinate represents a specific radioactivity percentage (Y) as a function of insulin concentration (X). With this, patient insulin levels can be precisely measured which guides physicians in diagnostics and treatment strategies for patients. Let's try a "mock" case:

Suppose a patient's blood sample yielded radioactivity of 20 percent using the competitive binding method. The lab technologist would next locate "20%" on the Y axis, draw a horizontal line until reaching the standard curve, then draw a vertical line until reaching the X axis. The insulin concentration on the X axis is the patient's insulin level, as indicated with the down arrow on the X axis in the mock graph below.

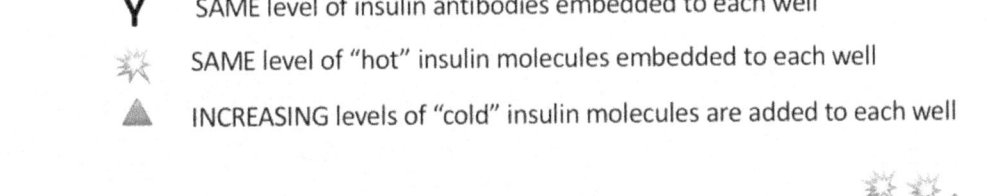
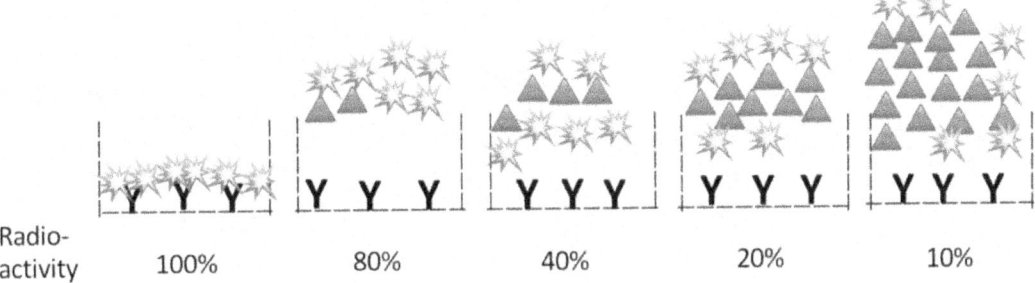

Image 103 Radioactivity quantified. By Nancy Liu-Sullivan.

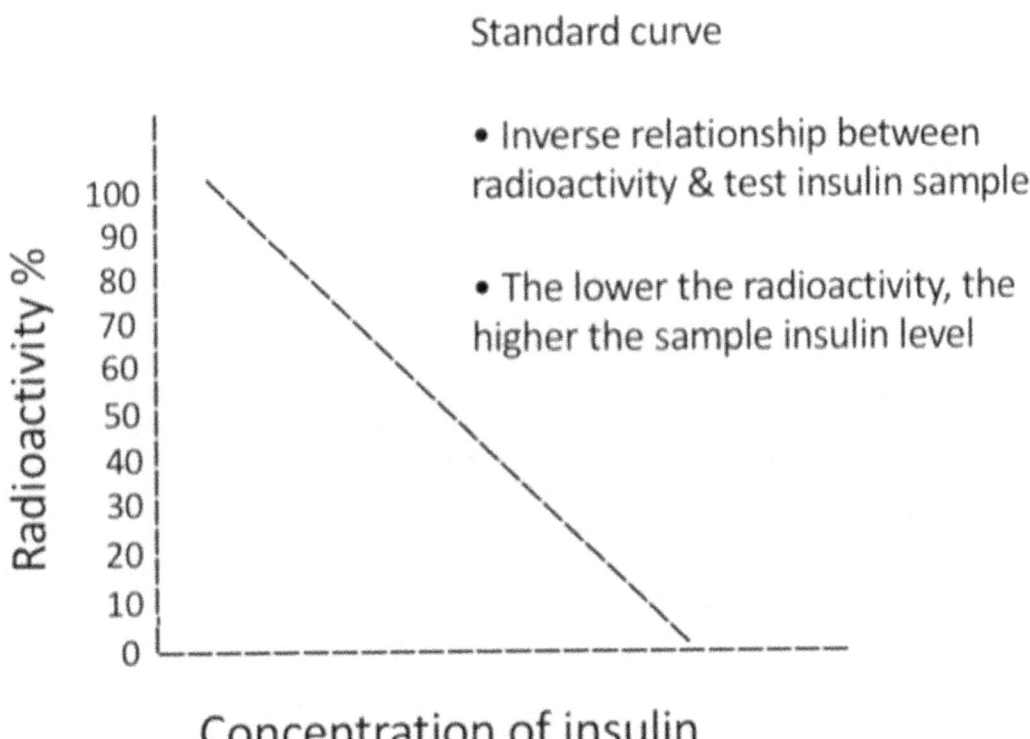

Image 104 Standard curve 1. By Nancy Liu-Sullivan.

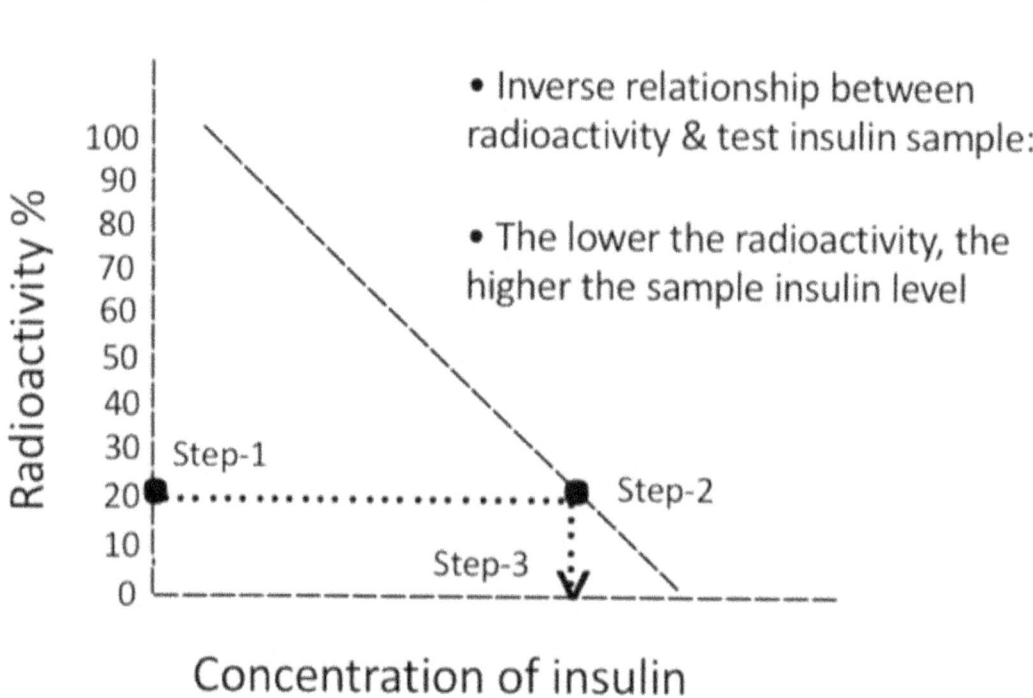

Image 105 Standard curve 2. By Nancy Liu-Sullivan.

The brilliant RIA method by Dr. Yalow and Dr. Berson allows medical technologists to determine levels of blood substances of insulin and beyond with *impeccable* precision. Despite potential safety concerns over radiation exposure, Radio-Immuno-Assay is still used today for the detection of hepatitis B and an extensive list of hormones and drugs.

Pride of CUNY! By following her passion in nuclear physics, Dr. Yalow did not become a full-time school teacher as her parents had planned for her. That said, Dr. Yalow did get to teach physics to American G.I.s who returned home from the Second World War and thoroughly enjoyed it! A women's college and tuition-free back in the 1940s and 1950s, Hunter College was extremely competitive for admissions. Today, as a leading senior college of the City University of New York (CUNY), Hunter College remains highly competitive as it continues to carry on the living legacy of Dr. Rosalyn Yalow.

Z

ZENITH OF SUCCESS NOT DEFINED BY A PRIZE

A graduate of McGill University, Montreal, Canada, Ralph Steinman moved south to Cambridge, MA, to attend Harvard University Medical School. A few scientific stints later, Dr. Ralph Steinman took a position at Rockefeller University, on the Upper East Side of Manhattan, New York, where he made a seminal discovery that has profoundly shaped the field of immunology. To gain a good grasp of the immune cell type discovered by Dr. Steinman, let's revisit the two arms of the human immune system.

"Street smart" or "Book smart." As discussed in *ATLAS OF IMMUNE BIG PICTURE* (page 5), all immune cells were born out of HSC cradled in the bone marrow. From there, the stem divides into two distinct but related *innate* and *adaptive* branches, which metaphorically harbor features of "street smart" versus "book smart." By the late 1960s, it was generally acknowledged that "book smart" adaptive immune cells such as T cells rely on "accessory immune cells" to mount an immune response. For years, macrophages (from the innate "street smart" camp) were speculated to be the likely immune candidates responsible for assisting adaptive immune T and B cells. Short of lines of supporting evidence, assertions are but assertions. Then came the moment of truth.

The hunt for the mysterious immune accessory cell. In 1970, having received his MD degree from Harvard Medical School, Dr. Steinman joined The Cohn Laboratory at Rockefeller University as a postdoctoral research fellow. His project was to decipher whether macrophages are the accessory cell. Using advanced microscopy and working through many a wee hour, Dr. Steinman stumbled upon an uncanny cell type under the magnifying lens. The cells manifested surface spikes in constant motion of extending and retracting that looked nothing like macrophages. After methodically checking, double-checking, and triple-checking, it finally dawned on Dr. Steinman that a brand new immune type was right in front of his eyes! Taken by the conspicuously wavy surface spikes, Dr. Steinman named the new discovery "Dendritic cell," inspired by *dendreon* for "tree" in Ancient Greek. More excitingly, Dr. Steinman had a strong instinctual feeling that the dendritic cell (DC) was *THE ONE*, the accessory cell on the hunt! Again, intuition in science does not fly very far. Scientific proof must be presented to make (or break) the claim.

A tall order. The first order of business for Dr. Steinman was to obtain purified dendritic cells (DC) from a mixture of entangled cells. Many more into-the-wee-hours workdays later, thanks to two collaborating laboratories equipped with state-of-the-art cell biology technologies housed at Rockefeller University, and countless trials, errors, and more trials, purified DC cells were finally obtained and unequivocally demonstrated as the master immune organizer capable of

- *Spotting foreign and dangerous "antigens" that stick out like a loud "antenna" on unwanted cells, whether they infected cells or cancer cells.*
- *Taking a slice of the telltale antigen and displaying it on a protein platter called HLA.*

- *Traveling with this cargo to a nearby lymph node to meet up with naive CD4-T cells to pass on the "foreign antigen intel," followed by another round of presentation by DC, this time to CD8-T cells how to spot and capture danger signs displayed on "enemy" cells.*
- *The rest of the story is all too familiar: CD8-T cells are mobilized to initiate a cascade of events that aim to eliminate unwanted cells while, at the same time, B cells are activated to become plasma cells that churn out antibodies specific to the antigenic antenna of the dangerous bug of interest. The joint venture by CD8-T and antibodies leads to total annihilation of substances that pose a danger to the host body.*

At the very immune center stage are dendritic cells (DCs) from the innate "street smart" arm coordinating communication between the two camps of "book-smart" and "street smart." The discovery of DCs has not only filled a void in basic immunology but has also timely translated into a milestone cancer immunotherapy med for prostate cancer patients. For a detailed description, please go to **CANCER VACCINES (4): PAP—A BAIT TO HARNESS PROSTATE CANCER** (page 42).

Long-distance call from Stockholm. Shockingly, Dr. Steinman was diagnosed with late-stage pancreatic cancer in March 2007 but kept on with his research endeavors until literally a few days before his passing on September 30, 2011, in New York City. Meanwhile, some 4,000 miles away in Stockholm, Sweden, the Nobel Assembly had finalized their decision to award Dr. Ralph Steinman the 2011 Nobel Prize for Physiology or Medicine. The phone call from Stockholm came on October 3, 2011, seventy-two hours after Dr. Steinman had passed away. By tradition, the Nobel Prize is not awarded to awardees posthumously. However, since the decision had already been finalized before learning about Dr. Steinman's passing, the prize stands. Deservedly so!

ZOOMING IN ON TUMOR: BENIGN VERSUS MALIGNANT

Tumors are healthy cells gone awry. The time taken for a normal cell to become a tumor cell is typically more than a decade or much longer. The diagram below illustrates key features that characterize a progressive process of normal cells "gone bad," with a summary after the figure starting from left to right, following the arrows:

- Step 1: Normal cells are orderly and disciplined. Assuming a regular shape, normal cells grow only when needed. For example, during the leading process of a wound, extra cells are produced to do the repair job.
- Step 2: Hyperplasia cells are organized with a regular cell shape, akin to normal cells. However, cell growth picks up speed during the state of hyperplasia. The excess growth does not serve a useful purpose such as for tissue repairing; on the contrary, hyperplasic cells expand as a result of mutations in genes that normally control growth but turned unruly. Word Anatomy: hyper = excess; plasia = growth.
- Step 3: Dysplasia is a state where cells appear out of shape and grow out of control. Dysplasic cells also harbor an edging front. Dys = not functioning properly.

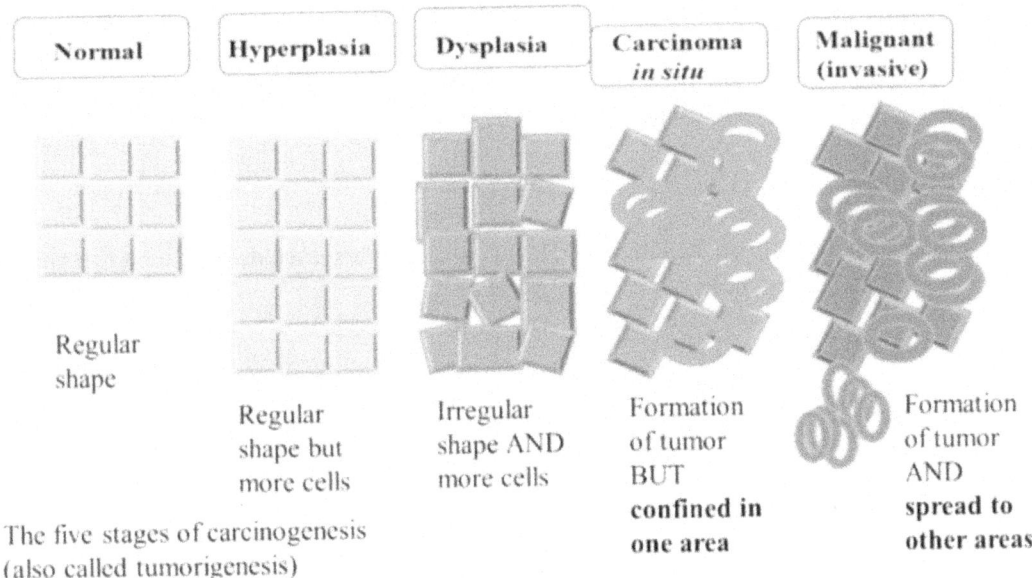

- A benign tumor stays
- A malignant tumor metastasizes

Image 106 How normal cells degrade to cancer cells. By Nancy Liu-Sullivan.

Step 4: Carcinoma in situ is the next step along the continuum of tumor development. At this stage, the tumor, also called "carcinoma," stays immobile, hence in situ, Latin for "at its original location." Carcinoma in situ is usually not defined as "cancer" because it does not spread to invade neighboring healthy cells. However, this is the "prelude" of cancer. Still, tumors detected at this stage are usually treatable owing to the absence of metastasis.

Step 5: Malignant tumor is synonymous to cancer. Malignant denotes the invasive and aggressive nature of tumor at this stage. Invasion is carried out via two routes: (1) Blood vessels and (2) lymphatic vessels. These two types of vessels also maintain a constant and intimate communication with each other. Tumor cells that jump onto the bandwagon on these routes are destined to arrive at distal cells, tissues, and organs. It is generally known that breast cancer cells can spread to the liver, the lungs, and the brain; pancreatic cancer cells tend to spread to the liver; and melanoma tends to metastasize to the brain.

Science has come a long but productive way: More people survive cancer and live with cancer, thanks to remarkable progress made in diagnostics and therapeutics. One of many compelling examples is Tom Brokaw, the iconic NBC anchor and accomplished writer who portrayed a heroic account of how his MM was battled against and arrived at a manageable state in *A Lucky Life Interrupted: A Memoir of Hope*.

The best hope is built with willpower and hope, by all means, but there is one more ingredient for the victorious recipe: early detection. The earlier the detection, the less the probability for a carcinoma *in situ* to be confined within the primary tumor without metastasizing to healthy tissues or, worse, to lymph nodes. Accordingly, early detection remains the first order of cancer care success. Cancer screening continues to serve as the bedrock for early detection! Follow guidelines recommended by professional agencies such as the National Institutes of Health (NIH), National Cancer Institute (NCI), and Food and Drug Administration (FDA). And it is always a wise idea to consult your family physician. To health and a long, happy, productive life!

Food for thought:

1. A malignant tumor is not built in a day; rather, it takes years, even decades for a hyperplasia mass to deteriorate to become metastatic cancer.
   A. True
   B. False

2. The best deterrence of cancer is early detection!
   A. True
   B. False

ZOOMING OUT ON HOW CANCER IMMUNOTHERAPY SHAPES EFFECTIVE TEACHING: AN EPILOGUE

As an added pillar of cancer treatment based upon unleashing patient inner immune power, cancer immunotherapy continues to evolve. From a teaching perspective, cancer immunotherapy serves as an ideal subject for instructors to help students connect the dots of several essential life science disciplines ranging from immunology, bioengineering, cell biology, and molecular genetics.

On multiple occasions throughout this book, core concepts in cancer basics and immune fundamentals appear more than once. This is done intentionally to help students and readers grasp a thorough understanding of topics of interest through topic visiting and revisiting. As an added effort in the 101 essays presented in this book, theoretical concepts are placed in real-world contexts and clinical settings—a teaching methodology highly appreciated by my students.

Speaking of teaching, having been recruited to the City University of New York College of Staten Island continues to be a professional honor. Watching my pre-medicine and first-generation-college students tirelessly juggle between job and school while never wavering their aspirations for medicine to help the needy has, in no uncertain terms, served as a driving force for me to dedicate utmost best to teaching and research mentorship. Reflecting upon how research students start out being terrified at giving a lab meeting presentation to gradually mastering research matters to ultimately wearing the proudest smile on their face at medical school White Coat Ceremony cements in me the noble meaning of *teaching to make a difference*—coined by a respected colleague. Carry on!

Welcome to Cancer Jeopardy in Memory of Alex Trebeck

1. Derived from a normal cell but gained capacity to grow uncontrollably.
   WHAT IS A _____ CELL?

2. Excess in cell growth but confined within the site of first appearance or *in situ*.
   WHAT IS A _____ TUMOR?

3. Aggressive in both cell growth and invading healthy cells, tissues, and organs.
   WHAT IS A _____ TUMOR?

4. A simple sugar that cancer cells constantly rely on to produce ATP, the cellular gasoline.
   WHAT IS _____?

5. A type of acid produced as a byproduct of breaking down glucose in the absence of oxygen.
   WHAT IS _____ ACID?

6. The tumor village surrounding the tumor core.
   WHAT IS _____ _____?

7. The hard fence at the outermost edge of the tumor village.
   WHAT IS _____?

8. The two arms of immunity: one being "street smart" with quick response but no memory, and the other "book smart" with a delayed immune response but long-lasting memory.
   WHAT ARE _____ IMMUNITY AND _____ IMMUNITY?

9. Immune cells that ingest and fragment infectious bugs and unwanted cells.
   WHAT ARE _____?

10. Mast cells and basophils overlap in the same immune reaction that leads to this medical condition.
    WHAT IS _____?

11. When UV or higher-energy radiation passes through cells, it breaks down water molecules to produce a class of unrestrained harmful chemicals capable of damaging DNA.
    WHAT ARE _____ _____?

12. The female nuclear physicist who discovered two radioactive elements and coined the very term "radioactivity."
    WHO IS _____?

13. The German physician who was the first to report a close link between cancer and immune response.
    WHO WAS _____ ?

14. The first pediatric leukemia patient who received an experimental CAR-T therapy and who has remained cancer-free for more than one decade.
    WHO IS _____ _____ ?

15. The molecular biologist who reported the very first form of oncogenic (cancer-causing) Ras in humans.
    WHO IS _____ _____ ?

16. Lymph, the toxin-cleansing clear liquid that circulates in the lymphatic system; it cannot be pumped like blood being pumped by the heart. This activity facilitates lymph movement which helps expedite clearance of unwanted substances out of the body.
    WHAT IS _____ ?

17. Aspirin, the inflammation-curbing and pain-reducing genetic drug, was originally isolated from this tree and subsequently chemically modified by German scientists to remove corrosiveness.
    WHAT IS THE _____ TREE?

18. Currently, there are two FDA-approved cancer preventive vaccines that work by clearing these two types of viruses that cause cancer-prone chronic infections.
    WHAT ARE _____ AND _____ ?

19. This type of antibody is found richly embedded in our nasal cavity and in the appendix, ready to hit the ground running when encountering harmful bacteria or viruses.
    WHAT IS IMMUNOGLOBULIN _____ ?

20. This type of radiation therapy spares 60 percent of healthy tissue from radiation damage compared to the conventional high-dose X-ray photon therapy.
    WHAT IS _____ _____ THERAPY?

21. Among a few options, this type of colon cancer screening approach is the most recommended for being the most sensitive test, in addition to allowing physicians to remove pre-cancerous polyps during the procedure.
    WHAT IS _____ ?

22. There are three aliases for the most fierce fighter cell in our immune system against unwanted cells such as infected cells or cancer cells. Aside from *cytotoxic T cell* (CTL) and *CD8 T cell*, this particular type of T cell has a third name.
    WHAT IS _____ T CELL?

23. This gene has multiple functions, including being a tumor suppressor gene and a DNA repair gene. Mutations of this gene are found in more than 50 percent of all cancers.
    WHAT IS _____ ?

24. This type of skin cell is responsible for replacing old skin cells with new ones.
    WHAT ARE _____ CELLS?

25. This type of recreational station has met with vehement criticism from dermatologists for being the culprit of the increased incidence of skin cancer in young people.
    WHAT IS A _____ STATION?

26. CRISPR/Cas9 is found in bacteria as an immune defense apparatus against this type of infectious agent that invades and infects bacteria.
    WHAT IS _____?

27. These two molecular biologists solved the structure of DNA as a double-helical structure.
    WHO ARE _____ AND _____.

28. Two Japanese physician-scientists repeatedly painted this chemical onto rabbit ears that gave rise to skin cancer and demonstrated unequivocally that carcinogens cause cancer.
    WHAT IS _____ _____.

29. This brilliant physician-scientist from MSKCC established the foundation that anti-TB vaccine BCG can treat early-stage bladder cancer.
    WHO IS _____ _____?

30. This determined physician-scientist ran the first physician-initiated clinical trial in which a mixture of modified infectious agents was used to treat inoperable sarcoma and laid the groundwork for cancer immunotherapy.
    WHO IS _____ _____?

31. This institute, quartered a few blocks from the Empire State Building, Manhattan, New York, is the one-and-only organization dedicated solely to research and development of cancer immunotherapy.
    WHAT IS _____ _____ _____?

32. This coveted prize was awarded for the first time in a line of clinical therapy that uses antibody drugs to liberate subdued Killer T (KT) cells for killing cancer cells.
    WHAT IS THE _____ PRIZE?

33. This physician-scientist innovated the method of collecting patients' own immune cells from the tumor, culturing them in the laboratory in the presence of important cytokine signaling molecules, followed by returning these modified cells to the patient, achieved great progress and saved many lives.
    WHO IS _____?

34. This medical condition describes an overreaction of one's immune system.
    WHAT IS _____?

35. HIV preferentially attacks this type of T cells in humans.
    WHAT ARE _____ T CELLS?

36. This high-energy radiation can be blocked by a piece of paper or intact skin.
    WHAT IS _____ PARTICLE RADIATION?

37. This high-energy radiation can enter human skin but can be blocked by a thin sheet of aluminum.
    WHAT IS _____ PARTICLE RADIATION?

38. These two types of high-energy radiation can only be blocked by thick concrete or lead.
    WHAT ARE _____ RAY RADIATION AND _____ RAY RADIATION?

39. This high-energy radiation is emitted by certain rocks and can be absorbed by humans through inhalation, causing lung cancer even in non-smokers.
    WHAT IS _____ GAS?

40. Antigen binds to this type of protein receptor.
    WHAT IS _____ RECEPTOR?

41. All cells in our body stem from this immune organ.
    WHAT IS THE _____ _____?

42. Immune T cells receive boot camp training in this immune organ where they learn how to distinguish antigen IDs that are from the host body and non-host body sources.
    WHAT IS THE _____?

43. Immune B cells undergo development and selection in this immune organ.
    WHAT IS THE _____?

44. At the end of a successful immune battle, this type of immune cells take charge to make sure the immune system returns to baseline without overreactions.
    WHAT ARE _____ T CELLS?

45. This type of virus has evolved to have a special taste for cancer cells and has been engineered for cancer treatments.
    WHAT IS AN _____ VIRUS?

46. Good bacteria of different sorts in our guts are called beneficial microbiota. A secret stash of this prized immune possession is stored in this immune organ.
    WHAT IS _____?

47. This type of cell found in the guts harbor microfoils on their surface that trap infectious bugs for processing and relay the important immune intel to macrophages for destruction.
    WHAT ARE _____ CELLS?

48. This female nuclear physicist, together with her science partner, innovated a high-precision laboratory measurement protocol that measures minuscule-level substances, including insulin.
    WHO IS _____?

49. CAR-T therapy, with the full name of CAR-T cell therapy, engineers a molecular GPS and an Energizer that dispatches this type of immune cells to find and kill cancer cells.
    WHAT ARE _____ CELLS?

50. This type of cancer therapy is tailor-designed as a unique molecular arsenal against the cancer in each patient.
    WHAT IS _____ CANCER THERAPY?

Cancer Jeopardy Answers

1. Acquired from a normal cell but gained capacity to grow uncontrollably.
   WHAT IS A **CANCER** CELL?

2. Excess in cell growth but confined within the site of first appearance or *in situ*.
   WHAT IS A **BENIGN** TUMOR?

3. Aggressive in both cell growth and invading healthy cells, tissues, and organs.
   WHAT IS A **MALIGNANT** TUMOR?

4. A simple sugar that cancer cells constantly rely on to produce ATP, the cellular gasoline.
   WHAT IS **GLUCOSE**?

5. A type of acid produced as a byproduct of breaking down glucose in the absence of oxygen.
   WHAT IS **LACTIC** ACID?

6. The tumor village surrounding the tumor core.
   WHAT IS **TUMOR MICROENVIRONMENT**?

7. The hard fence at the outermost edge of the tumor village.
   WHAT IS **DESMOPLASIA**?

8. The two arms of immunity: one being "street smart" with quick response but no memory, and the other "book smart" with a delayed immune response but long-lasting memory.
   WHAT ARE **INNATE** IMMUNITY AND **ADAPTIVE** IMMUNITY?

9. Immune cells that ingest and fragment infectious bugs and unwanted cells.
   WHAT ARE **PHAGOCYTES**?

10. Mast cells and basophils overlap in the same immune reaction that leads to this medical condition.
    WHAT IS **HYPERSENSITIVITY**?

11. When UV or higher-energy radiation passes through cells, it breaks down water molecules to produce this class of unrestrained harmful chemicals capable of damaging DNA.
    WHAT ARE **FREE RADICALS**?

12. The female nuclear physicist who discovered two radioactive elements and coined the very term "radioactivity."
    WHO IS **MADAM CURIE**?

13. The German physician who was the first to report a close link between cancer and immune response.
    WHO IS **RUDOLF VIRCHOW**?

14. The first pediatric leukemia patient who received an experimental CAR-T therapy and who has remained cancer-free for more than one decade.
    WHO IS **EMILY WHITEHEAD**?

15. The molecular biologist who reported the very first form of oncogenic (cancer-causing) Ras in humans.
    WHO IS **ROBERT WEINBERG**?

16. Lymph, the toxin-cleansing clear liquid that circulates in the lymphatic system; it cannot be pumped like blood being pumped by the heart. This activity facilitates lymph movement which helps expedite clearance of unwanted substances out of the body.
    WHAT IS **EXERCISE**?

17. Aspirin, the inflammation-curbing and pain-reducing genetic drug was originally isolated from this tree and subsequently chemically modified by German scientists to remove corrosiveness.
    WHAT IS THE **WILLOW** TREE?

18. Currently, there are two FDA-approved cancer preventive vaccines that work by clearing these two types of viruses that cause cancer-prone chronic infections.
    WHAT ARE **HEPATITIS B VIRUS (HBV)** AND **HUMAN PAPILLOMA VIRUS (HPV)**?

19. This type of antibody is found richly embedded in our nasal cavity and in the appendix, ready to hit the ground running when encountering harmful bacteria or viruses.
    WHAT IS IMMUNOGLOBULIN **A** (IgA)?

20. This type of radiation therapy spares 60 percent of healthy tissue from radiation damage compared to the conventional high-dose X-ray photon therapy.
    WHAT IS **PROTON BEAM** THERAPY?

21. Among a few options, this type of colon cancer screening approach is the most recommended for being the most sensitive test, in addition to allowing physicians to remove pre-cancerous polyps during the procedure.
    WHAT IS **COLONOSCOPY**?

22. There are three aliases for the most fierce fighter cell in our immune system against unwanted cells such as infected cells or cancer cells. Aside from *cytotoxic T cell* (CTL) and *CD8 T cell*, this particular type of T cell has a third name.
    WHAT IS **KILLER** T CELL?

23. This gene has multiple functions, including being a tumor suppressor gene and a DNA repair gene. Mutations of this gene are found in more than 50 percent of all cancers.
    WHAT IS **P53**?

24. This type of skin cell is responsible for replacing old skin cells with new ones.
    WHAT ARE **BASAL** CELLS?

25. This type of recreational station has met with vehement criticisms from dermatologists for being the culprit of the increased incidence of skin cancer in young people.
WHAT IS **TANNING** STATION?

26. CRISPR/Cas9 is found in bacteria as an immune defense apparatus against this type of infectious agent that invades and infects bacteria.
WHAT IS **PHAGE**?

27. These two molecular biologists solved the structure of DNA as a double-helical structure.
WHO ARE **JAMES WATSON** and **FRANCIS CRICK**?

28. Two Japanese physician-scientists repeatedly painted this chemical onto rabbit ears that gave rise to skin cancer and demonstrated unequivocally that carcinogens cause cancer.
WHAT IS **COAL TAR**?

29. This brilliant physician-scientist from MSKCC established the foundation that anti-TB vaccine BCG can treat early-stage bladder cancer.
WHO IS **LLYOD OLD**?

30. This determined physician-scientist ran the first physician-initiated clinical trial in which a mixture of modified infectious agents was used to treat inoperable sarcoma and laid the groundwork for cancer immunotherapy.
WHO IS **WILLIAM COLEY**?

31. This institute, quartered a few blocks from the Empire State Building, Manhattan, New York, is the one-and-only organization dedicated solely to research and development of cancer immunotherapy.
WHAT IS **CANCER RESEARCH INSTITUTE**?

32. This coveted prize was awarded for the first time in a line of clinical therapy that uses antibody drugs to liberate subdued Killer T (KT) cells for killing cancer cells.
WHAT IS THE **NOBEL** PRIZE?

33. This physician-scientist innovated the method of collecting patients' own immune cells from the tumor, culturing them in the laboratory in the presence of important cytokine signaling molecules, followed by returning these modified cells to the patient, achieved great progress and saved many lives.
WHO IS **STEVEN ROSENBERG**?

34. This medical condition describes an overreaction of one's immune system.
WHAT IS **HYPERSENSITIVITY**?

35. HIV preferentially attacks this type of T cells in humans.
WHAT ARE **CD4** T CELLS?

36. This high-energy radiation can be blocked by a piece of paper or intact skin.
    WHAT IS **ALPHA** PARTICLE RADIATION?

37. This high-energy radiation can enter human skin but can be blocked by a thin sheet of aluminum.
    WHAT IS **BETA** PARTICLE RADIATION?

38. These two types of high-energy radiation can only be blocked by thick concrete or lead.
    WHAT ARE **GAMMA** RAY RADIATION AND **X**-RAY RADIATION?

39. This high-energy radiation is emitted by certain rocks and can be absorbed by humans through inhalation, causing lung cancer even in non-smokers.
    WHAT IS **RADON** GAS?

40. Antigen binds to this type of protein receptor.
    WHAT IS **ANTIGEN** RECEPTOR?

41. All cells in our body stem from this immune organ.
    WHAT IS THE **BONE MARROW**?

42. Immune T cells receive boot camp training in this immune organ where they learn how to distinguish antigen IDs that are from the host body and non-host body sources.
    WHAT IS THE **THYMUS**?

43. Immune B cells undergo development and selection in this immune organ.
    WHAT IS THE **SPLEEN**?

44. At the end of a successful immune battle, this type of immune cells take charge to make sure the immune system returns to baseline without overreactions.
    WHAT ARE **REGULATORY** T (Tregs) CELLS?

45. This type of virus has evolved to have a special taste for cancer cells and has been engineered for cancer treatments.
    WHAT IS AN **ONCOLYTIC** VIRUS?

46. Good bacteria of different sorts in our guts are called beneficial microbiota. A secret stash of this prized immune possession is stored in this immune organ.
    WHAT IS THE **APPENDIX**?

47. This type of cell found in the guts harbor microfoils on their surface that traps infectious bugs for processing and relay the important immune intel to macrophages for destruction.
    WHAT ARE **M** CELLS?

48. This female nuclear physicist, together with her science partner, innovated a high-precision laboratory measurement protocol that measures minuscule-level substances, including insulin.
    WHO IS **ROSALYN YALOW**?

49. CAR-T therapy, with the full name of CAR-T cell therapy, engineers a molecular GPS and an Energizer that dispatches this type of immune cells to find and kill cancer cells.
WHAT ARE **T** CELLS?

50. This type of cancer therapy is tailor-designed as a unique molecular arsenal against the cancer in each patient.
WHAT IS **PERSONALIZED** CANCER THERAPY?

Bibliography

Agilent. From the Warburg Effect to the Latest in Cancer Research. https://www.agilent.com/about/features/en/warburg-effect.

American Association for Cancer Research (AACR). https://www.aacr.org/.

American Cancer Society. Viruses that Can Lead to Cancer. https://www.cancer.org/cancer/risk-prevention/infections/infections-that-can-lead-to-cancer/viruses.html.

American Chemical Society. Alexander Fleming Discovery and Development of Penicillin – Landmark. https://www.acs.org/education/whatischemistry/landmarks/flemingpenicillin.

American Chemical Society. Insulin Development and Commercialization. https://www.acs.org/education/whatischemistry/landmarks/insulin.html.

Anassi, E. and Ndefo, UA. 2001. Sipuleucel-T (Provenge) Ibjrction: The First Immunotherapy Agent (Vaccine) For Hormone-Refractory Prostate Cancer. *PT* 36(4): 197–202.

ASCO Connection. The Stories of the Scientists Behind Immuno-Oncology, in Their Own Words. https://connection.asco.org/magazine/features/stories-scientists-behind-immuno-oncology-their-own-words.

ASCO Hub. American Society of Clinical Oncology. https://www.asco.org/

Bar-Sagi, D. and Fermisco, JR. 1985. Microinjection of the Rasoncogene Protein Into PC12 Cells Induces Morphological Differentiation. *Cell* 42: 841–8.

Becker's Hospital Review. Healthcare News & Analysis. https://www.beckershospitalreview.com/.

Berg, JHVD., Heemskerk, B., Rooij, NV. et al. 2020. Tumor Infiltrating Lymphocytes (TIL) Therapy in Metastatic Melanoma: Boosting of Neoantigen-Specific T Cell Reactivity and Long-Term Follow-Up. *J Immunother Cancer* 8: e000848. https://jitc.bmj.com/content/8/2/e000848.

Best Immunology Scientists. http://research.com/scientists-rankings/immunology.

BioNTech. https://www.biontech.com/int/en/home.html.

Blumenthal, S. 2009. The Insulin Immunoassay After 50 Years: A Reassessment. *Perspective Bio Med.*

Bouche, G., Vandeborne, L., Pantziarka, P., and Van Nuffel, AMT. 2021. Repurposing Infectious Diseases Vaccines Against Cancer. *J Clin Oncol.* 39: e14564. https://ascopubs.org/doi/10.1200/JCO.2021.39.15_suppl.e14564.

Brea, EJ., Ou, CY., Manchado, E. et al. 2016. Kinase Regulation of Human MHC Class I Molecule Expression on Cancer Cells. *Cancer Immunol Res.* 4(11): 936–47.

Bristol Myers Squibb. Global Biopharmaceutical Company. https://www.bms.com/.

Cancer Disparities. http://www.cancer.gov/about-cancer/understanding/disparities.

Cancer Research Institute. Cancer Research Institute Announces New Lloyd J. Old STARs Class. https://www.cancerresearch.org/media-room/2024/cancer-research-institute-announces-new-lloyd-j-old-stars-class.

Cancer Research Institute. CRI Funded Scientists. http://www.cancerresearch.org/cri-funded-scientists.

Cancer Research Institute. CRI Lloyd J. Old STAR Program. https://www.cancerresearch.org/lloyd-j-old-star-program.

Cancer Research Institute. Dr. Michel Sadelain, MD, PhD. https://www.cancerresearch.org/scientific-advisory-council/michel-sadelain-m-d-ph-d.

Cancer Research Institute. Helen Coley Nauts Monographs. https://www.cancerresearch.org/helen-coley-nauts-monographs.

Cancer Research Institute. James P. Allison, PhD. https://www.cancerresearch.org/scientific-advisory-council/james-allison.

Cancer Research Institute. William B. Coley Award. https://www.cancerresearch.org/william-b-coley-award.

CDC. Food Allergies in Schools Toolkit. Healthy Schools. https://www.cdc.gov/healthyschools/foodallergies/toolkit.htm.

Chaffer, CL and Weinberg, RA. 2015. How Does Multi Step Tumorigenesis Really Proceed? *Cancer Discov.* 5(1): 22–4.

Chen, H., Li, Y., Li, H. et al. 2024. NBS1 Lactylation is Required for Efficient DNA Repair and Chemotherapy Resistance. *Nature* 631: 663–9.

Chiche, J., Brahimi-Horn, MC., and Pouyssegur, J. 2010. Tumourhypoxia Induces a Metabolic Shift Causing Acidosis: A Common Feature in Cancer. *J Cell Mol Med.* 14(4): 771–94.

CIDRAP. Life-Threatening Cancer Drug Shortages are Result of a Cascade of Troubles. https://www.cidrap.umn.edu/resilient-drug-supply/life-threatening-cancer-drug-shortages-are-result-cascade-troubles.

City of Hope Cancer Treatment Centers. https://www.cancercenter.com/.

Cold Spring Harbor Laboratory. CSHL Ranks in Top One Percent of Institutions Impacting Future Biomedical Diagnoses and Treatments. https://www.cshl.edu/cshl-ranks-in-top-one-percent-of-institutions-impacting-future-biomedical-diagnoses-and-treatments/.

Collis, J., Das, S., and Bar-Sagi, D. Kras and Tumor Immunity: Friend or Foe? *Cold Spring Harb Perspect Med.* doi: 10.1101/cshperspect.a031849.

Columbia University Irving Medical Center. NewYork-Presbyterian #1 Hospital in New York City and Among Top 10 of U.S. Hospitals. https://www.cuimc.columbia.edu/news/newyork-presbyterian-1-hospital-new-york-city-and-among-top-10-u-s-hospitals.

Dana-Farber Cancer Institute. https://www.dana-farber.org/.

Depleted Uranium, Devastated Health: Military Operations and Environmental Injustice in the Middle East. https://hir.harvard.edu/depleted-uranium-devastated-health-military-operations-and-environmental-injustice-in-the-middle-east/.

Diamantis, A., Magiorkinis, E., Sakorafas, GH., and Androutsos, G. 2008. A Brief History of Apoptosis: From Ancient to Modern Times. *Onkologie* 31: 702–6.

Division of Biology & Biomedical Sciences. Immunology. https://dbbs.wustl.edu/programs/immunology/.

Eil, R., Vodnala, SK. et al. 2016. Ionic Immune Suppression Within the Tumour Microenvironment Limits T Cell Effector Function. *Nature* 537(7621): 539–543.

Emily Whitehead, First Pediatric Patient to Receive CAR T-Cell Therapy, Celebrates Cure 10 Years Later. https://www.chop.edu/news/emily-whitehead-first-pediatric-patient-receive-car-t-cell-therapy-celebrates-cure-10-years.

Ercolano, E. Water Nymphs and Divine Madness: The Surprising Etymology of "Lymphedema". https://thelymphielife.com/2017/07/20/water-nymphs-and-divine-madness-the-surprising-etymology-of-lymphedema/.

FDA-Approved AI Trends for Your Medical Practice in 2024. https://www.medscape.com/viewarticle/999838.

FDA Approves Casgevy, the First CRISPR Therapy, for Sickle Cell Disease. http://www.geneengnews.com/topics/genome-editing/fda-approves-casgevy-the-first-crispr-therapy-for-the-sickle-cell-disease/.

Fighting Cancer on a Fixed Income: How MSKCC Helps Patients Cope Financial Uncertainty. https://www.mskcc.org/news/fighting-cancer-on-fixed-income-how-msk-helps-patients-cope-with-financial-uncertainty.

Find a Treatment Center. http://www.yescarta.com/fl/find-a-treatment-center/.

Fred Hutchinson Cancer Center. Dead to Me? Insights Into a Tumor's Necrotic Core. https://www.fredhutch.org/en/news/center-news/2023/02/new-research-insights-into-cancer-tumor-necrotic-core-.html.

Fred Hutchinson Cancer Center. https://www.fredhutch.org/en.html.

Galleri® for Employers. Offer a Cancer Screening Test as a Benefit. https://www.galleri.com/employer.

Genetically Modified Herpes Virus Delivers One-Two Punch Against Advanced Cancers. http://www.icr.ac.uk/news-archive/genetically-modified-herpes-virus-delivers-one-two-punch-against-advanced-cancers/.

Gilead Sciences, Inc. https://www.gilead.com/.

Greenup, RA., Rishing, C., and Fish, L. et al. 2019. Financial Costs and Burden Related to Decisions for Breast Cancer Surgery. *J Oncol Pract.* 15(8): e666–e676.

Hanahan, D. 2022. Hallmarks of Cancer: New Dimensions. *Cancer Discov.* 12: 31–46.

Hanahan, D. and Weinberg, RA. 2000. The Hallmarks of Cancer. *Cell* 100: 57–70.

Hanahan, D. and Weinberg, RA. 2011. The Hallmarks of Cancer: The Next Generation. *Cell* 144: 646–74.

Harvard Health. Fever. https://www.health.harvard.edu/a_to_z/fever-a-to-z.

Hatton, IA., Galbraith, ED. et al. 2023. The Human Cell Count and Size Distribution. *Proc Natl Acad Sci USA* 120(39): e2303077120.

Hombach, A., Weiczarkowiecz, A., Marquardt, T. et al. 2001. Tumor-Specific T Cell Activation by Recombinant Immunoreceptors: CD3ζ Signaling and CD28 CostimulationAre Simultaneously Required for Efficient IL-2 Secretion and Can Be Integrated Into One Combined CD28/CD3ζ Signaling Receptor Molecule. *J Immunol.* 167(11): 6123–31.

IARC Monographs on the Identification of Carcinogenic Hazards to Humans. Agents Classified by the IARC Monographs, Volumes 1–136. https://monographs.iarc.who.int/agents-classified-by-the-iarc/.

Inside Precision Medicine. First Engineered T Cell Therapy for Solid Tumors Approved by the FDA. https://www.insideprecisionmedicine.com/topics/patient-care/first-engineered-t-cell-therapy-for-solid-tumors-approved-by-the-fda/.

Jhunjhunwala, S., Hammer, C., and Delamarre L. 2021. Antigen Presentation in Cancer: Insights Into Tumour Immunogenicity and Immune Evasion. *Nat Rev Cancer.* 21: 298–312.

Karnoub, AE. and Weinberg, RA. 2008. Ras Oncogenes: Split Personalities. *Nat Rev Mol Cell Biol.* 9: 517–351.

Kastenhuber, E. and Lowe, S. 2017. Putting p53 in Context. *Cell* 170(6): 1062–78.

Kite Pharma. Changing the Way Cancer Is Treated. http://www.kitepharma.com/.

Lasek, W. 2022. Cancer Immunorditing Hypothesis: History, Clinical Implications, and Controversies. *Cent Eur J Immunol.* 47(2): 168–74.

Levine, AJ. 2020. P53 and The Immune Response: 40 Years of Exploration—A Plan for the Future. *Int. J Mol Sci.* 21(2): 541.

Levy, B. Dying Tumors Suppress Anti-Cancer Immune Response. http://irp.nih.gov/blog/post/2023/04/dying-tumor-cells-suppress-anti-cancer-immune-response.

Liu-Sullivan, N. A Carcinogen in Bread? https://www.mcgill.ca/oss/article/carcinogen-bread.

Liu-Sullivan, N. Bunnies and Cancer. https://www.mcgill.ca/oss/article/history-general-science/bunnies-and-cancer.

Liu-Sullivan, N. Cancer's Sweet Tooth. https://www.mcgill.ca/oss/article/health-and-nutrition-contributors/cancers-sweet-tooth.

Liu-Sullivan, N. Edison's Inadvertent Folly. https://www.mcgill.ca/oss/article/medical-history/edisons-inadvertant-folly.

Liu-Sullivan, N. Get that Lymph Going! https://www.mcgill.ca/oss/article/medical-contributors/get-lymph-moving.

Liu-Sullivan, N. Hallmarks and Signaling of Cancer Cells. https://www.medialab.com/hallmarks_and_signalling_of_cancer_cells.aspx.

Liu-Sullivan, N. HLA and Cancer Immunotherapy. https://www.labce.com/hla_and_cancer_immunotherapy.aspx.

Liu-Sullivan, N. Nobel's Sugar Twist. https://www.mcgill.ca/oss/article/medical-contributors/nobels-sugar-twist.

Liu-Sullivan, N. Non-Smoker's Lung Cancer and the Hidden Link. https://www.mcgill.ca/oss/article/health-and-nutrition/non-smokers-lung-cancer-and-hidden-link.

Liu-Sullivan, N. "Pasteur's Bacterial Culture" and "Coley's Toxins": Anomalies and Landmark Discoveries. https://www.mcgill.ca/oss/article/contributors-history-general-science/pasteurs-bacterial-culture-coleys-toxins-anomalies-and-landmark-discoveries.

Liu-Sullivan, N. Splendid Rays and Skin Cancer. https://www.mcgill.ca/oss/article/environment-general-science/splendid-rays-and-skin-vancer.

Loizou, E., Banito, A., Livshits, G. et al. 2019. A Gain-of-Function p53 Mutant Oncogene Promotes Cell Fate Plasticity and Myeloid Leukemia through the Pluripotent Factor FOXH1. *Cancer Discov.* 9(7): 962–79.

Marks, L. 1998. *Between Silk and Cyanide*. New York: The Free Press (Simon and Schuster) p454z.

Mayo Clinic. Colonoscopy. https://www.mayoclinic.org/tests-procedures/colonoscopy/about/pac-20393569.

MD Anderson Cancer Center. Are Swollen Lymph Nodes in Your Neck a Symptom of Lymphoma? https://www.mdanderson.org/cancerwise/swollen-lymph-nodes-and-other-symptoms-of-lymphoma.h00-159464790.html.

MD Anderson Cancer Center. MD Anderson Cancer Center: Cancer Treatment & Cancer Research Hospital. https://www.mdanderson.org/.

Mechanism of Action for Sipuleucel-T PROVENGE. https://provenge.com/hcp/sipuleucel-t-mechanism-of-action/.

MediaLab. HLA and Cancer Immunotherapy. https://www.medialab.com/hla_and_cancer_immunotherapy.aspx.

Medscape. Upadacitinib Improves Giant Cell Arteritis in Phase 3 Trial. https://www.medscape.com/viewarticle/upadacitinib-improves-giant-cell-arteritis-phase-3-trial-2024a1000b4r.

Memorial Sloan Kettering Cancer Center. Can Tattoos Hide Skin Cancer? Advice from MSK on How to Stay Safe. https://www.mskcc.org/news/can-tattoos-hide-skin-cancer-advice-msk-how-stay-safe.

Memorial Sloan Kettering Cancer Center. Ginger. https://www.mskcc.org/cancer-care/integrative-medicine/herbs/ginger.

Memorial Sloan Kettering Cancer Center. Investigational mRNA Vaccine Induced Persistent Immune Response in Phase 1 Trial of Patients With Pancreatic Cancer. https://www.mskcc.org/news/can-mrna-vaccines-fight-pancreatic-cancer-msk-clinical-researchers-are-trying-find-out.

Memorial Sloan Kettering Cancer Center. Managing Hair Loss with Scalp Cooling during Chemotherapy for Solid Tumors. http://www.mskcc.org/cancer-care/patient-education/managing-hair-loss-scalp-cooling.

Memorial Sloan Kettering Cancer Center. Mouth Care During Your Cancer Treatment. https://www.mskcc.org/cancer-care/patient-education/mouth-care-during-your-treatment.

Memorial Sloan Kettering Cancer Center. Sloan Kettering Institute Scientists Retool CAR T Cells to Serve as 'Micropharmacies' for Cancer Drugs. https://www.mskcc.org/news/sloan-kettering-institute-scientists-retool-car-cells-serve-micropharmacies-cancer-drugs.

Memorial Sloan Kettering Cancer Center. The ABCs of BCG: Oldest Approved Immunotherapy Gets New Explanation. https://www.mskcc.org/news/oldest-approved-immunotherapy-gets-new-explanation.

Meo, C., Palmer, G., Bruzzese, F., et al. 2023. Spontaneous Cancer Remission After COVID-19: Insights from the Pandemic and Their Relevance for Cancer Treatment. *Journal of Translational Medicine* 21: 273.

Mount Sinai. Colorectal Polyps Information. https://www.mountsinai.org/health-library/diseases-conditions/colorectal-polyps#:~:text=Polyps%20are%20benign%2C%20meaning%20that,than%20polyps%20under%201%20centimeter.

National Association for Proton Therapy. Find a Proton Center. https://proton-therapy.org/findacenter/.

National Institutes of Health (NIH). An mRNA Vaccine to Treat Pancreatic Cancer. https://www.nih.gov/news-events/nih-research-matters/mrna-vaccine-treat-pancreatic-cancer.

National Institutes of Health (NIH). National Cancer Institute (NCI). https://www.nih.gov/about-nih/what-we-do/nih-almanac/national-cancer-institute-nci.

Nature Immunology. Lloyd John Old 1933-2011. http://www.nature/com/articles/ni.2209.

NCBI Bookshelf. Histology, M Cell. StatPearls. https://www.ncbi.nlm.nih.gov/books/NBK534232/.

NCI. CAR T Cells: Engineering Immune Cells to Treat Cancer. https://www.cancer.gov/about-cancer/treatment/research/car-t-cells.

NCI. FDA Approves T-VEC to Treat Metastatic Melanoma. http://www.cancer.gov/news-events-blog/2015/t-vec-melanoma.

NCI. Lifileucel First Cellular Therapy Approved for Cancer. https://www.cancer.gov/news-events/cancer-currents-blog/2024/fda-amtagvi-til-therapy-melanoma.

NCI. OEEB Research on "Forever Chemicals". https://dceg.cancer.gov/news-events/news/2023/pfas-research.

NCI. Steps to Find a Clinical Trial. http://www.cancer.gov/research/participate/clinical-trials-search/steps.

NCI. Targeted Therapy Drug List by Cancer Type. http://www.cancer.gov/about-cancer/treatment/types/targeted-therapies/approved-drug-list.

NIAID: National Institute of Allergy and Infectious Diseases. Severe Combined Immunodeficiency (SCID). https://www.niaid.nih.gov/diseases-conditions/severe-combined-immunodeficiency-scid.

NIH Record. Rosenberg Receives Presidential Medal. https://nihrecord.nih.gov/2023/11/24/rosenberg-receives-presidential-medal.

NIH Record. Rosenberg's Research Spans a Half-Century and Counting. http://nihrecord.nih.gov/2023/10/13/rosenberg-s-research-spans-half-cent-and-counting.

Northwell Health. Children's Cancer Center – Staten Island University Hospital. https://siuh.northwell.edu/pediatrics/childrens-cancer-center.

Northwell Health. Manhattan Cancer Care – Northwell Campaign. https://www.northwell.edu/manhattan-cancer-care.

NRC.gov. Doses in Our Daily Lives. https://www.nrc.gov/about-nrc/radiation/around-us/doses-daily-lives.html.

NRC.gov. High Radiation Doses. https://www.nrc.gov/about-nrc/radiation/health-effects/high-rad-doses.html.

NSAIDs (Nonsteroidal Anti-Inflammatory Drugs): Uses. https://my.clevelandclinic.org/health/treatments/11086-non-steroidal-anti-inflammatory-medicines-nsaids.
NYU Langone Health. https://nyulangone.org/.
O'Sullivan, E., Keogh, A., Hendersen, B. et al. 2023. Treatment Strategies for KRAS-Mutated Non-Small-Cell Lung Cancer. *Cancers* 15(6): 1635.
Penn Medicine. Drug Allergy – Symptoms and Causes. https://www.pennmedicine.org/for-patients-and-visitors/patient-information/conditions-treated-a-to-z/drug-allergy.
Penn Medicine. University of Pennsylvania Health System. https://www.pennmedicine.org/.
PMC. From Bench to Bedside: The History and Progress of CAR T Cell Therapy. https://www.ncbi.nlm.nih.gov/pmc/articles/PMC10225594/.
PMC. Recent Advances in Cancer Immunotherapy with a Focus on FDA-Approved Vaccines and Neoantigen-Based Vaccines. https://www.ncbi.nlm.nih.gov/pmc/articles/PMC10675687/.
PMC. Role of IL-2 in Cancer Immunotherapy. https://www.ncbi.nlm.nih.gov/pmc/articles/PMC4938354/.
Poetry Foundation. Water by Ralph Waldo Emerson. Original source: Poets of the English Language (Viking Press, 1950).
ProteoGenix. From the First to the Fifth Generation of CAR-T Cells. http://www.proteogenix.science/scientific-corner/car-t/car-r-generations/.
PROVENGE® (sipuleucel-T). https://provenge.com/
PROVENGE (sipuleucel-T). Immunotherapy. https://provenge.com/immunotherapy-prostate-cancer/.
Quianzon, CC. and Cheikh, I. 2012. History of Insulin. *J Community Hosp Intern Med Perspect.* 2(2): 10.
Raskov, H., Orhan, A., Christensen, J.P. et al. 2021. Cytotoxic CD8+ T Cells in Cancer and Cancer Immunotherapy. *Br J Cancer* 124, 359–67.
Recognizing and Responding to Anaphylaxis. www.cdc.gov/COVID-19.
Remembering Jackie Kennedy. http://lymphomanewstoday.com/social-clip/2016/05/26//9175.
Sahin, U. 2023. CLDN6-specific CAR-T Cells Plus Amplifying RNA Vaccine in Relapsed for Refractory Solid Tumors: The Phase 1BNT211-01 Trial. *Nat Med.* 29: 2844–53.
Schultz, M. 2008. Rudolf Virchow. *Emerg Infect Dis.* 14(9): 1480–1.
Schwartz, IL., Berson, SA., and Rosalyn, S. 1973. Yalow: A Scientific Appreciation. *Mt Sinai J Med.*
Science History Institute. Rosalyn Yalow and Solomon A. Berson. https://www.sciencehistory.org/education/scientific-biographies/rosalyn-yalow-and-solomon-berson/.
Secondary Malignancies. http://www.hoafredericksburg.com/secondary-malignancies/.
Shih, C., Shilo, B-Z., and Goldfarb, MP. 1979. Passage of Phenotypes of Chemically Transformed Cells via Transfer Ion of DNA and Chromatin. *Proc. Natl. Acad. Sci USA* 76(11): 5714–18.
Shih C. and Weinberg, RA. 1982. Isolation of a Transforming Sequence from a Human Bladder Carcinoma Cell Line. *Cell* 29(1): 161–9.
Shimizu, K., Goldfarb, M., Perucho, M., and Wigler, M. 1983. Isolation and Preliminary Characterization of the Transforming Gene of a Human Neuroblastoma Cell Line. *Proc Natl Acad Sci USA* 80(2): 383–7.
Sloan Kettering Institute. https://www.mskcc.org/research/ski.
Soengas, M., Capodieci, P., Polsky, D. et al. 2001. Inactivation of the Apoptosis Effector Apaf-1 in Malignant Melanoma. *Nature* 409: 207–11.
Sousa LG, McGrail DJ, et al. (2022). Spontaneous Tumor Regression Following COVID-19 Vaccination. https://pubmed.ncbi.nlm.nih.gov/35241495/
Stony Brook Cancer Center. https://cancer.stonybrookmedicine.edu/.
Tasuku Honjo – Biographical. NobelPrize.org. Nobel Prize Outreach AB 2024. Tue. 21 May 2024.
The City University of New York. https://www.cuny.edu/.
The Lancet Oncology. Chimney-Sweeps' Cancer—Early Proof of Environmentally Driven Tumourigenicity. https://www.thelancet.com/journals/lanonc/article/PIIS1470-2045(19)30106-8/abstract.
The New Yorker. How 3M Discovered, Then Concealed, the Dangers of Forever Chemicals. https://www.newyorker.com/magazine/2024/05/27/3m-forever-chemicals-pfas-pfos-toxic.
The New Yorker. What's Wrong with Me? https://www.newyorker.com/magazine/2013/08/26/whats-wrong-with-me.
The Nobel Prize. Women Who Changed Science. https://www.nobelprize.org/womenwhochangedscience/stories.

The Nobel Prize in Physiology or Medicine. 2018. James P. Allison. https://www.nobelprize.org/prizes/medicine/2018/allison/facts/.

The Nobel Prize in Physiology or Medicine. 1977. Rosalyn Yalow. https://www.nobelprize.org/prizes/medicine/1977/yalow/facts/.

The Nobel Prize in Physiology or Medicine. 2018. Tasuku Honjo. https://www.nobelprize.org/prizes/medicine/2018/honjo/facts/.

The Rockefeller University. Clinical Research at the Rockefeller University Hospital. https://www.rockefeller.edu/research/clinical-research/.

The Rockefeller University. Nobel Laureate Ralph Steinman Dies at 68. https://www.rockefeller.edu/news/1816-nobel-laureate-ralph-steinman-dies-at-68/.

Tilden C Emerson and arren H Cole (1956). Spontaneous Regression of Cancer: Preliminary Report. https://pmc.ncbi.nlm.nih.gov/articles/PMC1465423/

Torgovnick, A. and Schmacher, B. 2015. DNA Repair Mechanisms in Cancer Development and Therapy. *Front Genet.* 6: 157.

Trial Details. https://trials.modernatx.com/study/?id=mRNA-4157-P201.

Trump, DL. and Rosenthal, ET. 2021. *Centers of the Cancer Universe: A Half-Century of Progress Against Cancer.* Rowman & Littlefield.

Tun, ZT. Theranos: A Fallen Unicorn. https://www.investopedia.com/articles/investing/020116/theranos-fallen-unicorn.asp.

Vecchio, I., Tornali, C. et al. 2018. The Discovery of Insulin: An Important Milestone in the History of Medicine. *Front Endocrinol.* 9: 613.

Vogelstein, B., Sur, S. and Prives, C. 2010. p53: The Most Frequently Altered Gene in Human Cancers. *Nature Education* 3(9): 6

Weill Cornell Medicine. https://weillcornell.org/.

Weinberg, RA. 2024. It Took a Long, Long Time: Ras and the Race for a Cancer Cure. *Cell* 187(7): 1574–7.

Weyand, CM. and Goronzy, JJ. 2016. Aging of the Immune System. Mechanisms and Therapeutic Targets. *Ann Am Thorac Soc.* 17(5): S422–8.

Xie, N., Shen, G., Gao, W. et al. 2023. Neoantigens: Promising Targets for Cancer Therapy. *Sig Transduct Target Ther.* 8: 9. https://www.nature.com/articles/s41392-022-01270-x.

Yalow, RS. 1978. Radioimmunoassay: A Probe for the Fine Structure of Biologic System. *Science.*

Yuan, S., Stewart, K.S., Yang, Y. et al. 2022. Ras Drives Malignancy through Stem Cell Crosstalk with the Microenvironment. *Nature* 612: 555–63.

Zeng, M., Kikuchi, H., Pino, MS., and Chung, DC. 2010. Hypoxia Activates the K-Ras Proto-Oncogene to Stimulate Angiogenesis and Inhibit Apoptosis in Colon Cancer Cells. *PLoS One* 5(6): e10966.

Zhang, Y. and Zhang, Z. 2020. The History and Advances in Cancer Immunotherapy: Understanding the Characteristics of Tumor-Infiltrating Immune Cells and their Therapeutic Implications. *Cell Mol Immunol.* 17: 807–21.

Index

4-1BB   50–3, 55, 117

ABECMA   62–6
adaptive immunity   7, 22, 129
adenine   114, 151, 164
adenosine triphosphate (ATP)   25–7, 29, 34–5, 138, 163, 184–5, 215, 225, 230
adjuvant   45
allergens   12–14, 106
Allison, James   109–10
anaphylaxis   9, 14–15
antibiotics   14, 125, 179
antigen   6, 8–9, 11–13, 35–6, 39–40, 43–5, 47–50, 59, 64, 81, 115–16, 131, 136–7, 181–2, 187–8, 190, 193, 195, 216–17, 221–2, 228, 233
antigen presentation cells (APC)   40, 115
aplastic pernicious anemia   125–6, 156
apoptosis   6, 26, 43, 51, 87, 135, 137–9, 151, 191–2, 209–10
autoimmune diseases   115

Bacillus Calmette-Guerin (BCG)   37–8, 71, 196, 211, 227, 232
Bar-Sagi, Dafna   31–2, 159
basophils   8–9, 14, 91, 225, 230
B cells   5–7, 9, 21–4, 27, 40, 51, 57–9, 61–3, 91–4, 116, 131, 136, 183, 189, 193, 221–2, 228, 233
benign tumor   134, 168, 230
BioNTech   47, 181
bladder cancer   37–8, 42, 71, 136, 161, 179, 196, 211, 227, 232
bone marrow   6–7, 9, 23, 57, 63, 85, 91–2, 125–6, 154–6, 187–8, 209, 221, 233
breast cancer   27, 36, 71, 99–100, 178–9, 185, 223
BREYANZI   61–4
Brokaw, Tom   65, 223
Bursa of Fabricius   21

cancer-associated fibroblasts (CAF)   30, 32, 105
cancer hallmarks   74
cancer immunotherapy   38, 42, 54, 63, 66, 100, 109–10, 115–19, 181, 184, 191, 196, 222, 224, 227, 232
Cancer Research Institute   71, 110, 232
cancer tricks and traps   25–36, 44, 73, 90, 185, 188, 191
cancer vaccine   37, 39–48, 114, 141, 181, 196, 222
carcinogen   123–4, 138, 167–70, 173–4, 207, 211–12, 227, 232

carcinoma *in situ*   223
CARVYKTI   65–6
CD4-T   32–3, 38, 40, 61–3, 83–5, 87, 181, 222
CD8-T   32–4, 51, 61–2, 181, 189–92, 195, 222
CD19   50–1, 53, 55, 61, 63, 65, 67, 115–16
CD28   50–1, 53, 115–17
cell cycle   124, 134–5, 160
cervical cancer   39–41, 105, 139, 141
Chimeric antigen receptor T cell therapy (CAR-T)   22, 37, 48–68, 94, 100, 105, 115–17, 181, 191, 226, 229, 231, 234
Class Switch Recombination (CSR)   10–11
clinical trial   37–8, 40, 43, 47–8, 54, 65–6, 70, 105, 109, 116–17, 119–21, 165–6, 181, 227, 232
coal tar   106, 167–70, 232
Coley, William   69–71, 110, 182, 196, 232
colon cancer   15–18, 51, 71, 100, 165, 226, 231
Cooper, Max   21
corticosteroids   87–8
COVID-19   8, 13, 41, 47, 114, 116, 127, 182, 190
CRISPR   74–85, 125, 227, 232
crRNA   75–6
CTL   6, 226, 231
CTLA-4   109
cytokines   52, 56, 66, 87, 96, 115, 182–4, 190–1, 211
cytosine   114, 164

dendritic cells   8, 27, 34, 40, 44, 46, 106, 130–2, 136, 183, 189, 221–2
desmoplasia   30–2, 230
DNA damage   124–5, 134–5, 137, 143, 154, 168–9, 174, 185, 196, 205
DNA repair genes   134, 143
dysplasia   222

elephants   133–4
eosinophil   88, 91–2
epitope   12
Epstein-Barr Virus (EBV)   23–4
Extracellular Signal-Regulated Kinase (ERK)   160

Food for Thought   7, 9, 11, 13, 15, 18, 20, 22, 24, 26–7, 29, 32–3, 35, 37–8, 41, 44, 46, 48, 51, 53, 57, 61, 65–6, 68, 71–2, 78, 80, 85, 88, 90, 94, 96, 98, 102, 106, 123–4, 126, 128, 132, 134, 136, 139, 141, 146, 148, 153, 155, 158, 161, 163, 166, 168, 170, 173, 175, 177, 179, 182, 184, 186, 188, 190–2, 195, 202, 207, 209, 213, 224 free radicals   124, 143, 145–6, 169, 179–80, 206–9, 230

Gardasil   39–40, 45
Gardasil 9   39–40
ginger   97–8
glioblastoma multiforme (GBM)   28, 32
glucose   25–7, 29, 34, 162, 177, 184–5, 205, 215, 225, 230
glycolysis   25–7
Granulocytes macrophage colony-stimulating factor (GM-CSF)   43
gRNA   75–6, 80
guanine   114, 164

happy hormones   176–7
hematopoietic stem cells (HSC)   91–2, 98, 154, 221
hepatitis B virus (HepB)   44–6
Herpes Simplex Virus (HSV)   41–2
histamine   8–9, 14–15
Honjo, Tasuku   109, 203
H-Ras   159, 161
human immunodeficiency virus (HIV)   23, 83–5, 227
human leukocyte antigen (HLA)   6, 36–7, 43–4, 49, 115, 136, 189–90, 195, 221
Human papilloma virus (HPV)   39–41, 45, 105, 139–41, 231
hydrogen peroxide (H2O2)   205
hyperplasia   222, 224
hyperplasia   222, 224
hypoxia   28–9, 161–2, 184

IgA   8–9, 11, 195, 231
IgG   8–11
IgM   7–11
infection   5, 7, 12, 21–4, 26, 37, 39–42, 44–8, 52, 57–8, 63, 69–70, 74, 83–4, 88–8, 92–96, 105–7, 116, 125, 127–8, 130, 140, 154–5, 182–4, 190–1, 193, 196, 212, 226, 231
inflammation   5, 17–19, 74, 87–8, 95, 97, 105, 106, 147, 183–5, 194, 226, 231
innate immunity   129, 195, 230
interferon (IFN)   38, 182
Interleukin 1 (IL-1)   87–8, 106, 182, 184
Interleukin 2 (IL-2)   118–19
Interleukin 6 (IL-6)   52–3, 88, 182
ionizing radiation (IR)   143, 145, 154–5, 169, 171, 205
Ipilimumab   109

June, Carl   50, 52, 55, 105, 116–17

Kariko, Katalin   46–7, 113–14
Keytruda   101

Killer T cell (KT)   6, 18, 26, 33–5, 37, 43, 46, 48, 51, 59, 61, 66, 87, 90, 109, 118, 131, 136, 181, 187, 190, 196, 227, 231–2
K-Ras   134–5, 165–6
Kymriah   54–8, 61, 117

lactic acid   26–7, 29, 49, 90, 185, 230
leukemia   22, 50–2, 54, 59, 62, 65, 67, 72, 85, 92–4, 100, 105, 115–16, 153, 159, 179, 210, 226, 231
leukotrienes   9, 14
liver cancer   44–6
Lowe, Scott   134, 139, 196
lung cancer   36, 38, 51, 72, 136, 159, 165, 167, 170–3, 185, 211, 228, 233
lymph nodes   6, 34, 40, 43, 47, 59, 92, 127, 131, 152, 190, 223
lymphoid   91–2
lymphoma   23, 50, 57–62, 67, 92–3, 127, 153, 157, 182

macrophage   6, 8, 27, 30, 87, 91–2, 106, 130–1, 183, 221, 228, 233
malignant tumor   1, 28, 32, 68, 123, 134, 183–4, 203, 223–4, 230
Mayo Clinic   20, 121–2
MD Anderson   72, 103, 110, 127
MEK   160
membrane attack complex (MAC)   81–2
Memorial Sloan Kettering Cancer Center (MSKCC)   28, 38, 46, 48, 68–9, 71–2, 90, 103, 109, 115, 121, 123, 134, 139, 153, 161–2, 181, 183, 193, 196, 211, 227, 232
Merck   39, 101
messenger RNA (mRNA)   9–10, 46–8, 113–14, 177, 181
metastasis   1, 17, 27, 30, 223
methylation   139
MHC-I 35–7, 43–4, 189–90
MHC-II 189–90
monocyte   91
multiple myeloma   53, 62–3, 65–6, 92–4, 100, 153
myeloid   91–2, 98

National Cancer Institute (NCI)   16, 38, 70, 72, 89, 99, 117, 119, 161, 174, 184, 224
National Institute of Health (NIH)   70, 99, 117, 136, 161, 224
neutrophil   30, 88, 91, 97–8, 106, 183, 195
N-Ras   159, 161

O'Donnell-Tormey, Jill   71, 110–12
Old, Lloyd   38, 71, 196
oncogenes   136, 143, 161
Osso buco   125–6

P53   133–41, 168, 196, 231
pancreatic cancer (pancreatic ductal carcinoma, PDA)   27, 30–2, 46–8, 159, 161, 165, 181, 222
PAP   39, 42–4, 46, 222, 228, 231
paratope   12
Patient #67   118
PD-1   203–4
phagocytosis   8, 63, 130–1
plasma cells   7–8, 40, 62–4, 91–4, 116, 131, 222
prostaglandins   8, 14, 95, 97, 106
prostate cancer   42–4, 46, 178, 222
proton beam therapy   121–3, 157–8, 231
PROVENGE (Sipuleucel-T)   42–4
pyruvate   25–6

Quick Word Anatomy   8, 28, 30, 33, 39, 41, 43, 45, 76, 91, 135, 162, 191

radiation and cancer   147–53, 155–6
radiation sickness   125, 153–5
radium   155–6, 170, 200
radon gas   124, 138, 167, 170–3, 233
Raf   160–1
RIA   216–17, 220
risk reduction of cancer   166–75
Rosenberg, Steven A.   117–19, 232

Sadelain, Michel   50, 115, 117
salicylic acid   19–20, 97
severe combined immunodeficiency (SCID)   22–4
skin cancer   41, 72, 118, 137, 147–53, 168, 227, 232
spleen   5–6, 9, 21–2, 57, 63, 233
spontaneous tumor remission   118, 182–3
standard curve   218–20
Steinman, Ralph   132, 221–2

T cell memory   192–3
T cell receptor (TCR)   35, 63, 83, 115, 190
T cell selection   187–8
Tecartus   59–61
thymine   151
thymus   5, 21–2, 187–8, 233
tocilizumab   52
tracrRNA   75–6
Tregs   26–7, 30, 49, 119, 187–8, 233
tumor-associated macrophages (TAM)   30–1
tumor microenvironment (TME)   27, 29–30, 66, 163, 185, 192, 230
tumor necrotic factor (TNF)   183, 196
tumor suppressor genes (TSG)   124, 134
T-VEC   41–2

ultraviolet (UV)   149–52
uracil   114, 164
uranium   148, 155–6, 170, 172–3, 199–200, 202

Virchow, Rudolf   32, 230

Warburg effect   26
water (H_2O)   82, 90, 110, 123, 127, 135, 143, 146, 150, 152, 154, 156, 162, 167, 183, 190–1, 199, 203–7, 209, 225, 230
Weinberg, Robert   74, 161, 231
Whitehead, Emily   51–4, 57, 65, 103, 105, 231

X-Ray   121, 123, 143–4, 146–50, 154–6, 170–1, 205, 226, 231, 233

Yalow, Rosalyn   215–16, 220, 233
Yamagiwa, Katsusaburo   168
Yescarta   57–9, 61, 100–1

About the Author

Nancy Liu-Sullivan holds a PhD in molecular and cellular pharmacology, an MS in molecular genetics, and a BA in English literature. Prior to joining the biology faculty at the City University of New York (CUNY) College of Staten Island (CSI) where she teaches immunology, radiation biology, cancer biology, and general biology, Dr. Liu-Sullivan served as a senior research scientist at Memorial Sloan Kettering Cancer Center (MSKCC) with a specialty in cancer genomics and drug discovery. An avid author of a series of online courses published by MediaLab and approved for continuing education credits by the American Society of Clinical Laboratory Sciences (ASCLS) for practicing medical laboratory scientists and pathology fellows, Dr. Liu-Sullivan has covered a wide range of well-received topics highlighted in *Cancer Cell and Signaling*, *HLA and Cancer*, *CRISPR/Cas9*, *Cancer Vaccines*, and *Cell Therapy Coming of Age*. In addition to being an *at-times* contributor to the McGill University Office of Science and Society (OSS) Weekly Digest on cancer, Dr. Liu-Sullivan has also served on the faculty advisory board in immunology for Macmillan Learning and Oxford University Press.